Praise for *The Great Oom* by Robert Love

Top Ten Biographies of 2010, *Booklist*

Best Books of 2010, *Kirkus Reviews*

"Exemplary popular history, tracing the intersection of influence, taste, and charisma in the propagation of practices that were originally esoteric, tantalizing, and scandalous."　　　　　　　　　　*—The New Yorker*

"A story of scandal, financial shenanigans, bodily discipline, oversize egos, and bizarre love triangles, with a few performing elephants thrown in for good measure."　　　　　　　　　　*—The Wall Street Journal*

"As entertaining as a good novel . . . This is a jaw-dropping story unearthed from our recent history, full of sex and scandal and outrage, and its central figure, Pierre Bernard, is the equal of any schemer we Americans have yet given rise to."
　　　　　—T. C. Boyle, author of The Women and The Road to Wellville

"Lively and idiosyncratic . . . [about] a headline-making swami-entrepreneur who defied his bland Iowa origins to become one of the most renowned eccentrics of the Jazz Age. And the legacy of his program and his acolytes is still with us."　　　　　　　　*—Janet Maslin, The New York Times*

"Entertaining and enlightening."　　　　　　　　　*—Yoga Journal*

"Robert Love's entertaining biography depicts a bold and successful liar . . . [who] learned well the lesson of all successful purveyors of self-help from the Buddha to Bikram Choudhury . . . target the very rich."
　　　　　　　　　　　　—The New York Times Book Review

"Part cultural history, part biography, part yarn—Love brings a suitably irreverent eye to Bernard's story and his less than purely spiritual appeal."
　　　　　　　　　　　　　　　　　　　—Slate

"Fascinating, eminently readable, and eye-opening at many levels."
　　　—Scott Turow, author of Presumed Innocent and the sequel Innocent

"Love writes with all the zest, wit, and empathy his protean subject deserves as he tells this dazzling tale of a self-made man of holistic convictions and archetypal flaws."　　　　　　　　　*—Booklist (starred review)*

"Entertaining . . . [Love] strikes just the right note of amused admiration for this P. T. Barnum in tights."   —*Milwaukee Journal Sentinel*

"Love's work proceeds with a thoroughgoing vitality [as] American guru Bernard garners an evenhanded new consideration."   —*Kirkus Reviews*

"This is a great book and never mind that I'm personally more interested in getting out of uncomfortable positions than into them. Bob Love fascinates me with *The Great Oom*."
    —P. J. O'Rourke, author of *Parliament of Whores* and *Give War a Chance*

"Thoroughly researched, vividly written, and often fascinating."
    —*The New Republic*

"A guru, a mystic, a con artist, a prophet, an aviator, a charismatic Casanova, Pierre Bernard is as iconic an American operator as Harry Houdini or Howard Hughes or Elvis. Robert Love deploys an unflagging wit and verve as he chronicles the ways in which we attempt to assuage our insatiable cravings for inner peace and carnal pleasure."
    —Mark Leyner, author of *Why Do Men Have Nipples?* and
    Why Do Men Fall Asleep After Sex?

"A striking reminder of the strange worlds to be found when traveling no farther than your own backyard."
    —Robert Sabbag, author of *Snowblind* and *Down Around Midnight*

"Over the last few decades, historians have realized the central role that Tantric yoga has played in America's embrace of Asian religions. What we didn't know was what a great love story it was. With *The Great Oom*, Robert Love has given us a marvelous early chapter of this American epic—in delightful, careful, and critical detail."
    —Jeffrey J. Kripal, professor of religious studies, Rice University, and
    author of *Esalen: America and the Religion of No Religion*

"Placing Bernard within the context of new spiritual trends, occultism, and the fascination with India in the early twentieth century, Love has shed important new light on the birth of yoga as a spiritual industry in modern America. It's a terrific read."
    —Hugh Urban, professor of religious studies, Ohio State
    University, and author of *The Economics of Ecstasy*

PENGUIN BOOKS

THE GREAT OOM

Robert Love was the managing editor of *Rolling Stone* and executive editor of *Best Life*. He is an adjunct professor at the Columbia University Graduate School of Journalism. His articles have appeared in the *New York Times*, the *New York Observer*, and the *Utne Reader*. He lives with his wife in Nyack, New York.

The GREAT OOM

THE MYSTERIOUS ORIGINS OF AMERICA'S FIRST YOGI

Robert Love

PENGUIN BOOKS

For Nichol

PENGUIN BOOKS

Published by the Penguin Group

Penguin Group (USA) Inc., 375 Hudson Street, New York, New York 10014, U. S. A. • Penguin Group
(Canada), 90 Eglinton Avenue East, Suite 700, Toronto, Ontario, Canada M4P 2Y3 (a division of Pear-
son Penguin Canada Inc.) • Penguin Books Ltd, 80 Strand, London WC2R 0RL, England • Penguin
Ireland, 25 St Stephen's Green, Dublin 2, Ireland (a division of Penguin Books Ltd) • Penguin Books
Australia Ltd, 250 Camberwell Road, Camberwell, Victoria 3124, Australia (a division of Pearson
Australia Group Pty Ltd) • Penguin Books India Pvt Ltd, 11 Community Centre, Panchsheel Park,
New Delhi – 110 017, India • Penguin Group (NZ), 67 Apollo Drive, Rosedale, North Shore 0632, New
Zealand (a division of Pearson New Zealand Ltd) • Penguin Books (South Africa) (Pty) Ltd, 24 Sturdee
Avenue, Rosebank, Johannesburg 2196, South Africa

Penguin Books Ltd, Registered Offices:
80 Strand, London WC2R 0RL, England

First published in the United States of America by Viking Penguin,
a member of Penguin Group (USA) Inc. 2010
Published in Penguin Books 2011

1 3 5 7 9 10 8 6 4 2

Photograph credits
Bernard Collection, Historical Society of Rockland County, New York, New York: all photographs
except those cited below
Nyack Library Local History Collection: pp. 18, 94, 203
Personal collection of Joan Wofford: pp. 120, 220
Library of Congress: p. 192
Viola W. Bernard Papers, Archives and Special Collections, Columbia
University Health Sciences Library: pp. 260, 324

THE LIBRARY OF CONGRESS HAS CATALOGED THE HARDCOVER EDITION AS FOLLOWS:
Love, Robert, 1951–
The great oom : the improbable birth of yoga in America / Robert Love.
p. cm.
Includes bibliographical references and index.
ISBN 978-0-670-02175-8 (hc.)
ISBN 978-0-14-311917-3 (pbk.)
1. Yoga.   2. United States—Religion.   I. Title.
B132.Y6L64 2010
294 3'44360973—dc22   2009044784

Printed in the United States of America
Set in Bodoni Std with Bodoni BE   Designed by Daniel Lagin

Contents

Preface

hen I was in college, I found myself with a copy of *Richard Hittleman's Introduction to Yoga*, a little paperback that promised "peace and physical fulfillment." I'd seen the loose-limbed author on our local PBS-TV station, and something about what he was teaching spoke to me on a deep level. I lay on the floor in my bedroom in "deep relaxation" pose, practicing abdominal breathing, hoping to feel the prana stream out from my torso to my fingertips. I tried and mastered a few of the beginning poses and kept at it for a while, but soon enough, yoga was just another one of many passing interests to a young man.

In the ensuing decades, I hit the yoga mat from time to time—at a retreat in the Catskill Mountains, at the Kripalu Center in Massachusetts, at health clubs—wondering how it came to pass that this foreign practice, with its Sanskrit terms, chanting, and incense, had become so American. I blithely presumed that the news of yoga had arrived in this country with the Beatles—attached to their fleeting affiliation with the Maharishi Mahesh Yogi—after which it had been subsumed in the countercultural hunger for all things Eastern.

But in 1998, when my wife and I moved to a stone cottage in South Nyack, New York, we found evidence of a wildly different story. The walls and fixtures of our home were decorated with mystical symbols. Over the front door, an Egyptian ankh carved in granite stood above the architect's initials and the year of construction, 1927. The entryway keyhole was circled with an escutcheon of lotus leaves. On the front wall of the house a brass bell dropped from the mouth of a winged dragon, and inside, a brass door hook was rendered in the shape of a lion-headed snake—the gnostic *chnouibis* it's called, as I later found out. In the middle of the snake's body was a tiny bas-relief of a tiger, the beast reputed in Tantric mythology to carry the goddess Kali on its back. I was a little jealous of my next-door neighbor, whose entranceway was ornamented with a heavy brass door knocker in the shape of a coiled snake eating its tail—the *ouroboros*—an ancient symbol of eternal life. It was from this neighbor that I first learned about the history of our houses, the yoga club that flourished for decades down the hill from us, and its founder, Pierre Arnold Bernard, whom my neighbor called "the father of yoga in America." There were rumors of sex and romance at Bernard's club, whispers of heiresses and great wealth. But our combined curiosity far surpassed the accumulation of known facts about Bernard and his followers. My wife, Nichol Hlinka, suggested we look more closely at this father-of-yoga guy.

In my initial research I discovered, to my shock, that the Beatles were not at all involved in yoga's American beginnings. Like rock and roll before the 1960s, yoga was for decades feared and loathed by mainstream authorities. It slowly crept from the margins of society into its safe, warm center. But no biography had been written about the man who seemed to be responsible for its journey there. In fact, most histories of yoga in the West completely bypassed his contribution. When Nyack College, which had long ago taken over the largest share of Bernard's property, hosted a lecture on its previous occupants, the place was packed—standing room only. That night, I realized that here was a story that needed to be told in full.

In seven years of research, I've spoken to more than one hundred sources, some of whom had parents or grandparents who played a major role in Bernard's club. I've talked to a growing cadre of scholars who have been tracing the threads of Bernard's influence on New Age spirituality and the yoga boom that's still growing. We have traded facts and corrected one another on sources and details.

One fact is indisputable, though, since I see its proof through my back windows: on football nights in the fall, the sky above Nyack literally glows with Pierre Bernard's legacy. The old high school athletic field lights up like a landing strip, courtesy of the Great Oom—as he was called by some—who bequeathed the community seven sixty-foot stanchions and 100,000 watts of illumination before his death in 1955. Just what a yogi was doing with stadium-quality lighting requires some explanation, but that will come later in our story.

First some definitions, terms, and clarifications: The word *yoga* has several meanings in its modern use, but at bottom it is a system of beliefs and practices, a guided philosophy whose goal is to merge the individual's soul with the ultimate reality, divinity, or God. In India, its birthplace, yoga is the name of an ancient philosophical system and remains entwined with Hindu and Buddhist religious traditions. In the West, however, it has become virtually synonymous with a single component of the Indian yogic traditions: the hatha yoga system of postures, breathing exercises, and meditation.

Pierre Bernard taught hatha yoga, the yoga familiar to more than 100 million Americans today. But he didn't stop there. He taught the philosophy behind hatha yoga as well as other paths and variations that will be mentioned in this book. When used alone in these pages, though, the word *yoga* should be taken to mean hatha yoga.

I have relied on standard English spellings for Sanskrit words, save for a few exceptional cases. Bernard and his followers tended to employ Hindi variations of Sanskrit words; they called themselves Tantrikas or Tantriks and used the word *Tantrik* to describe their organization, beliefs, and activities, and I've preserved this spelling in references to them. On the other hand, I've used the modern spelling of *Tantric* to describe the practices and practitioners of Tantra, the Indian religious philosophy adopted—and adapted—by Pierre Bernard.

Since this is a story that involves a multitude of families, there were instances where using last names alone produced more confusion than clarity. In these cases, I thought it better to rely on first names for identification. Many of the people in this story went by three or four identities in their lifetimes—some more than that. Bernard and his wife, Blanche DeVries, altered their birth names and took pseudonyms. Some of their followers relied on stage names or went by their secret lodge names, by which they were identified at the yoga club. A few women then abandoned those to take married names. To prevent confusion, I have adhered to either first names or club names, whichever seemed the more effective identifier for the individual.

The locus for much of this story is Nyack, New York, which is popular shorthand for the combination of incorporated villages and hamlets that includes Nyack, South Nyack, Upper Nyack, Central Nyack, and West Nyack. In this book "Nyack" encompasses them all, unless a specific village or hamlet is named.

The Great Oom is a work of nonfiction. No facts, scenes, or dialogue have been invented. Quotations are verbatim, from documents, diaries, memoirs, lecture notes, and transcribed interviews. All supporting material is sourced and enumerated in chapter notes at the end of the narrative.

THE GREAT OOM

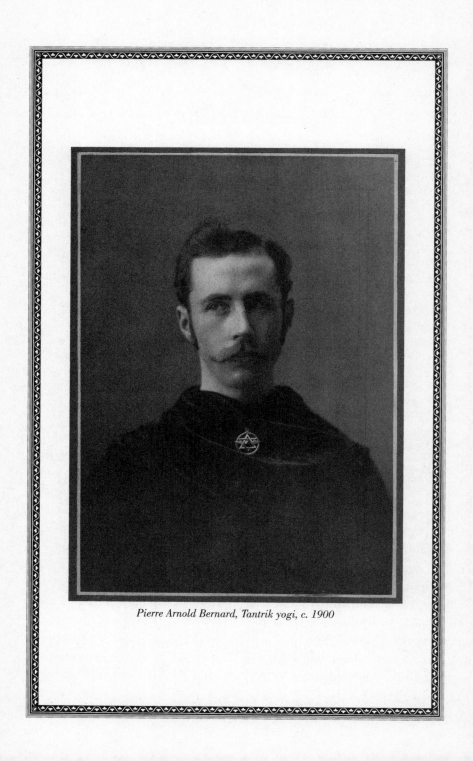

Pierre Arnold Bernard, Tantrik yogi, c. 1900

Prologue

A MAN IN LOVE WITH BEAUTY

I look out at it and I think it is the most beautiful history in the world. . . . It is the history of all aspiration, not just the American dream but the human dream.

—F. Scott Fitzgerald

ierre Arnold Bernard, the first American yogi and a spiritual hero to members of the Lost Generation, was conducting a tour of his property for Joseph Mitchell of the *New York World-Telegram*. "A place of mystery," Mitchell called it. "On summer afternoons townspeople crowd about the estate and look through the edges as the solemn students of Sanskrit go through their Oriental calisthenics. Small boys dare each other to go through the gates."

In 1931, when Mitchell trained his eyes on him, Bernard was fifty-five years old and at the pinnacle of his influence, commanding the loyalty and devotion of four hundred elite, educated followers. These men and women came to his ashram on the Hudson River, two hundred acres of leafy real estate in Nyack, New York, that included a zoo, a yacht, airplanes, and a dozen mansions that Mitchell could only describe as the "English countryside estates one sees in the moving pictures." Bernard had made his fortune teaching yoga, and his students made up a who's who of American life: college presidents, medical doctors, ministers, a spy or two, theologians, heiresses, a future congresswoman, famed authors and composers—some of the wealthiest and most influential people in the world. *Doctor* Bernard, they called him, and like a benevolent physician he ministered to their needs, body and soul. He sheltered them, entertained them, and gathered them together to teach them the art of living. They stood on their heads for him, worked in his fields, sang in his theatrical productions, and performed in elaborate, professional-level circuses for his approval. Some of them came to delve deeply into hatha yoga and the philosophy behind it, some for romance and fresh air, some for the Bernard cure, having been abandoned by hospitals and mental institutions. These he literally led back from ruination—from ledges of despair, lethal addictions, and Great War nightmares. How he managed to do this has remained his closely guarded secret. Bernard's gravitational pull was far more powerful than his appearance. His gray-blue eyes, close-set above a long, tapered nose, gave his countenance a perpetually skeptical cast. He was not classically handsome, but a natural athlete, at ease on the tumbling mats and baseball diamond and possessed of fantastic stores of energy. He could be learned or crude or nineteenth-century courtly, but to shake his hand was like touching a high-voltage current. To Joe Mitchell, Bernard looked like nothing less than an American success story, a hero of the Great Depression, rambling over his landscaped acres in his tweeds.

Pierre Bernard may have been one of the more celebrated Americans of the 1920s and 1930s, but early in the century he bore the burden of notoriety as "the Omnipotent Oom, Loving Guru of the Tantriks," the very model of the licentious, greedy Svengali. In those days he was labeled a big-city charlatan, a fraud, a seducer of young girls, a spiritual con artist. He was accused of orchestrating sexual orgies, performing abortions, hypnotizing wealthy female benefactors (and beautiful poor ones, too), and fleecing veterans of their savings. The police raided his yoga schools and clubs on numerous occasions, and the federal government kept his dossier on file. His nickname, the Great Oom, was an epithet that would stay with him for life.

Still, that was then, twenty years past, and now, in the first terrible years of the Great Depression, Bernard was as wealthy as a maharaja. His name appeared in the social pages next to Katharine Hepburn's. His American yoga school, the weird, wonderful creation he called the Clarkstown Country Club, was just as famous as he was.

When Bernard led Mitchell up the staircase of the just-completed, million-dollar clubhouse, the latest addition to his sprawling Nyack empire, he turned to the young man and announced, "You are the first newspaper man ever to enter these rooms and I don't want you to overlook the opium dens and the orgy rooms." Mitchell acknowledged the twinkle in Bernard's eyes and took down his words in his notebook. On this sunny day, Bernard did not conceal his pride in this vast operation as he guided Mitchell around, showing off his glass-covered swimming pool, his gymnasium and theater, his seven-thousand-volume library, and his herd of trained elephants.

Duly impressed by the sprawling grounds and Bernard's lavish eccentricity, the reporter had one final question. A sly and sophisticated observer even at twenty-three, Mitchell wanted to know if Bernard wasn't perhaps "more concerned with money than metaphysics?"

Bernard turned to face him directly, smiled, and answered, "I wouldn't care to say."

What intrigued newsmen like Mitchell—indeed what intrigued America about Bernard—was not merely the Oom notoriety and the flamboyant weirdness. It was the question of whether these trappings of wealth, this fantastic life—elephants, tigers, circuses, Vanderbilt heiresses, and everywhere the scent of sex—might actually be the result of an intense and authentic spiritual pursuit. Was Pierre Bernard a real mystic? The Hindu scholars who'd come to meet "the Guru of Nyack," as *Town & Country* called Bernard, had praised their host as the most learned and generous Sanskrit student in America. In India, his reputation as a gifted theologian never went into eclipse; he had befriended and sponsored more than a few Brahmin students who had come to the United States to study. In return they sent him a wall of honorary degrees from Indian universities. The Reverend Charles Francis Potter, who was Clarence Darrow's Bible expert at the legendary Scopes trial, said Bernard possessed "all the earmarks of a genius. He is the greatest authority in this country on Yoga teaching and practice."

But who was he *really*, this uneducated savant who could lecture extemporaneously for three hours on the similarities between the philosophies of ancient India and the gnostic heresies of the early Christians? This same man was known to stage a three-ring circus, manage a semipro baseball team, train a world-class heavyweight boxer, repair a Stanley

Steamer automobile, and whoop it up on fight nights at Madison Square Garden with nicotine-stained reporters. This last was where he was most at home, some said, shouting, swearing, happily chomping on a cigar. Who was this man of such wild contradictions, a name as familiar to headline writers of the 1920s as Charles Lindbergh's? The answer depended to a large degree on who was doing the asking.

"Dr. Bernard seems to delight in being a surprising person," wrote *Fortune* magazine in 1933, applauding him as a "shrewd, level headed businessman," whose banks and businesses were thriving while the nation descended into economic depression and panic. "Dr. Pierre Bernard, one of the outstanding citizens of Nyack, a classical scholar of considerable attainment," wrote the *New Yorker*, was a supremely talented teacher known for his ability to break down complex philosophical tenets into man-in-the-street advice. The Great Oom was so thoroughly embroidered into every aspect of American life, in fact, that he inspired film villains and a cartoon character. To describe the box-office magic of W. C. Fields, the *New York Times* invoked Bernard's nickname and hailed the film comedian as "the Omnipotent Oom of one of the screen's most devoted cults."

"Of all the natural forces, vitality is the incommunicable one," Fitzgerald wrote in "The Crack-Up." Yet transmitting vitality to those in need of it was the very task that Bernard had set for himself and his followers. Joining his club, with its elysian grounds and pretty yoga teachers, was like sipping from an energy drink of Roaring Twenties fizz. "We take sufferers from melancholia, old boys threatening to commit suicide and build them up," he told Mitchell. How did he do it? He patched them up using midwestern common sense and the principles of hatha yoga. Yoga was the path to a better life, he said, and teaching its virtues to Americans was his single greatest talent.

From Philadelphia, Chicago, Pittsburgh, and Cleveland, wise and successful people came to the little river town of Nyack to witness this authority for themselves at Bernard's wild Saturday night lectures. He was a thoroughly entertaining speaker. He shouted and whispered, swooped from orotund formality to gutter lingo, mashing Sanskrit with flapper slang—always in confident pronouncements and warnings: "The safety valve of this age for repressed, suppressed emotion is hooch, sex and drugs," he declared in 1927. He guided his students through the concepts of maya, Brahma, and the application of yoga as a counterbalance to what he called "the modern 'jazz' life."

In his more relaxed moments, Bernard's speech fell into a kind of vaudevillian patois. "There's nothing high-brow about me, my boy," he told Mitchell that day. "I'm a curious combination of the business man and the religious scholar . . . a man of common sense in love with beauty."

But ultimately, no individual had yet succeeded in accessing that combination and revealing the one true Bernard. His commitment to secrecy and privacy was born of necessity—for his own safety and that of his followers. In his lifetime, yoga was labeled a criminal fraud and an abomination against the purity of American women. It was associated with sexual promiscuity and kicked to the fringes of society. Today, when some 20 million Americans of all ages routinely practice yoga and accept its benign spirituality, these statements may seem impossible to believe.

Believe them: There was once an American war against yoga, a decades-long conflict waged by the media, clergy, and even the government. During Bernard's early years, the perception of yoga morphed from a queer imported pastime to an evil cult—uncivilized, heathen, and anti-American. The nation's press lords waged an endless campaign against anyone who taught it; even the word *yoga* became a synonym for secret doorways and sex worship. Yogis were seen as swindlers and seducers. Bernard and his band of Tantriks were chased from San Francisco in 1906 and fled Seattle in 1909; they were banished from New York City in 1911 and again in 1918.

Not that he wasn't a rogue. Pierre Bernard was far from faultless in his personal conduct, and his enemies found plenty of sins to tar him with. But he endured—as a man, as a teacher and philosopher—for more than a half century. Because of his efforts and energy, yoga morphed again from an ascetic practice to the healthy, vital activity we know today. He was a general in the campaign to defend yoga, and he lived to see it become tolerated, then accepted, and finally praised.

In Bernard's life story is the untold tale of how yoga became American, how it grew in influence as it intersected with Freemasons, hypnotists, vaudeville doyennes, modern dancers, English spies, and Gilded Age families. They all sought out the Great Oom and came to study at his ashram at Nyack, where he presided over great love affairs and terrible betrayals. There in a little Hudson River village, he engineered the rescue of many tortured souls and witnessed the savage, inevitable decline of others.

Here, then, is the life of Pierre A. Bernard, the Great Oom, in three acts: an unlikely rise to prominence, a ghastly fall from grace, and the long road back from dishonor. In reexamining his days and nights, in calling forth the women he loved and the men who revered him, we will also bear witness to the strange, scandalous, and entertaining tale of yoga's journey in the West.

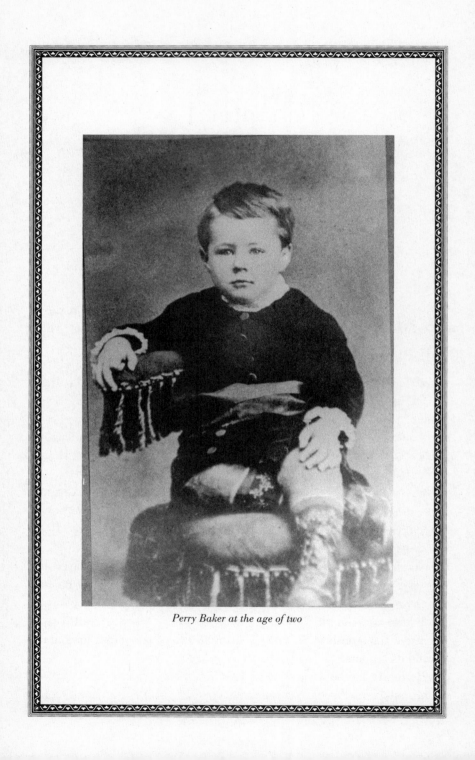

Perry Baker at the age of two

Chapter 1

FIRST SON OF
A FIRST SON

ike most self-made men, Pierre Bernard was never at ease with the facts of his origins. Asked where he was born, he volunteered Paris, Chicago, or even Des Moines, but never, ever Leon, Iowa. Leon, the provincial capital of Decatur County, was the true and actual birthplace of the Omnipotent Oom, who arrived in this world as Perry Arnold Baker in the year of America's centennial, 1876. This small town of 1,300 souls never measured up to Bernard's inflated sense of himself. "May be alright to die in, but never thought much of it as a place in which to live," he wrote to his cousin Martha Hoffman. "From my angle it has nothing to offer."

On most days Perry Baker's hometown smelled like woodsmoke and horse manure; the adults planned their activities according to the train schedule and bore on their clothing the scent of kerosene and strong soap. Chickens prowled the yards, even in downtown Leon, and roosters awoke the populace. Church bells rang on Sunday and pianos or organs played in most every parlor, but the music that caught the ear of young Perry Baker was the whistle of the steam locomotives that promised a way out of town. His boyhood was marked by the great expansion of America's railroads, when new lines pushed out every year in all directions across Iowa and beyond its borders.

Bernard's forebears arrived in Iowa following the westward sprawl of the nation in the early nineteenth century. They came from England, Ireland, and Germany, hardy souls compelled to take risks, cross borders, and vault obstacles in pursuit of freedom and better lives. The Iowa soil was rich, after all, and the railroads brought trade and prosperity to the hardworking, independent-minded men and women who settled there, Bernard's kin among the first to do so. The Bakers, Warners, and Hoffmans were a driven bunch, and they made up several of Iowa's original landed families. They built some of the original log cabins in the state and the first house in Decatur County to feature wooden floors.

Some say it was Dr. George Washington Baker, Perry's brainy, frontier-toughened grandfather, who provided the genetic spark to the man who would scandalize a great part of the civilized world as Pierre Arnold Bernard. G.W., a tall, imposing figure of grim mien, completed a two-year medical apprenticeship in 1847 and called himself a doctor. By the time he arrived in Leon in 1861 to establish his practice, he had already developed hardheaded, contrarian views on health. Dr. Baker insisted on boiling drinking water for typhoid fever sufferers, and he prescribed fresh air and open windows day or night, this at a time when conventional sickrooms were as dark and airless as tombs. His naturopathic philosophy cut against the conventional wisdom of the time, and he was accused of killing some of his patients, which naturally brought opprobrium and a few death threats to his door. Doc Baker, with his huge head of white hair and flowing white beard, was too busy for threats. He bought land, plenty of it, made his fortune in Iowa, and raised four sons.

G.W.'s firstborn, Erastus Warren Baker, took his time settling down, but he eventually did, getting his law degree and courting Catherine C. Givens, a dark-haired twenty-one-year-old known as Kittie. Ras and Kittie married on September 24, 1875; thirteen months and one week later, on October 31, 1876, their first and only child, Perry Arnold Baker, was born. Even before Perry arrived, however, his parents' marriage appeared to be headed for trouble. Erastus had hit the road soon after the ceremony, and he deserted his wife for good before their son turned four years old. By 1880, Kittie was a divorced single mother with a three-year-old, living back at home with her parents in Leon.

Perry's paternal grandfather looked after Perry's early education, teaching the boy natural history and science. It was Doc Baker's commonsense approach to medicine that resonated with Perry, who decades later preached a variation on the same gospel to wealthy, indolent apartment dwellers from New York City.

In 1881, Kittie married again, this time to John C. Bernard, a man with an even brow, a guileless face, and a tree trunk of a body that appeared to be incapable of a fast getaway. Here was a man who looked like he could put down roots—a first-generation American whose French parents had landed in nearby Wayne County, Iowa. J.C. and Kittie bought a home some twenty miles to the northeast of Leon, in the even smaller town of Humeston, Iowa. There he opened a barbershop on the south side of Broad Street, and the young couple set about creating their own family. Glen, Ervin, Clyde John, and Ray Bernard were all born in Humeston, and Perry, once an only child, now struggled to find his place in an increasingly crowded house.

He was a small-boned, delicate-looking boy—elfin in appearance—and a voracious reader. Though his formal education never progressed beyond grade school, he once bragged that as a teenager he buried his face in books "eighteen hours a day," retreating into the world of occult literature to escape from the crush of John Bernard's growing brood.

From time to time, he was trundled off to his Aunt Ina's—Kittie's younger sister—in Lamoni, Iowa, a thirty-six-mile trek. Lamoni had become the home and headquarters of the Reorganized Latter Day Saints under chief prophet and president Joseph Smith III, and Perry grew up in close contact with the followers of these frontier mystics. Through his youthful eyes, he was witnessing the formative days of a new American religion, and he was drawn to tales of the Mormons' persecution and flight west. But it was a chance meeting in Lincoln, Nebraska, that would change his life irrevocably, setting him on a steady course for the next sixty-five years.

Perry had been shipped off to Lincoln when he was thirteen, with arrangements to stay with a cousin of John Bernard's, who was said to be an architect and millwright contractor. The elders had no doubt decided that Kittie's son, inclined as he was to keep his pointy nose buried in books, might apprentice at an actual moneymaking trade. Lincoln was the right place for that; it was a city literally bursting its seams with opportunity in the 1880s, having grown in population from 13,000 to 52,000 during the previous decade.

The ensuing building boom meant plenty of work for the construction trades Perry was meant to apprentice in, but that kind of activity held little interest for him. He stuck to his reading, which naturally had expanded with the availability of Lincoln's eighteen newspapers and magazines. The city was a metropolis compared to Leon. Circuses and chautauqua moved through in good weather, and there was a brand-new opera house. At the state university, a world-class Sanskritist was translating ancient Hindu literature, and there flourished an intellectual and spiritual fervor that sustained thirty-eight churches and fifty-three secret societies, including nine Masonic lodges, where the allure of the "Orient" was transmuted nightly into elaborate rituals, rites, and costumes.

One day in 1889, Perry Baker found himself drifting deep in conversation with a boy who lived across the street from his cousin's house. This young neighbor was also intensely interested in the occult—the hidden powers of hypnotism, magic, and mind reading—and he had come into contact with an actual teacher of such things. The young man, whose name is lost to history, was studying with a jovial-looking Syrian Indian named Sylvais Hamati.

***

It is a maxim among spiritual seekers that when the student is ready, the teacher will appear. And so, as if plucked from a candlelit cave in the foothills of the Himalayas and materialized on the muddy streets of the frontier town of Lincoln, this dapper Asian émigré stood before the skinny, wide-eyed kid from Iowa. The odds against this meeting are not just long, they are nigh impossible; fewer than eight hundred Indians *in total* immigrated to the United States between 1820 and 1900.

Who was Sylvais Hamati? In appearance, he was a handsome, dark-skinned man with a direct, penetrating gaze—heavy lids over wide-set pecan-colored eyes. He styled his hair like a modern American gent of the time, parted straight down the middle and slicked to the sides, though his curls resisted the pomade in places. More successfully, his waxed handle-bar mustache defied gravity, turning up proudly over full lips.

Hamati came to America from Calcutta, and may have arrived in the United States as a freelance tutor or an entertainer in a traveling show—a mind reader or a hypnotist, like "Professor Craig of Hebron, the boy prodigy" who promised Nebraskans he could place a subject in a "cataleptic state" for five days. Or perhaps he worked first for the western railroads, where many South Asians were employed. There were few options other than those in the 1880s. Whichever the case, by the time Perry met him in 1889, Hamati had attained a measure of success, living in the West by his wits and earning his keep as an itinerant tutor of what he termed "Vedic philosophy"—the Vedas being the oldest sacred Hindu texts of India.

When the two were introduced in a park in Lincoln, Perry was barely into his teens. The bookish Iowan was immediately transfixed by what transpired there. "Hamati made it very clear to me that his knowledge of human nature and life was so far superior to mine that he gained my confidence," he later wrote. From that day on, Perry Baker would remain under Hamati's tutelage for eighteen years, working directly with him for up to three hours every day, diligently pursuing the exact course of study Hamati proposed.

In 1893, the year Perry turned seventeen, guru and student hit the road for an extended journey to California, where they stayed in various towns over the next few years. Kittie, who had moved there with her husband and children at about the same time, supported her eldest son in his yoga studies, giving him a small stipend to live on. Perry attended no formal educational institution, but designed his own curriculum with the help of his tutor and his books. "The time that I did not spend with Hamati was with my studies, or spent in what I term practice in advanced physical culture," he wrote later.

What Perry called with pursed-lipped propriety "advanced physical culture" was code for hatha yoga, which includes the postures—called asanas—so familiar to Westerners today in their practice of lotus position, headstand, and so on. He also meant breath-control techniques, known as pranayama, which adepts use to slow heart rate, lower blood pressure, cleanse the body of toxins, and even alter their psychological state. And he included the meditative arts, the ancient Indian techniques used to deepen the concentration first attained by breath control. This triad of skills was conveyed to him firsthand, skin-to-skin, the only way that such knowledge can be truly transmitted—by a practicing master yogi.

Hamati provided not only hatha yoga training for breath and body; he also gave his young *chela*—Sanskrit for "student"—the same healthy dose of Vedic education that any son of Hindu Brahmin parents would encounter in Sikkim, India: ethics, psychology, philosophy, religion, and natural science. The two of them pored over a mass of Sanskrit literature in translation, including, Perry later boasted, "every authoritative Tantra Yoga text."

Hamati, it turned out, was a Tantric yogi, who provided Perry with a living link to an ancient, secret tradition. Older and more closely guarded than the canons of Western esotericism, the Tantras—the texts and their preliterate knowledge—were believed by some experts at the time to represent a connection to the bedrock of all religions, the original spiritual wisdom of the human species. Americans had been reading Indian texts in translation for decades, but not a single seeker on record had been lucky enough to have found an authentic guide to the experience hinted at between the lines of the sacred writings. Perry Baker proved himself the perfect pupil, pliable and smart enough to absorb what he was being taught at a rapid rate; physically strong enough to withstand the rigors of the early years of yoga training; and, most surprising of all, perfectly content to assume the submissive role of the student in the relationship, knowing his day would come. Perry later referred to the transmission of wisdom from Hamati to himself as nothing less than a "blood transfusion."

During the early years of Perry's time with Hamati, Eastern mysticism had joined an enlarging menu of spiritual alternatives for Americans. The young Iowan became part of an avant-garde—an early counterculture—that rejected the traditions of the West. His absorption in this world was total. "To the very best of my knowledge and belief, I have lived those studies and in the manner prescribed by your traditional teacher," he later wrote. "As a small boy, I was placed in the hands of Hamati to mold as he might see fit and proper, and the ideal to reach was the Yoga in its fullness and that means to live the study, and that I have done to date and expect to do it to the end." He would carry his guru's photograph with him for the rest of his life, keeping it in a place of honor wherever he traveled, taught, and meditated.

In 1895, Perry turned up in the news after an incident that would have killed an ordinary young man unschooled in the art of pranayama. Swimming in a millrace, a canal that directs a river's flow to a mill's waterwheel—Perry must have misjudged the force of the strong spring runoff, for he was sucked down and pinned beneath the gate that kept debris from damaging the wheel. The force of the water began dragging him deeper, pulling him toward the mill wheel and certain death. A hero named H. H. Rollins rushed to Perry's aid and tried to pull him out from the other side of the gate, but he was stuck fast under the rushing water. Minutes went by and more neighbors gathered and tried to lift the gate but made matters even worse by dropping it on him. Finally, someone turned up an old iron bar, pried the gate upward, and dragged him out of the current. He was laid out on the ground, "apparently more dead than alive," as the local stringer for the *Los Angeles Times* reported. "He appeared to be unconscious, but his companions pounded his chest, turned him over and brought him back to the land of the living." Evidently, Perry's mastery of pranayama had not only saved his life but also given him his first taste of publicity.

A year later, Kittie and John Bernard decided to make the long journey back east to Iowa, taking with them eight-year-old Glen and his three brothers. Perry remained with Hamati on the West Coast, forming a working relationship with his paternal uncle, Dr. Clarence Baker. The brother of Perry's biological father, Erastus, Dr. Baker had established a medical practice in Oakland, and employed his nephew's unusual set of therapeutic techniques to address patients' lingering ailments, using yoga or mental suggestion or both. In fact, Dr. Baker thought highly enough of Perry's skills to begin referring patients to him. This arrangement with Uncle Clarence, as well as other ties to the Baker clan that would reveal themselves later in Perry's life, suggests Perry had some contact with Erastus, who had by this time fathered five more children on his own westward flight from Iowa with his new wife. But there is no record of the two ever reuniting in person.

In fact, Perry dropped his Baker birth name—his father's legacy—in favor of his stepfather's and began the process of re-creating himself in his newly adopted home of San Francisco. He changed Perry to Pierre, and began adding a title or two when he deemed it necessary. He continued his studies with Hamati and set out to explore the city, hoping to figure out what he might do with the rest of his life. Developing a set of skills that augmented what he had learned from his teacher, Pierre Arnold Bernard soon found his calling as a teacher of hypnotism, yoga, and other occult practices—not just to medical men like Dr. Baker, but to those well-off enough to pay his exorbitant fees. He roomed with Hamati in a succession of boardinghouses and began to develop a substantial network of followers who wanted yoga training.

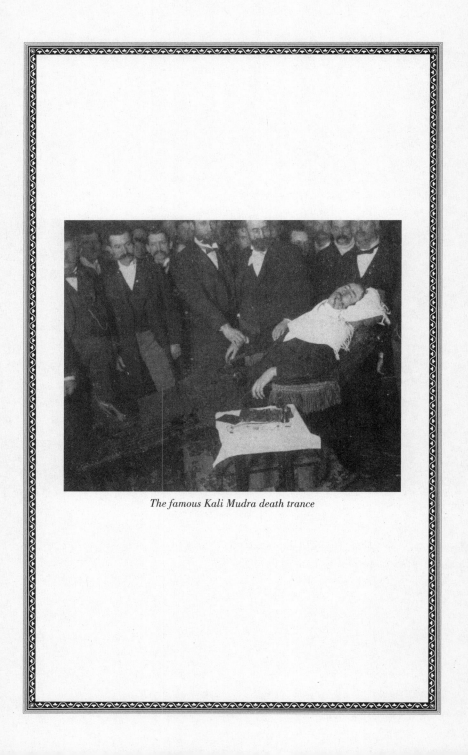

The famous Kali Mudra death trance

Chapter 2

KALI MUDRA

t was January 26, 1898, four days into San Francisco's party of the century. The city had been buffed to a glow for its weeklong Golden Jubilee, the fiftieth anniversary of the discovery of gold in California. The streets were awash in golden bunting; banners and flags hung from window, pillar, and post; everywhere there were portraits of James Marshall, the lucky handyman who found the first gold nugget in 1848. Tons of yellow poppies, California's state flower, decorated the city's doorways, and the Stars and Stripes—folded and sewn into various shapes and sizes—billowed alongside the flags of all the great nations. The city's parks were illuminated by strings of electric lights and Chinese lanterns, and in the drunken shivaree that went on around the clock, frequent booms and blasts shattered the air—from naval cannons and twenty-one-gun salutes to elaborate fireworks that contributed to the wildest week San Francisco had ever known.

But on this cool winter evening, a more dignified assembly had gathered itself at a quiet location a few blocks from the festivities. The San Francisco College of Suggestive Therapeutics had invited some forty doctors and other distinguished guests to 325 Ellis Street to witness a groundbreaking demonstration. As gentlemen of science, the guests were dressed formally for the occasion in wing collars and frock coats, and they hushed themselves as they turned their attention to the thin young man seated before them.

Professor Pierre Arnold Bernard was twenty-one years old and looked it: sandy-haired and pink-skinned, he could nearly be described as boy-ish, save for a lush reddish mustache and intense gray-blue eyes that defied his elders to doubt him. He informed the gallery that they were about to see a rare simulation of death by mental power, a self-imposed anesthetic trance that he, Professor Bernard, called the Kali Mudra in honor of the fierce Hindu goddess. Two reporters took down his words and witnessed the feat as it unfolded. A sketch artist and a photographer, authorized to make "flashlight portraits" of the proceedings in the dark-ened room, worked quietly.

"Ready," said the subject. He closed his eyes, while an elderly man named Dr. D. McMillan prepared the surgical tools. Dr. McMillan knew it would take three minutes before he could begin. His subject, whose physi-cal attributes the older man described as "sensitive in nature, contrary to what one would expect in such work," had even now fled the realm of sensation and was drawing his thoughts inward. Hamati, who was not there that night physically, had taught him well. Bernard lengthened his respiration, slowed it, stretched it, thinned it to a near nothing. His chest gradually stopped moving, and he slid his eyes up beneath the lids. He burrowed his consciousness down, down, down—deep inside the muck and thud of his pulsing blood and organs—and shrank it to a pinpoint less than the size of a cell before he pushed it out through this portal into a vast, undulating, ethery peace the yogis called samadhi. He was gone.

Drs. McMillan and Semple Turman of the college turned to the on-lookers, who watched with intense curiosity. Bernard now appeared to be as still as a corpse. McMillan then brandished for the gallery a steel surgi-cal needle, nearly a foot or so in length. He stepped up to his subject and pushed it slowly through one of Bernard's earlobes. The doctors watched as he pushed another needle through the young man's cheek. He inserted a third through Bernard's upper lip and then ran a fourth through his nostril, sewing the ends of the metal together with thread. A bit of blood began running into the swaddling wrapped around the subject's neck.

The surgery continued, but there was no movement from the patient, whose rosy features had turned white. His hands were cold and clammy to Dr. McMillan's touch. The surgeons finished their work and stepped back. The assembled group were invited to come close for a better look, but . . . Wait, they were told. This was not yet the culmination of the demonstration. McMillan gently opened Bernard's mouth. In one hand he brandished a large ladies' hat pin and slowly ran it through the center of Bernard's tongue, which no doubt caused a few in the room to wince, but produced not even a flutter of reaction from the tongue's owner. The assembled doctors were beckoned to come close once again to inspect the man in the trance, and they did.

The doubters among them were convinced by their own eyes. This was not a carnival sideshow or a magician's trick. The young American yogi had successfully put himself into a trance state deep enough to induce anesthesia to the degree that he slept when an instrument cut through his tongue like a fork through a beefsteak. Dr. McMillan snipped the threads and removed the needles and pins from Bernard's flesh; the towel around his neck had turned dark with his blood. Though Bernard appeared to be somewhat dazed when he came to, he quickly regained himself and assured the crowd he was perfectly fine. He felt well enough in fact to stand up and demonstrate his own powers of suggestion on a professional subject named E. Mansfield Williams, whose head dropped into a trance without Dr. Bernard employing any of the objects and hocus-pocus of the performing hypnotist.

Bernard, a reporter noted with awe, did it "telepathically."

The evening edition of the *San Francisco Call* went for the obvious gruesome details, but didn't miss the larger point of the Kali Mudra demonstration. The headline read:

SEWED HIS LIP TO HIS NOSE
SOME STARTLING EXPERIMENTS IN THE STATE OF
SELF-INDUCED HYPNOTISM.
TORTURED WHILE ASLEEP.

The tens of thousands in town for the Golden Jubilee must have lingered on the description of the bizarre event. "Professor P. A. Bernard, of Des Moines, Iowa," was relatively new to the city, they learned, and very young indeed. His extraordinary display of mental powers had demonstrated once and for all that "the administration of an anesthetic for the performing of a surgical operation is totally unnecessary," as one reporter attested. Most important, Professor Bernard's techniques could be passed along to anyone who wished to enroll at the College of Suggestive Therapeutics and learn the secrets of what he called "trained occultism."

By Saturday, Bernard's feat was a topic of breakfast-table discussion across the nation. He shared the front page of the *New York Times* on that day with William Kissam Vanderbilt, grandson of the Commodore, who was moving quietly to assume control of the family's New York Central Railroad—and it wouldn't be the last time their names appeared together. At Harvard Medical College, Dr. T. B. Keyes, founding chair of hypnotism studies at the school and one of the country's leading experts, conveyed his approval of the San Francisco experiment: "The use of hypnosis in medical work is always satisfactory, much more so than drugs, and it may be used with perfect safety in many cases where anesthetics would almost surely have fatal results. I am thoroughly convinced that Professor Bernard's experiments will prove of great value to the medical and scientific world."

In Chicago, a panel of esteemed physicians bickered among themselves about the technicalities of Bernard's method; in the end they refused to be impressed. Dr. H. N. Moyer, the city's famous specialist in nervous disorders, dismissed the experiment and said, "Self-induced hypnosis . . . will never be of real value to medical science, until suggestive hypnosis is more thoroughly understood."

The public just wanted to know more. From the man in the street to intellectuals like William James of Harvard, Americans were fascinated with hypnosis, autosuggestion, and other forms of mental power. Nearly eight hundred books on hypnotism were published from 1894 to 1897, and schools teaching mind-control techniques and theory sprang up in major cities on the East and West coasts.

The San Francisco College of Suggestive Therapeutics, founded by McMillan and Turman, had been in operation for some time before Bernard signed on to lead the school's fourth course of hypnosis demonstrations in early 1898. For Dr. McMillan, a local surgeon who had maintained a thirty-year fascination with hypnotism, witnessing the formidable skills of Professor Bernard confirmed his deepest beliefs. As the young man had proved, anesthesia could indeed be produced naturally by the properly trained human mind. But McMillan had also been campaigning to prevent what were politely called "premature burials"—when still living people were accidentally buried or cremated—which he insisted took place every week in the United States. Bernard's cataleptic trance would prove to his colleagues once and for all that only advanced electrical testing or decomposition could reasonably ensure that a corpse was really a corpse. And the young man clearly showed he could consistently put others under with little effort. Bragging about his prodigy's "wonderful" ability, McMillan could barely control his enthusiasm. Bernard's talent "outclasses anything I have ever seen," he told a reporter.

McMillan gladly took on the role of Bernard's assistant and helped the twenty-one-year-old cultivate a public persona as a man of science—a great boon to the young man's career. At this time, the nation was embroiled in a roiling debate over the uses of hypnotism, which was considered a powerful, dangerous tool—a human narcotic. In San Francisco, a majority of medical experts polled by a local paper came to the conclusion that hypnotism's potential for evil "far outweighs the good." Seeking to protect the public from quacks and frauds, lawmakers wanted hypnotism's use outlawed or limited to physicians. For Bernard, his association with MDs like his uncle Clarence Baker and McMillan granted him cover and legitimacy.

In May 1898, four months after their first public demonstration, McMillan and Bernard were still working together. McMillan, responding to what he said were requests to provide more information on his experiments, wrote in the *Washington Post* of Bernard's uncanny consistency and accuracy in his feats of bodily control. "I will say first of all he regulates the sleep by having some physician suggest how long it shall last, and in his sleep of forty minutes, I have never seen him miss it more than for six to ten seconds."

McMillan's imprimatur in the national press turned out to be a publicity coup for Bernard, who then repeated the Kali Mudra demonstration for physicians and surgeons at other medical schools in San Francisco, building his reputation and gaining additional admirers. Bernard's lectures ultimately provided him with seventy-two private pupils, he said, all of whom were licensed physicians and surgeons who each paid $100 to learn his skills. The fee was more than twice the average American worker's monthly salary at the time, so it goes without saying that Bernard quickly became a rich young man.

<hr>

San Francisco at the turn of the twentieth century was the preeminent port of the West Coast, a freewheeling metropolis of grand opera and great wickedness—the "Paris of the Pacific," in its planners' eyes. The wealthy, cosmopolitan class had produced its first generation of heirs, and on cool evenings the cable cars filled with these young men in tall silk hats, escorting young ladies wearing furred opera coats and kidskin gloves. It was a youthful city enjoying long days and nights—a city in love with its own limitless energy.

Bernard had set himself down among an emerging middle class, living among busy salesmen and merchants and their growing families. He had established a firm footing with his teaching job at the College of Suggestive Therapeutics, but his real bread and butter came from ministering to those wealthy young heirs moving in societal strata high above his neighbors and even the doctors he taught in his day job. This clientele he cultivated in his second, parallel career as a personal guru—life coach, in modern terms—to the rich and famous young people of the city. He made a fortune teaching them, as Hamati had taught him, "Vedic philosophy and the physical training peculiar to that branch of work in India."

San Francisco also provided Bernard with a front-row seat—and backstage pass—as the first wave of Indian swamis arrived in the United States, following the success of the World Parliament of Religions in Chicago in 1893. Actually these men (and one woman) came to the United States as reverse missionaries, Hindu monks spreading the word of a new and modern version of their faith. These were highly educated, English-speaking emissaries for a reformed, westernized Hinduism—monotheistic and service oriented—that shared its God, Brahma, with Christians, Jews, and Muslims.

The most famous of the first wave was Swami Vivekananda, the noted spokesman for this new "practical" Hinduism. He was of average height and somewhat stout in physical appearance, but so dynamic at the podium that reporters nicknamed him "the Cyclonic Monk" and scrambled for his rhetorical offerings. Bernard befriended Vivekananda when the swami passed through San Francisco in the spring of 1900 to appear at Washington Hall, where he delivered his signature modern message that *everyone can do it.* "The science of Yoga tells us that we are all geniuses if we try hard to be," Vivekananda told his audience. "Some will come into this life better fitted and will do it quicker perhaps. We can all do the same. The same power is in everyone."

Following in his footsteps came a group of youthful, attractive yogis, in particular Ram Tirath, a thirty-year-old Hindu intellectual and practicing Tantric priest whom Bernard took under his wing and gave a place to live. Swami Ram was so impressed with the young Iowan that he told a San Francisco reporter that Bernard possessed a "perfect understanding of Tantrik doctrine, principles, and practice," and that the young American was "most earnest, sincere, and zealous for the cause."

Bernard later recalled this time with affection as the period when he was, in essence, assembling his own curriculum from the teachers he met. "I always made it a point to assure myself that they had nothing that I was not already familiar with," he said, "or I devoted the time necessary to get what they had."

But the work of the westernized swamis differed from Bernard's on a fundamental point: their yoga was *not* of the body, but rather an ascetic, Christianized yoga, influenced by British Victorian morals and the ideas of the Theosophical Society. Following the prejudices of his upbringing, Vivekananda in fact criticized hatha yoga as dangerous and unnecessary to enlightenment. The nascent network of Vedanta schools he built as he traveled around the country all subscribed to this nonphysical notion of yoga.

Bernard read Vivekananda's work and took from it what he needed, but he stuck fast to his opinion about the value of physical yoga, which he had already begun to explore for its therapeutic potential. To that end, he added to his résumé by opening a free clinic for the treatment of nervous disorders, and from this office he expanded the arrangements he'd enjoyed with Dr. Baker, referring patients to the doctors he had trained in hypnosis. They in turn made referrals back to his private practice for the well-off. In effect, Bernard had created a personally branded business, a sturdy three-legged enterprise that nourished its own growth and was based entirely on his renown as a master of mental and physical powers.

It turned out that there were plenty of wealthy takers. Nervous disorders were a common ailment, particularly among the rich, and these maladies had long proved quite amenable to treatment by hypnotic suggestion. Bernard, an obviously skilled hypnotist, made an excellent living treating these patients.

But he was restless by nature, always on the lookout for the next opportunity—a good thing, since his uncle, Dr. Clarence Baker, was none too pleased to discover that Bernard had taken to misrepresenting his medical credentials—a habit that would lead to Bernard's arrest in April 1902 for practicing medicine illegally. By the time these setbacks transpired, however, he and Hamati had already embarked on a new joint venture, developing plans for a brotherhood of Tantrik lodges that would, they projected, stretch across America and around the world.

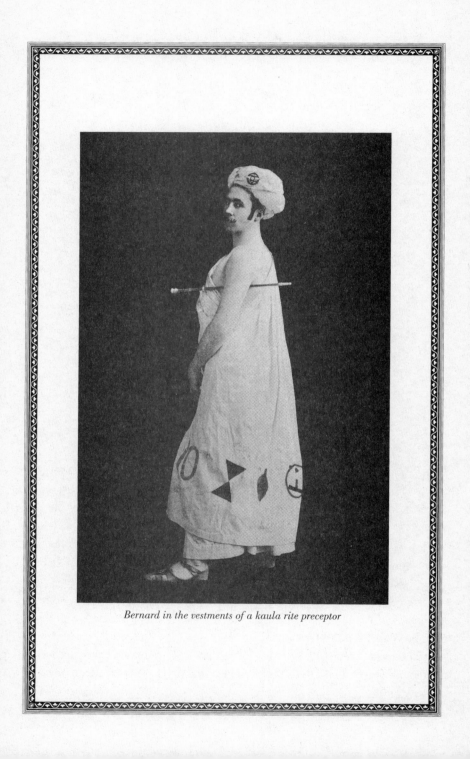

Bernard in the vestments of a kaula rite preceptor

Chapter 3

TANTRIK NIGHTS

KAULA rite, Chakra Ring, or Full Initiation, with 7 M's begins midnight October 8th; Siva festival following. Tantriks sojourning on coast must first register for examination with attendant.

–W. TORMES, 1411A GOLDEN GATE AVE.

alling all Tantriks! The snake-encircled logo of the Tantrik Order, which appeared with this ad in the classified section of a San Francisco newspaper circa 1900, was an "eyes only" message. Its meaning was understood by devotees, initiates, and other parties interested in Bernard's brand of yoga on the West Coast. He and Hamati were teaching the secret stuff: hatha yoga and its philosophical underpinnings from the Tantras, a set of sacred scriptures containing beliefs, rituals, and practices that maintain that enlightenment can be obtained through body practices. What exactly was being offered with the use of such strange and unfamiliar language will soon become obvious, but first meet Bernard's new followers, the free spirits who joined him body and soul on October nights like this.

The most prominent members of the Tantrik Order were the brothers Hugh and Harry Tevis, sons of the richest man in California, Lloyd Tevis. The elder Tevis was a cold, hard, and successful businessman: a president of Wells Fargo Express Co., vice president of the Southern Pacific

Railroad, and a principal of Anaconda Copper Mining Company. He'd had a hand in nearly every booming business in San Francisco from the gold rush onward and left his descendants great wealth and impeccable social connections. But the Tevis heirs also encountered a large share of misfortune: suicide, illness, early death, and accidents—tragedies that befell the family in swift succession after the century's turning.

Bernard attended to the Tevis men personally, teaching them yoga and philosophy two hours per day for a year and a half. He also boasted of his friendships with society party boy Lansing Kellogg and Major Henry Farnsby Bulwer, well known throughout the state as a rich and flamboyant British ex-pat who was doing his best to elevate California from a circuit of dirt-street oil towns to an industrial power.

Adding a bit of bohemian color to this group of well-heeled followers, Bernard mixed in artists like Winfield Jesse Nicholls, the handsome son of a well-to-do family who lived on Eddy Street. Nicholls was just nineteen years old when he met the man he would follow for the next forty years. The teenager was so impressed with Bernard that he quit his job as an illustrator for the *San Francisco Chronicle,* abandoning career and family to live and study full-time with the Tantriks, taking the lodge name of "Tormes" for the time being.

Another adult runaway was Florin Howard Jones, the tall, soft-spoken son of a prominent real estate broker whose office on Montgomery Street dealt in turn-of-the-century McMansions. Jones was an earnest young seeker, and he carried himself with the dignity of a very old soul. He had recently begun his own business, a merchandising operation on Fillmore, but it soon enough took second place to his yoga studies with Pierre Bernard.

These young people stepped away from their straight middle-class lives and virtually disappeared into Bernard's Tantrik Order. They discarded their given names and took up new identities—in some cases more than one. Joined by musicians, actors, and other performers, they formed an appealing group of free spirits—a band of dashing gypsy occultists who traveled in a pack, lived together in communes, and conducted their mystical business late in the evenings. They dwelt among Irish and German immigrants on Ellis Street and Golden Gate Avenue, as well as on Pine and Jones streets, where they rented rooms and apartments—always requesting the top floor for a little more privacy and unobstructed views of the night sky. Clusters of up to three domiciles formed what Bernard insisted they call lodges, where they performed their rituals after midnight, the most solemn of these under a full moon.

The training he gave them was divided into seven departments, or degrees—Bernard called it a "life school"—requiring blood oaths and vows of lifetime silence and obedience. Initiates were warned that much hard work lay ahead: to reach the seventh degree, Bernard's ranking, a newcomer would need to dedicate himself to "seven years working at fourteen hours a day." To teach others and lead a lodge required further study of four to six years in hatha yoga, Sanskrit, and medicine. All interested parties were welcome, except those with chronic disease, "blood taints, those deformed or stiff of limb, intellectually short sighted or impure at heart."

Nicholls's former colleague at the *Chronicle*, L. C. Pedlar, became a peripheral member of the group and witnessed firsthand their rites and rituals. "Bernard seemed to have considerable knowledge of 'Brahmanism,' as he called it," Pedlar told a reporter some years later. "He and [Nicholls] engaged in most curious performances. They called their tricks 'self hypnosis.' They could sew their lips close together, drawing the strands of silk back and forth through the living flesh, without apparent pain. This man Bernard could slice a finger deeply with a knife or razor—so deep that the blood spurted. He would then, without the application of apparent external pressure or the use of a tourniquet, stop the flow of blood instantly."

Bernard and Hamati continued to expand their network of lodges in San Francisco. Bernard called for a committee to raise funds for new buildings and worldwide expansion. Hamati's connections in his native land gave the group an international claim, and documents from the early days of the Tantrik Order (T.O.) consistently mention three other associates building Tantrik lodges in Europe, but no further evidence has ever been found of their existence. In the United States, Bernard traveled to Chicago, St. Louis, New York, and other cities to plant the seeds of his secret society, but at this point his plans were probably bigger than the brotherhood itself. His vision for the future, however, was elaborate and meticulous: he formulated rules and standards to be applied to everything from the governance of the membership to the design of the physical buildings, their furnishings, and the curriculum. Each lodge must maintain a large library, he declared, containing "thousands of all the best standard texts both in original Sanskrit and in translation aside from works cover-ing all collateral studies from the scientific, ethical, and philosophical sides."

In every lodge, Sanskrit study would be available as an elective, but hatha yoga was a *required* course, taught in classrooms in the modern Western style, using room-sized mats of his own design. "Our yoga rooms are padded with four-inch hair mats," he advertised, "and an equable temperature [is] maintained there in summer and winter. Our Lecture rooms are large and the walls entirely covered by black boards in constant use. All through the degrees, we carry the practice of Yoga to the highest point."

There were women who came along for the ride, too; a few perhaps mo-tivated more by romance than by spirituality. These were brave souls, or foolish to a fault, as women risked severe recriminations in Victorian America for even a perceived stain on their character. Purity was the current watchword for an entire social movement, and society painted a bright line between women who kept their reputations pure and those who had fallen.

So what kind of woman would dare join Bernard and his dashing band of yogis? Some came to improve their health, both mental and physi-cal, some were curious seekers who wished to understand his philosophy, even if they did not commit to full participation. There also came into the Tantriks' circle a few freethinking intellectuals or members of the "woman movement," as the feminist parlance had it. These ladies proclaimed prop-erly that it was their right to worship or love as they chose and to vote for whom they wished. So among the membership there were trysts and romances, as evidenced by the paper trail left behind. Howard Petterson, for example, was arrested at one of the Tantrik lodges and not released until he agreed to marry seventeen-year-old Alma Sylvester. Bernard himself applied for a license to marry twenty-two-year-old Eugenie Charbonnier, though the couple didn't go through with it. Young as these women were, however, most of Bernard's female followers seemed well aware of the perils that their association with the Tantrik Order could bring about.

The entire nation—women and men alike—feared especially the bony finger of U.S. Postal Inspector Anthony Comstock, still at the height of his power after more than four decades terrorizing those who dared to write, speak—or even think—freely about sex. Comstock, the founder of the New York Society for the Suppression of Vice, had gained a position in the postal service and used it to turn himself into the nation's top morals cop. He organized a vice-sniffing apparatus of undercover agents, burned by his own count 73,000 pounds of books, and prosecuted more than two thousand people for distributing "obscene, lewd and/or lascivious" information through the mail. Any hint of sensuality was thought to be potentially illegal in Comstock's America, where the legion forces of conformity and puritanism occupied the highest reaches of government, law enforcement, the press, and the clergy. They terrorized novelists, printers, artists, publishers, moviemakers, Theosophists, Orientalists, physical culture buffs, and church lottery operators, and they remained Bernard's mortal enemies as he campaigned to make yoga acceptable for Americans. Comstock's heirs would pursue him and his followers across the United States for the next thirty years.

America was also in the midst of a nativist backlash against the massive influx of immigrants. Nearly 12 million foreign nationals had come to the United States between 1870 and 1900, and this flood of humanity reached its peak in the decade between 1900 and 1910, during which time some one million immigrants per year entered the United States. On the West Coast a growing xenophobia, aimed first at the Chinese and Japanese, slowly turned toward "East Indians," as South Asians were called. The Chinese Exclusion Act, the first of a series of laws passed in the 1880s to control Asian immigration, was extended in 1902. Its sentiments were nowhere more explicitly displayed than in San Francisco, where the proudly racist Asiatic Exclusion League now turned its attention to dark-skinned immigrants from India. By 1906 all Asian Indians would be denied U.S. citizenship.

So wherever Bernard, Hamati, and the Tantriks went, they were viewed with suspicion by a nosy troika of landlords, policemen, and reporters. At their lodge at 1411A Golden Gate Avenue, snitches told the press, there was a dark-skinned "turbanned Syrian"—Hamati, no doubt—who made frequent appearances. A Japanese-American woman could be found at their evening gatherings. Thinly veiled race-based attacks provided a foundation for a series of allegations made against the Tantriks, never proved, of course, that their organization was a den of opium, free love, and prostitution.

But there *was* something going on that kept suspicions raised. "The neighbors complained of the racket and the undesirable class of men and women who frequented them," said Nicholls's friend Pedlar. "Complaint was made to the police and they were forced to move."

Bernard himself seemed unfazed by these setbacks. He'd begun the grand work of his life: to spread the knowledge of yoga in his native land, organizing devotees and initiates into an ambitious national network of lodges. In New York City, he established a fledgling publishing firm called the Tantrik Press. During his New York journeys, he cultivated writers and editors for the press and had begun to personally coach Broadway actresses, a practice that would become a mainstay of his business in the years to come.

In the winter of 1904, Bernard left San Francisco on a grimmer task, making his way to Plainview, Nebraska, to meet the remains of his step-father, John C. Bernard, who had died at the age of fifty-four. Then, as the eldest of his mother's sons, Pierre began to assume the role of pater-familias, taking charge of the funeral arrangements. When he left, he brought his half brother Glen back to California to take care of him, while Kittie remained in Nebraska with the other boys.

Glen was welcomed into this new family and handed over to Hamati, who undertook the task of training another member of the Bernard clan. Pierre accepted the responsibility of keeping his brother fed, clothed, and housed, as he would for others in his extended family, and in return, Glen was put to work writing and researching for publications of the Tantrik Press. Glen was greatly influenced by these years, especially by Hamati, who instilled in the younger Bernard the same great love and curiosity for yoga that he had inspired in Pierre.

While Hamati worked with Glen, Bernard labored to build the Tantrik Order into an influential secret society akin to the Freemasons, of which he himself was a rising member. If the T.O. seems exotic by today's social standards, it was not very far from the mainstream of American life at the time. Every night in cities large and small, bewhiskered fraternal broth-ers and their sisters in veils and gloves scurried across the cobblestones from meeting to meeting, carrying rule books, manuals, pins, badges, and feathers. During the first decade of the century, membership in all such societies ran into the millions, so most Americans were familiar with—and even drawn to—the ideas of inner and outer circles, passwords, initiations, tests of allegiance, and degrees of initiation.

In his use of symbols, codes, and rituals, Bernard borrowed liberally from the Freemasons, the Theosophists, and other groups, religious as well as secular. Beneath the pomp and plumes, however, he detected a genuine hunger for mystical experience—a direct connection to the divine—that many Americans failed to find in church. This was a time of great spiritual upheaval in the nation, what has been called alternately the Third Great Awakening or the first New Age, depending on your point of view. Revivals abounded and mainstream Christian churches struggled to confront the fresh miseries of the teeming cities, where crime, violence, and vice were rampant. Missionaries for a new "muscular Christianity" shipped out for heathen lands to make converts, while social movements for sexual purity, temperance, and universal suffrage grew in strength at home.

There arose in these days the first serious scientific challenges to the average American's religious convictions, primarily that the world was created in seven days. Darwin's evolutionary theories had undermined received truths about religious faith, fomenting the mighty rift between dogma and science that gave rise to Christian fundamentalism. Addressing the rift, Theosophy, Mormonism, Christian Science, New Thought, spiritualism, and Mind Cure had erupted into the culture during Pierre Bernard's coming of age. Occult groups such as the Hermetic Brotherhood of Luxor and the Hermetic Order of the Golden Dawn (the latter an English offshoot of the Freemasons) also developed fledgling networks in the United States, as did clusters of believers in Eastern philosophies. These new religions grew and morphed and borrowed from one another in the process. And they flourished so fast that they came to be seen as threats by mainstream pastors, who demonized the new spiritualities as cults.

Meanwhile, a number of individuals emerged as self-proclaimed mystics bent on fashioning their own religions. G. I. Gurdjieff, P. D. Ouspensky, Edgar Cayce, Aleister Crowley, Father Divine, Aimee Semple McPherson, H. P. Lovecraft, and more than a dozen others all came to national attention around the turn of the century, eager to take part in one of the other prevailing debates of the times: spirit versus matter. All of them, Bernard included, grew into their spiritual inclinations during the height of this debate.

Though it sounds so esoteric today, the question of which is superior, spirit or matter, engaged Americans from all levels of society. The discussion spilled over from the pulpits into newsrooms and economic societies, social clubs and political organizations. The ancillary questions went like this: "Is the nation in need of male rationality or female spirituality?" And was male desire or feminine virtue the better path to hasten human evolution, to perfect "the race" (which at the time meant white Anglo-Saxons)? And perhaps most important of all, could spirit, in the form of the human mind, actually influence the physical world?

Bernard believed it could—had even proved it with his own body for the medical establishment—and he taught his followers how to harness the power of the mind. His system was an American adaptation of Hindu Tantrism, a mix of religious rituals, beliefs, and practices, based on sacred scriptures called Tantras, which teach that the material world is an expression of the divine. Linking the many diverse sects of Tantrism is their worship of the feminine power of procreation, and Hindu Tantric ritual revolves around the worship of the goddess Shakti (sometimes spelled Sakti), the female principle of regeneration. From this platform the Tantric masters later arrived at the idea of the human body as potentially pure and godlike, and in India's tenth century, Tantrism gave birth to hatha yoga, the science of postures and breathing that Bernard taught and that is familiar to twenty-first-century Americans. By the time Hamati had exported the philosophy to Lincoln, Nebraska, Tantrism had been suppressed for centuries in its mother country, functioning as a kind of underground to the westernized Hindu society imposed on India by British rulers and Western missionaries.

Tantrikas divide themselves along two very different paths. The right-hand path takes a conservative approach, interpreting the Tantric texts symbolically. A right-hand Tantric, for example, could pursue the worship of Shakti through reverence for his wife, without violating the bonds of his marriage. Those taking the left-hand path, however, are willing to flout society's traditional norms and revel in mixing the sacred and the so-called profane. This path utilizes taboos—drugs, alcohol, and extramarital sex—and engages in the ritual known in India as the five M's, which refer to the Sanskrit words for wine, meat, fish, parched grain (perhaps a psychotropic substance or drug), and sexual intercourse.

The first four are used to rouse the sexual instinct, which is then channeled in order to rouse the serpent power, the kundalini, granting the adept great powers and knowledge. In the ascetic traditions of Indian religion, all of the five M's are forbidden fruit, so a left-handed Tantric ritual could be a shameful, heart-pounding excursion into outlaw behavior.

The ritual of sacramental sexual intercourse, performed by two young initiates in the midst of a solemn circle of chanting devotees and choreographed by a high priest, has captured the human imagination forever. It harks back to Ice Age rituals of female fertility worship and the Eleusinian mysteries of the Greeks, and it has found its way into the plot of the modern best seller *The Da Vinci Code*.

In several cities, according to witnesses, Bernard's group reserved secret rooms for such worship, and he gave many hints that sex as a sacrament was part of the Tantric practices he taught. In San Francisco, Bernard and the young Tantrikas were at least dabbling in the hard-core left-handed stuff. The evidence for this lies in the coded classified ad for the kaula ceremony, which is generally considered one of the most extreme forms of Tantra. In kaula rites, the sexual act is performed in a chakra "circle" of worshippers, always late at night in a deserted place in order to maintain the privacy necessary to perform the five M's.

And just so that there was no confusion about who was licensed to be at the center of the sacred sex, Bernard quoted to his followers from a translation of the Mahanirvana Tantra, which noted that only a worshipper who possesses a seventh-degree certification in the Tantrik Order—in this case Bernard himself—"may marry by mutual choice another, in the assemblage of the Sakti-worshipers, when a circle is formed." Bernard, it seems, could choose his own partner for sacred sex or act as a matchmaker for willing initiates.

Much of what we know about Bernard's thinking is contained in a remarkable book-length document called *Vira Sadhana: International Journal of the Tantrik Order*. This publication, whose title translates roughly to "the way of the hero," was the bible of the Tantrik Order, written and compiled during the San Francisco years by the Bernard brothers, Hamati, and other followers. The debut publication of the Tantrik Press, the book was an oversize, lavishly produced affair, using the best photographic reproduction obtainable by the printers of the day. On its cover, printed in gold on a field of deep red silk, were the group's mystical symbols: the two intersecting triangles (for the union of male and female), the winged globe (symbol of the cosmic egg), and a snake devouring its tail (the *ouroboros*, representing completion, perfection, and totality). In its pages were abstracts of texts from the Tantras and the Vedas, India's holy literature, as well as instructions for Tantrik rituals, quotations, exhortations, comparisons to Western religions, and a bibliography for further study.

The *Vira Sadhana* makes the case for Tantrik Yoga, as Bernard sometimes called his practice, proclaiming it to be the most scientific and up-to-date way to worship and live. In an essay called "The Basis of Religion," he makes the case for a more elevated discussion of love and sex.

> In this day and age, when matters pertaining to the sexes are generally avoided, and we are taught that the sexual appetite is an animal craving that should be subdued and concealed as unworthy of man's superior nature, it is not surprising that the great majority of persons are blind to the vast importance and significance of the sexual nature in its relation to the affairs of the world . . . not only is it the cause of our individual existence, but it is the foundation of society and the well spring of human life and happiness.

This erotic manifesto, which Bernard left unsigned for legal protection, was written with the kind of linguistic assurance that came through in his lectures. "The animating impulse of all organic life is the sexual instinct," he writes. "It is that which underlies the struggle for existence in the animal world and is the source of all human endeavor and emotion." Sex, Bernard goes on to attest, "is the most powerful factor in all that pertains to the human race and has ever been the cause and the subject of man's most exalted thought."

Not a bad start for the Tantrik Press, which Bernard said would next publish English-language translations of the most important Vedic and Tantric works. This first book, however, appears to be a mash-up of everything Bernard knew, read, believed at the time, or at least deemed important enough to print. It is a helter-skelter affair, mixing biblical passages with maxims from Hindu, Buddhist, and Christian philosophy, salted with Freemasonry references, sensual illustrations, and photography. All truth is sacred, Bernard said many times, and the pages of the *Vira Sadhana* are the quintessential embodiment of his agglomerative brand of Tantrism. Strangely, many of the quotations and commentary in the marginalia are attributed to friends and followers and even to his half brothers.

To the Tantrikas, discussion of the sex instinct was not merely theoretical. The success of the club relied on initiates like Jones and Nicholls drumming up new customers to come to the meetings and take the courses. The tall, blue-eyed Nicholls was the band's preferred female bait. He was so handsome and devastatingly soulful of nature, admirers said, that his sexual magnetism was legendary.

But his youth and inexperience soon proved to be a liability for the club. On June 4, 1905, Nicholls was arrested and thrown in jail for embezzlement, over a slew of unpaid bills from local merchants. The next day the *San Francisco Call* published a portrait of the boyish Nicholls on the front page, along with the headline "Police Are Looking into Occult Affairs: Nichols [*sic*] Tells of Mystic Class." Nicholls had apparently been augmenting his appeal to women by offering baubles—opera glasses, silver brush sets—to help land prospective clients. He was held in jail for a few days, left there by his father, who hoped that this tough-love experience would turn his son against Bernard.

Instead Bernard came to Nicholls's aid, and spent an entire afternoon with his attorney, D. W. Burchard. He explained to the lawyer that the club was doing serious work in mystical and spiritual matters, and that Nicholls was never sent out to do anything criminal. Nor did they ever smoke opium, as some neighbors had charged.

Burchard came away so convinced of Bernard's goodwill that he defended him to a reporter from the *San Francisco Call* as "a rare student" who had given up his practice as a physician to become an occultist and hypnotist. Nicholls was eventually released; the charges against him were dropped two weeks later, after his parents paid his debt.

But the San Francisco police stepped up their investigations of the

Tantriks, especially of the bawdy gatherings Bernard called the Bacchante Club. An undercover police officer infiltrated the group and later told reporters that at a meeting he attended he found "men dressed in long black gowns sitting on the floor smoking Turkish water pipes, while girls danced before them."

In a city rife with crime and riddled with vice, the youthful Tantrikas stood apart for their upper- and middle-class origins. These were not reviled Chinese opium addicts and prostitutes who could be herded into slums, harassed, and prosecuted at will; they were mainly well-off white kids, acting up in the better parts of the city and embarrassing their parents on the front pages of the dailies. And they showed no signs of stopping their activities. Something had to give. As the police made it more and more apparent that their continued presence was unwelcome, Bernard and his Tantrikas began scouting for friendlier climes. By April 18, 1906, the day of the great San Francisco earthquake, the group had already left, heading north up the Pacific Coast in search of their next home.

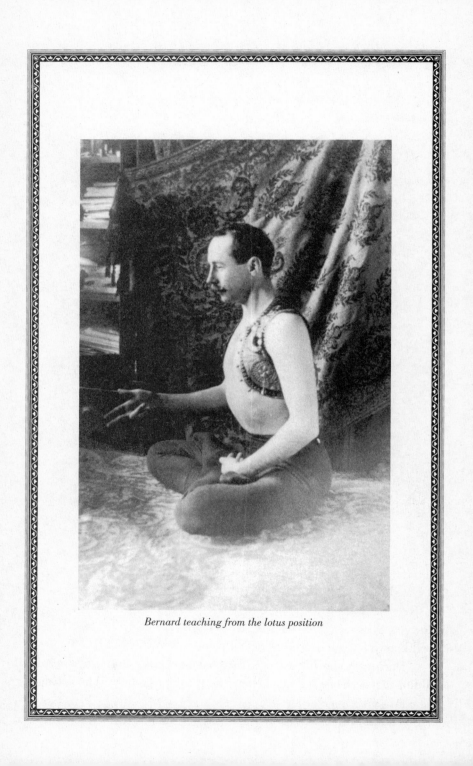

Bernard teaching from the lotus position

Chapter 4

DOWNFALL
AND DISGRACE

The whole man is approached and touched by yoga. Life becomes brighter, nobler, grander and happier; mind becomes
keen, calm, peaceful and emotionally satisfied and the body
clean, vital, strong.

—P. A. BERNARD, 1906

n Seattle, Washington, Bernard and Hamati made a fresh start. They quickly established a network of yoga schools and health clinics, there and in Portland, Oregon, recruiting followers from among the wealthy and powerful families of these cities. It was probably not a coincidence that the men who joined were not only pillars of propriety but also members of Masonic lodges, and thus familiar with rites, degrees, rituals, and the need for secrecy. Bernard boasted of his relationship with Judge John Stanley Webster, a respected Spokane jurist who would later serve three terms as a Republican congressman. He also counted among his flock Walter A. Keene, a well-known lawyer, as well as the oil pioneer W. W. French.

"During my stay in Seattle I had about 60 pupils," Bernard later said, adding that each one again paid him a hefty tuition of $100. Tantrik lodges were established on the shore of Lake Washington, on Third Avenue, and at two other prime locations. Expenses were shared by the newcomers, who were joined in these coed communes by the core group from San Francisco, including Nicholls and Jones.

Pierre's stepbrother Glen also came with them, but he would stay in Seattle only a short time. He'd begun to question his brother's outsize ego and use of hatha yoga for material gain—a violation of one of the *yamas*, the moral precepts of yoga. After a few months, he left the group, traveling across the country, and later settled in California, married, and had a son, Theos Casimir Hamati Bernard, whom he abandoned after a couple of years to devote himself to his yoga practice. Twenty-five years later he would return to Theos's life to pass along his well-tended grudges to his son, including one that burned hottest in his heart: that Pierre had stolen the credit for his work on the *Journal of the Tantrik Order.*

Back in Seattle, however, the open family slot among the Tantrikas was quickly filled by fifteen-year-old Ora Ray Baker, Pierre's shy, blond half sister, who'd left her father's home in Wenatchee and become Pierre's ward. Whether this handoff was arranged at a distance or in person is not known, but it appears to be the last contact Pierre had with his father, Erastus, who would die alone in a veterans' home in California fifteen years later. By that time Pierre and Ora Ray would both be long gone, settled into very different lives.

<hr>

Seattle provided a comfortable, multicultural haven for the Tantriks. The Queen City Theosophical Society hosted a Hindu lecturer that spring who spoke to packed houses for several weeks. There were Buddhists and Rosicrucians and other metaphysical iconoclasts settled in the hills around them. As a Pacific Coast port, Seattle was home to thriving Asian communities that supported at least one Zen temple and a judo school. Here the group cooked and ate their meals together, made music, fell in love, studied yoga and Hindu philosophy, and carried on in their freewheeling ways. Nicholls attracted the amorous attention of a young actress named Jennie Leo, who joined the group and agreed to sign her novitiate's oath in blood, pledging heart and soul to the Tantrik Order. His fellow San Franciscan, Florin Jones, had by this time married a young Tantrika known only by her lodge name, Duval.

From this home base in the Pacific Northwest, Bernard continued to make trips to New York City, where his roster of clients had expanded to include the legendary actress Lillian Russell. New York held great appeal for Bernard, drawn as he was to the electric lights of the Broadway marquees and the brassy but vulnerable ladies of the stage. He taught a few of these New York students personally; a few others he convinced to join him as employees of the Tantrik Press. In 1907 and 1908, he lingered in New York City for three months after befriending two Indian doctors, T. C. Iyengar and Major U. L. Desai, with whom he shared living quarters on the West Side of Manhattan. Iyengar and Desai were part of an early movement to resuscitate hatha yoga in India, where it remained verboten under the rules of Anglo-Indian society, and their friendship fortified Bernard's emotional ties to a land he'd never set foot in. Though he eventually circled back to the Northwest, he had begun to consider New York City the future home for the Tantrik Order.

Back in Seattle, Hamati and Bernard agreed that after eighteen years of association, the student had learned everything his teacher had to offer. It was time for Bernard to move on, and his teacher wished to go home. Together for one last formal occasion on the afternoon of October 26, 1907, they finalized matters. Before a notary public, Hamati signed over any legal rights he possessed to the intellectual material that made up the *Vira Sadhana*. He gave his home address as "Calcutta and other points in India" and testified that he was awarded $5,370 in gold coin, the equivalent of over $115,000 today.

Bernard was now officially on his own.

In 1908, the Tantriks' membership continued to grow in the Pacific Northwest—ultimately Bernard opened four lodges in Seattle and one in Portland. As happened in San Francisco, some of the members mingled romantically with the locals and a few had affairs that came back to haunt them. Jennie Leo made the mistake of giving her heart to Winfield Nicholls, who had never in his young life been known to settle down with one woman. In fact, he was at the time also seeing a woman named Daisy Mix, who was stuck in an unhappy common-law marriage with a wealthy Seattle businessman.

Watching from the sidelines was Jennie's younger sister, Gertrude, who was living with her in Seattle. Seeing her big sister dip in and out of this circle of wealthy and well-connected people, Gertrude wanted very much to be part of it. In January 1909, when she turned eighteen, she applied for membership and Bernard accepted her. Gertrude, a stenographer with a sweet, open face and blond, curly hair, had recently been hospitalized for a vaguely diagnosed heart condition. Bernard proposed to restore her to health with a series of yoga postures and breathing exercises that would slow down her metabolism and strengthen her heart. Both sisters consented, and soon Gertrude was living among the Tantriks in one of their lodges.

Bernard, meanwhile, was anxious to get back to New York, and he proposed that the others in the group move with him for good. He asked Gertrude to come along, suggesting that she'd be a good companion for seventeen-year-old Ora Ray. Gertrude could continue her studies and work for the organization as a stenographer and teacher of hatha yoga. The young woman agreed to the move, leaving her sister Jennie behind in the Pacific Northwest to nurse her heartbreak over Nicholls.

<hr />

Gertrude Leo arrived in New York on Monday, June 7, 1909. After she'd dropped her bags at the apartment Bernard had rented for everyone on West 171st Street, the two of them made their way down to Battery Park, at Manhattan's southern tip. The day grew sultry as it stretched on, and they sat for hours in a shady intersection of lawns, gardens, and promenades, watching the boats rounding the seawall: steamers, ferries, and sailing craft coming and going in the busiest harbor in the world. Battery Park was where New York had started its life, so it made a perfect spot to talk about new beginnings in their new home in the greatest city in the world.

Bernard told Gertrude about his vision for the Tantrik Order and the role he envisioned for her. She was to be a nautch girl, he said, like the girls in India who live at the Hindu temples and devote themselves to the priests. Gertrude probably knew very well what he was talking about. The idea of a sacred, sensual temple dancer, wrapped in precious jewels and worshipped by men, was well fixed in the popular imagination in 1909. The nautch girl had been westernized and glamorized by dancer Ruth St. Denis, who had become a raging success—critical as well as popular—on vaudeville stages across the United States and Europe. St. Denis performed solo and barefoot, her writhing yoga-inspired choreography accompanied by visiting Asian musicians. Moving across the stage through clouds of incense, St. Denis rippled her arms like cobras and swirled her sinewy abdomen in costumes that scandalously exposed four inches of bare midriff. Her choreography evoked a startling combination of spirituality and sensuousness that on several occasions stunned audiences into respectful silence at the end of her performance.

Bernard presented the nautch girl role as a new and modern means of feminine empowerment. "All priests," he told Gertrude, "have nautch girls. In my sacred capacity, I cannot marry, but our nautch girls serve us as wives. It is the duty of the priest to give her all the world's best goods. She is looked upon as sacred."

Bernard impressed upon Gertrude his knowledge of psychic powers, real and imaginary, and of the difference between simulative and real phenomena. The ability to produce deceptive appearances was a simulative phenomenon, he explained, common enough among occultists and magicians—Bernard himself was a talented magician who specialized in Hindu disappearing tricks. But the power to actually influence the bodies and souls of others with his mind was a real phenomenon and proof of his power. "I am not a real man," he told her, quoting ancient Hindu texts about yoga and supernatural powers. "I am a god, but I have condescended to put on the habit of a man, that I may perform the duties of a yogi and reveal true religion to the elect of America."

It was a pretty hard sell, and Gertrude told him she needed to think it over. That night she went back uptown and stayed with Ora Ray at the apartment.

The next day, she announced her decision to move to the next level of commitment. "I became a novitiate," she later said, just as her sister had before her. "The ends of my fingers were slit open and the blood was poured upon a pen. Then I signed my name on the document." This document, "The Tantrik Oath," begins with a fearsome warning: "As lightning from the womb of the clouds rends in twain the mighty oak, I pray that the relentless and exacting justice of the law of Brahma, which is as inexorable and all consuming as his love is inexhaustible, may shatter and torture me in agonizing pain beyond the power of speech to describe should I ever deviate from the following affirmations and declarations."

Then followed a call to fellowship and secrecy, vows to value education and trust in the hierarchy of the order, to submit to the teachers and to their ancient wisdom. Time and again, though, the oath cautions all who sign in their blood to "guard my speech and seal my mouth forever to those outside our ranks." Gertrude, assured of her special place in Bernard's life, became his nautch girl and his lover.

By July the Tantriks had moved to a beautiful new home in a posh neighborhood, an ivy-covered brownstone at 258 West Seventy-fourth Street. Jones arrived from Seattle with Duval, who was now pregnant with his child. Nicholls turned up, unattached, having dumped Jennie Leo and moved on from Daisy Mix. Other residents included an actress whose lodge name was Cornel and two single men who had come from the West Coast, Bradlaw, a banjo player, and an unremarkable follower named Richard Sanford.

The Tantrik Order's new headquarters was located a stone's throw from the luxurious apartment hotel the Ansonia on New York's swanky Upper West Side. This was a neighborhood recently favored by well-connected politicians as well as tycoons like Charles Schwab. Opulence was the order of the day, and Bernard saw to the interior decorations himself. The public rooms were done up in a typical Victorian cum "Oriental" manner—heavy drapes and dark-colored hangings and carpets. Upstairs, there were large padded rugs on the floor, covered in a painted canvas that displayed the order's mystical symbols. Once his growing spiritual library had arrived from Seattle, Bernard opened the doors of this well-kept townhouse as a yoga school and sanitarium.

Nicholls and Jones, Bradlaw and Sanford and others from Bernard's core group fanned out across New York in search of well-heeled, interested parties—doctors, patients, the sickly, occultists, spiritual seekers, and health-fad enthusiasts. The Tantrik heralds spread the news: There was a new guru in town. Come try our hatha yoga classes, offered several times a week in the evenings, along with instruction in yogic breathing, meditation, and philosophy. Or drop by on the weekends, on Bacchante evenings, when food and drink would be offered and the house was opened to respectful, curious seekers.

One of Bernard's first clients was a shy, dreamy young woman named

Zelia Hopp, who lived with her parents in the Bronx. Zelia was a sickly girl—a worry to her parents, who trundled her off to a succession of physicians, praying that she would get well and find a husband like her older sister, Esther. It was in fact Zelia's older sister, Mrs. Esther Betts, who'd heard the news about a famous and powerful healer named Dr. Warren, who had just arrived from the West Coast. Thus, Zelia and the Hopp family were introduced to this talented doctor, who was in fact Pierre Bernard, a specialist in the cure of heart troubles or what was called neurasthenia.

In the fall of 1909, Bernard visited the family for the first time, and he impressed Zelia's mother and father with his obvious erudition, his intentions, and the soundness of his methods. His fees were another matter. Though Zelia held a job as a milliner, she most likely worked for subsistence wages, and would never be able to move from her parents' home until she had married—an unlikely development if she remained ill. Surely her parents had this thought in mind as they scraped together the $40 initiation fee—a hefty sum considering the average American worker made about $13 a week at that time, for fifty-nine hours of labor.

The next day, with her parents' approval, Miss Hopp traveled alone to Manhattan and arrived at the brownstone, where Bernard, cigar in hand, ushered her into a back room and conducted a physical exam. He concluded that yes, he could help her; yes, she could regain her vitality and even flourish under his care . . . but it would take extreme measures and individual attention. He sent one of his associates to find a suitable place, and in November he installed her in his new "sanitarium," a rented apartment at 70 West 109th Street, near Central Park. Zelia's father visited the place to make sure it was on the up-and-up before allowing his daughter to move in.

Beneath the cloak of therapy, however, a powerful attraction developed between the worldly thirty-three-year-old Bernard and the nineteen-year-old Zelia. Her first night at the apartment, Bernard paid her a visit, and between boasts of his knowledge of spiritual domains, he kissed her until her breath gave out. She was a lucky woman, he told her—he was very powerful, very wealthy. He assured her of his commitment and his honorable intentions. She felt herself fall completely under his power, hypnotized to obey him. Several nights later, she surrendered to the most pressing of his wishes and the couple made love. Zelia stayed at the 109th

Street apartment for months, entertaining Bernard's visits until he could no longer manage the rent. She then returned home, cured of her heart trouble and in fine spirits, to her parents' great relief.

Money remained tight during the winter of 1909–1910. The weather was severe and the Tantriks were not bringing in enough cash to pay the bills in their new location. Clients like Zelia were few and far between, and Bernard grew angry at Nicholls and Jones for what he perceived as their lack of effort. There was little to eat, and the house grew cold; the gas and electric power were turned on only intermittently to economize. At one point, Bernard sold some of the furniture to buy food for his followers. The women in the group noted that Nicholls behaved like a slave around Bernard, bending to his whims, performing any task required without complaint. When Bernard needed cigars, Nicholls skipped meals to save enough money to buy them; he pawned his overcoat and spent the rest of the winter with newspapers stuffed inside his shirt to keep himself warm.

There was tragedy, too. The child of Jones and Duval was delivered by a physician forced to work by candlelight. The infant was often sick and would not eat, and Jones and Bernard were continually feuding over Jones's inability or unwillingness to turn his devotion into a means of support for the house. Bernard even threw him out for a time, and though Duval and the infant were allowed to stay, the baby died after only a few months. The doctor who'd delivered the child returned to certify the death, which he attributed to malnutrition.

With the arrival of spring came some much-needed good news. Bernard's mother had married a former Iowan named Robert D. Martin, a prosperous widower ten years her senior, and the couple had settled at his ranch in Fillmore, California. Kittie's nuptials brought relief to her worried son and auspicious tidings to the Tantrikas, as more and more pupils found their way to Bernard's brownstone. Suddenly there were some sixty new yoga students registered. By the time the weather had warmed, the place was hopping.

Jones and Nicholls took charge of administrative duties in the main-floor parlor. The enrollment contract they handed to potential students stipulated that the full $100 fee be paid at once for a discount or in three monthly installments of $40 each. For those seeking individual attention, a separate fee of $20 was charged for a physical examination with Bernard. Those seeking reading matter were sold the *Journal of the Tantrik Order* for $2. On Monday, Wednesday, and Friday, yoga classes, for ten to twelve students at a time, were held in the large mat rooms on the second floor, led by Ora Ray or Gertrude, who wore sexy "Yogi suits"—colored tights decorated with Tantrik symbols and formfitting blouses. Many of the customers were older men in search of rejuvenation, and the young women coached them to follow their movements in the asanas—and even to stand on their heads. Bernard stepped in to lead the group in the chanting of mantras and in between physical sessions would lecture on matters of health, nutrition, and spirituality. Despite the constant foot traffic and the late hours kept by its occupants, the house ran quietly, and neighbors knew next to nothing about the Tantriks, who they presumed were running a school for "ethical culture."

Zelia Hopp was holding out hope. She was very much in love with Bernard, and visited the busy West Seventy-fourth Street townhouse whenever she could. That spring she realized that parts of the house were kept off-limits to her. She also discovered that there were other young women on the premises—one of whom also had claims on her lover's heart. Her jealousy flaring, Zelia cornered Bernard and demanded that they marry immediately. Gertrude Leo, meanwhile, was living unhappily in one of those cloistered upper rooms, teaching and helping take care of the house, but receiving nothing for it but room and board. Soon enough she and Zelia met, and a triangle of sorts formed.

This was not entirely to Bernard's disliking. He soon convinced both women to put aside their jealousies—at least temporarily—and share a bed with him, an arrangement they carried out on at least a few occasions. But both women were in love with their guru, and he simply did not account for the chilling effect his broken promises would have on his fortunes. Several times that spring, Gertrude traveled up to the Bronx and visited the Hopp family home, and in early April stayed there for two weeks, both girls no doubt counting up their grievances. Gertrude had never been paid for her efforts after traveling cross-country to become his nautch girl, and Zelia was being thwarted in her attempts to marry Bernard.

Finally suspecting that in Gertrude's absence lurked rebellion,

Bernard sent Florin Jones up to the Bronx to patch things up, insisting that her presence was urgently required down at the Seventy-fourth Street house—on business matters, Jones told her. Though she agreed to return to Manhattan with Jones, she promised Zelia that she would be back.

When days passed with no word from Gertrude, Zelia became worried. She wrote to the girl's sister in Seattle. Jennie had by now married, but still harbored resentment at being dumped by Nicholls, so when Zelia suggested Gertrude was being held in Bernard's house against her will, Jennie decided to come east immediately.

On May 2, Mrs. Jennie Miller disembarked from her transcontinental train at Pennsylvania Station and hurried to her destination, not to see her sister but directly to the Hopp apartment in the Bronx. There she and Zelia finalized their elaborate extraction plan for Gertrude. They knew they had to be as swift and silent as Bernard was quick and canny and persuasive. They dressed to go out and made their way downtown to the West Side of Manhattan to meet with detectives at the Twenty-eighth Precinct.

<hr>

Bernard's students and staff were gathered at the house on that mild spring evening, a typical weekday in the life of the Tantriks. In a dimly lit room on the second floor, Gertrude Leo was leading a class of mostly older people, women and men, under the watchful eye of Bernard. The men wore gym clothes; the women students were in loose, divided skirts or bloomers. All were diligently following her directions, moving through yoga postures. When they needed a breather, Bernard stepped in and answered a question or two: yes, he said, it was beneficial to bathe every day, despite what some doctors said, and yes, there were strong and important connections between the body and the mind.

Outside, on West Seventy-fourth Street, the police and the two women stole up to the brownstone. It was close to midnight when Zelia stepped up to the door and rang the doorbell in the secret code: "a long, two short, a long, and a short ring, three times," as she told the detectives in her statement.

The lock snapped and the door opened a crack. With the two women following, the detectives rushed past the butler. The parlor floor was deserted, they determined, but upstairs the sounds of chanting could be heard. The men bounded up the staircase and into the darkened second-floor parlor, where they encountered a scene Detective T. J. Callanan later described this way: "A young man clad in filmy garments and squatting as a sort of presiding demigod among a dozen men and women strangely garbed in tight fitting gowns of one piece."

"What means this intrusion?" Bernard boomed out. Zelia and Jennie Miller rushed in behind the policemen, looking for Gertrude, whom they found dressed in a scanty swimsuit-like garment and in a highly emotional state. She fell into the arms of her sister, weeping. "For God's sake, take me away; get me out of this place."

Bernard surveyed the scene and glared coldly at Zelia. "So this is your revenge," he snapped. "You're sore because you're jealous of Gertrude."

One of the Tantrik women focused a menacing glare on Gertrude and began chanting ominously, *"Zim-zim-zim—Zee-zee-zee."*

Gertrude, who had been around these other women for some time, was obviously spooked. "She is *putting a curse* on me!" she screamed.

In the midst of all this, someone doused the lights, but it was clear even in the confusion and darkness that the young man in the filmy garments was the person the police were looking for.

"You're under arrest," said Callanan to Bernard.

Detective Joseph Leonard, the wise guy of the two partners, pointed at the symbols on Bernard's robe. "What are those things on your chest?" he demanded. When Bernard filled him in, the cop replied, "So that's the bunk."

After his initial indignation, Bernard stood calmly before the police. He confirmed his identity and that of the quivering girl in tights, Gertrude Leo. Then the detectives rousted the entire party and moved them down the steps of the brownstone and into the spring night: the officers, the irate witnesses, the young women in bathing suits, the others hissing curses, and finally, Bernard, wearing the elaborate ceremonial robe of a seventh-degree Tantrik priest, bearing the ancient symbols of birth, death, and regeneration. Together they set off from the brownstone in a comical-looking perp parade, headed for the West Sixty-eighth Street police station.

<hr />

Hours after the turmoil, in the middle of the night, Jones went racing back up to the Bronx. With tears running down his face, he begged the women not to follow through on legal action against Bernard. "I know all he has done," said Jones, "but I would like to see him freed. I consider I owe this to him for all he has taught me."

Mrs. Miller and Zelia were in no mood for reconciliation. They wanted to see Bernard punished. They wanted justice and not a little revenge. Jones measured their determination, and sensibly asked one more favor before departing in a hurry: "Keep my name out of it whatever you do."

As New York awoke on Tuesday, May 3, 1910, the morning papers carried the first news of the midnight raid. "Arrest Hindu Seer," the *New York Times* proclaimed. "Says He's a Swami," the *Herald* wrote. "His Students in Tights," added the *Tribune*. The night-desk editors had done their job, and now a fresh set of reporters arrived for work, reinterviewing the young women complainants, who in turn delivered a delicious new detail: Bernard had often referred to himself as "the great Om."

Somewhere between notebook and newsprint an extra *o* made its way into that already foreign-sounding name—rendering it as "Oom" in the afternoon editions. By the time newsboys were hawking the evening *World*, the story had migrated to the front page. The " 'Great God Oom' " was in jail, read the banner headline, charged with seducing young girls with his hypnotic powers. That Bernard looked nothing like what reporters thought a swami should look like only fueled their fire. They made fun of his worn suit, receding hairline, and wispy "sideboards." The city editors, in a spirit of one-upmanship—and gleefully aware that a hot one had landed on their desks—couldn't help heaping upon the defendant all the snide irony and condescension they could fit beneath the headlines. Before he had even faced a judge, Bernard was recast as "Oom, the Self-styled God," "Oom the Oriental," "the Great God Oom," "Hindoo Mystic," "Yogi Priest," "Head of Queer School," or just plain "the Oom."

Overnight, Pierre "the Omnipotent Oom" Bernard had become a creation of the powerful print media and one of the first twentieth-century examples of instant celebrity. In May 1910, there were thirteen daily newspapers in New York—publishing morning, afternoon, and special editions along with Sunday magazines—and their stories were picked up and syndicated nationally by news services. Juicy scandals sold tens of thousands of extra copies a day, and the biggest dailies, Joseph Pulitzer's *New York World* and William Randolph Hearst's *New York Journal*, fought savagely to get them first.

Bernard and his Tantriks were in fact merely the cult du jour for the yellow press, and the charges made against them were nearly identical to those leveled against any group that had the audacity to challenge mainstream beliefs. Quakers, Shakers, Mormons, Masons, Catholics, Theosophists, and lately Christian Scientists had all been scorned by the voracious print media, charged with sanctifying orgies and plural marriage, fraud, and even human sacrifice.

For Bernard, however, the woeful tale of Oom and his women—complete with Svengali, hapless heroines, and avenging angel—coincided with a moral panic that was sweeping New York City and the rest of the nation in the spring of 1910. The press had joined forces with police, purity reformers, and the state's vice commission to whip up the public's fear that a conspiracy of international cartels was selling white American women into sexual slavery with the willing cooperation of corrupt government officials. Even moguls like John D. Rockefeller lent his name to their efforts, and that spring the U.S. Congress passed, nearly unanimously, the Mann Act, still known as the "White Slave Traffic Act," which made it a federal crime to transport an unmarried woman across state lines for "immoral purposes."

Oom looked like the scapegoat everyone had been waiting for.

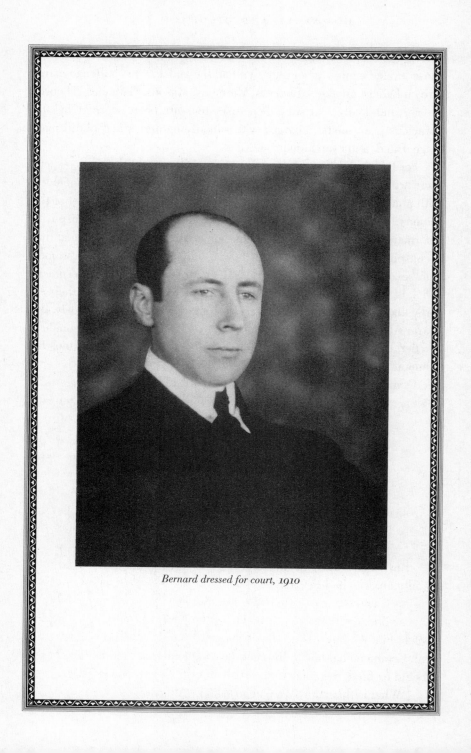

Bernard dressed for court, 1910

Chapter 5

"WHAT IS THIS MAN?"

ernard stood before city magistrate Matthew Patrick Breen in the crowded West Side courtroom. All eyes turned to special assistant district attorney James B. Reynolds, who read aloud from the affidavit in support of the indictment titled *The People of the State of New York v. Pierre A. Bernard, case number 77371.* The defendant, Reynolds said, was charged with having "inveigled and enticed" the complainant Miss Zelia Hopp "for the purpose of sexual intercourse."

If Bernard didn't feel a stab of cold fear at this moment, he should have. Reynolds was New York City's leading crusader against the white-slave trade and had just ended a lengthy undercover sting that culminated in a series of spectacular, headline-grabbing arrests. One low-life pimp, charged with luring teenage girls into sexual slavery on the Lower East Side, was at the moment being held on a record $25,000 bail.

Reynolds worked for the newly elected district attorney Charles A. Whitman, who had campaigned on a promise to root out white slavery in the city, a fact well known to magistrate Breen. With this scourge no doubt on his mind, the judge now turned his attention to Bernard, who appeared before him on May 3, 1910, having spent the rest of the previous night in jail. Commencing this preliminary hearing to determine whether charges should be filed, the magistrate set about establishing the facts.

"What is this man?" the judge asked. "A doctor?"

"No, he's not a doctor," said Detective Callanan. "He's a Hindu teacher; he claims to cure people by controlling spirits."

The judge squinted down at the small circus now assembled before him: five young women, ages fifteen to twenty-three, three police officers, two lawyers, and an Irish American–looking man in his thirties, balding on top, wearing side whiskers—obviously not a real Hindu, as anyone could see. Unfortunately for Bernard, the judge's indignation was just beginning to mount as he listened to the grim details.

"When we got upstairs, we saw eight elderly men and five women in tights and bathing costumes," Detective Callanan said. "They were just exercising. They were tumbling on a mat which had strange figures on it. The defendant was standing by a crystal ball and was clad in tights that came to his knees and a jersey on which there were some queer figures."

Where did all this take place? Breen wanted to know, and the detective responded, "It's a high-class place, Your Honor. Fixed up swell. It's next to Frank Platt's house."

At the mention of Platt's address, Judge Breen's limbic system fired up a storm of forty years of political associations. Frank Platt's father, Tom, had been the most powerful Republican boss in state politics. And then the judge knew that of all the miserable, low-life cases that would come before him this warm May morning, it would be this *sideshow* with its white-slave-and-Hindu-hypnotist angle that would attract the attention of his superiors, not to mention everyone who moved about in the expensive neighborhoods of the Upper West Side. He needed to sound not just wise but *magisterial*.

"This is a most serious condition of affairs," he began. "Public indignation may run very high in this matter," he added.

Bail was set at an unaffordable $15,000, and bailiffs led Bernard from the courtroom. Then, out of nowhere came sprinting a short man with a black beard, who stopped at the rail separating the spectators' area from the court. It was Zelia Hopp's father, who had once lent his blessing to Bernard's affections and who was now blind with rage about this treachery. "That man ought to be killed and I'd do it if I could," he shouted. "The dog ought to be shot."

Instead Bernard spent another night behind bars, mulling over the charge he was faced with: abduction of the deponent, Zelia Hopp, who was "unmarried and of chaste character," as noted by the judge. He was also charged with posing as a doctor to convince Miss Hopp to have sex with him as a therapy for her heart troubles. Asked to write down an explanation that might tend to his exculpation, he wrote only, "I am not guilty."

That night, a well-traveled reporter from the *Evening Mail* displayed enough professional empathy to elicit from Bernard the unvarnished truth. The yoga school started last August, he said, and then he added, "No, I never lived in India. . . . The whole scheme is physical culture, that's all. Only some of those nasty-tongued women got busy. You know, if you pay more attention to one than you do to another, she gets jealous. This whole white slave business was too much. Wonder they didn't hold me for murder."

He was lucky they didn't. On the same day and in the same courtroom where Bernard was arraigned, one Bernard Levinson, a twenty-seven-year-old salesman of Russian descent, confessed to actually selling young women with the assistance of "two negresses." The city gasped at the news of the confession, which seemed to prove the public's worst fears. The DA's office leaked to reporters that Levinson was about to spill the beans on the national scope of the slave trafficking. By dint of sheer timing, Bernard's story became intertwined with Levinson's in the press—and henceforth in public memory.

Jennie Miller was certainly determined to do everything she could to get Bernard a death sentence. She told the press that the Tantriks' yoga teaching was merely "a higher order of the white slave traffic than that in which such persons as Levinson are involved." She then dropped an even bigger bombshell, alleging that "wealthy women—women whose fortunes run high into the millions—are prime movers in this traffic." Finally she revealed that the Tantrik Order had branches in many cities, and "my sister has been at the house for months and knows all about the goings-on there."

For the next five days, morning and evening, there were fevered front-page headlines, stacked decks of type beneath wild graphics, and heavy-handed innuendo that would lead any reasonable reader to judge Bernard worthy of the gallows. The narrative was set: the victims, Zelia and Gertrude, were "comely" young girls, the seducer's house was "sumptuously furnished" and set in a "most exclusive" neighborhood, his slaves wore "scanty bathing suits," Bernard's hypnotic charms were "mesmerizing." Every large New York newspaper ran the updates, morning and evening, which then made the leap to national news. The wire services pushed the scandal out to the provinces, as did the syndicates for Sunday feature supplements and the New York offices of more than a dozen out-of-town newspapers. In Washington, Chicago, Los Angeles, Atlanta, Gettysburg, Pennsylvania, and Trenton, New Jersey—even Elyria, Ohio—Pierre Bernard was big news. The West Coast papers pursued the story particularly hard, since Bernard had once lived in San Francisco and the Northwest. The *San Francisco Chronicle* led off its coverage with this headline: "Wild Orgies in the Temple of 'Om.'"

There were new revelations by the hour, as the women revealed fresh details to special edition reporters. Bernard, they learned, used beautiful missionaries, female *and* male, to seduce initiates. The most reliable of them was his faithful servant Nicholls, who was routinely described as Oom's number one slave. Gertrude Leo, who'd had many opportunities to observe Nicholls in the flesh, said, "He was beautiful and had such a soulful manner that women fell fairly head over heels in love with him. Then he brought them to 'Oom' and by some strange power, 'Oom' transferred the power that [Nicholls] had over them to himself." She spoke with authority on this matter, she said, because both she and her sister, Mrs. Miller, had fallen under the spell of Nicholls—and then Bernard—on the West Coast.

Reports surfaced in the press on the most salacious details of Hindu Tantric practices. A diligent *New York World* reporter had turned up a copy of Bernard's *Vira Sadhana*, and published excerpts under the headline "Tantriks' Worship Calls for Dead Bodies and Young Girls." Since the *Vira Sadhana* was a compendium of abridged mystical tracts and translated Hindu writings that were long on metaphor and symbol, Oom's enemies found everything they wanted: they picked from a combination platter of yoga's alleged supernatural powers, sex rituals, phallic worship, and yes, even a mention of medieval Hindu rites that used dead bodies.

When apprised by a reporter that some of the texts he'd published were "salacious in nature," Bernard answered wistfully, "That's the trouble with people. They so readily misunderstand any true conception of the system."

On Thursday, May 5, the arraignment resumed. Bernard, confused and disheveled, was led into the courtroom again, wearing a worn black suit. "He didn't look very formidable," one reporter noted, "as he rested a shiny arm on his chair and from time to time pressed one hand over his small round pate where the scanty hair lay across it."

The courthouse was in a narrow building connected to the police station and jail. It was dark, not terribly well ventilated, and crowded night and day. Lawyers, clerks, defendants, attendants, and police jostled one another as cases streamed in and out. The close quarters upset the nervous systems of the young women, and when Gertrude Leo was called to testify, she appeared to be seconds from a full physical breakdown. She turned away from Bernard, who sat only a few feet from her, and clutched the arms of her chair as if to keep her body and soul together. "One of the court attendants stood at her elbow with a bottle of smelling salts," a witness noted. Gertrude paused often and placed her hands over her eyes as she related her story of how in the Seattle winter of 1909 she first met the defendant. She finished her story quickly and stepped down, and when she did, she walked the long way around the room rather than pass directly in front of Bernard.

Then Zelia Hopp, the refined girl from the Bronx, took the stand. Eyes cast downward and visibly trembling, she, too, could barely control her anxiety as she added further details to Gertrude's story. Zelia told of her move to the 109th Street apartment and her first night there. "Oom began kissing me. He told me he loved me desperately and wanted to marry me. He said I was so young and innocent. He told me then that his name was not Dr. Warren but Pierre Bernard. He told me if I knew who he really was I would be terribly afraid. . . . He said, 'You'd be frightened to death if you knew how important and awful a person I am. My influence . . . is unbounded. I can bring anybody to my feet.'"

Zelia paused and lowered her head and placed her arm on the magistrate's desk. Her shoulders began to heave, she became confused and, in the view of one witness, nearly collapsed. She then pointed at Bernard and said, "He embarrasses me. I don't think I can go on."

The lawyers began shouting. Bernard's attorney, Clark L. Jordan, objected to the implication that Bernard was doing anything to the girl, and Judge Breen asked that her chair be turned so that she wouldn't directly face the accused.

She began again, taking up the story of Bernard's pursuit of her, a self-admitted poor young woman with no education. She said he told her he "would rather have the raw material wrapped up on the back porch in burlap rather than one in shimmering silks, 'for then I can shape it as I wish.'"

Zelia was dismissed and Breen adjourned for the day. Outside the courtroom, the city's newspapers again picked up and ran with incendiary passages from Bernard's *Vira Sadhana* that dealt with the fiery combination of religion and sexuality. "Sex worship as a religion represents a stage in the development of the human mind," one passage read, "and the grand theologies of to-day are the outcome of this mode of worship. It constitutes the basis of all that is sacred, holy and beautiful." And finally this: "The whole world is embodied in the woman."

Arriving in court the next morning, Gertrude Leo, Zelia Hopp, and Jennie Miller posed for photographers in broad-brimmed hats decorated with bows, florets, and flowing ribbons. Mrs. Miller, a handsome woman with fine, straight features, turned out to be a newsman's dream. With her head cocked and chin slightly lifted, she projected an air of indignation and sisterly protectiveness toward Gertrude, who was a fragile, fine-boned copy of her. Zelia kept her brown eyes cast downward, her mien tragic and forlorn.

But when the court resumed its session, the fireworks began again. Zelia, although not a member of the Tantrik Order, spilled what secrets she knew, including allegations of blood oaths and sexual orgies. Bernard's attorney rose and startled the courtroom by shouting at Zelia that Bernard would indeed marry her, if that is what she wanted.

Her attorney shouted back, Zelia took to tears, and the court erupted into chaos until Judge Breen silenced them all and adjourned for the day.

The following morning, Gertrude Leo took the stand again, producing shocking new allegations: Bernard had threatened her on September 17, 1909, dosed her with morphine when she became hysterical, and kept her a prisoner with his hypnotic powers. "I both feared and loved him," she said. "He made me believe that he could communicate with priests of the order all over the world who would sit in council at his command and take away my mind if I did not obey him."

Gertrude managed to get out some description of a room fitted out with a raised bed for "kaula rites," or sex worship, before she started to lose her composure again. By admitting publicly and repeatedly to having had sexual relations with men before marriage, both she and Zelia were shattering any claim to respectability they once held. The *Atlanta Constitution* put the sentiment bluntly: "Ruin Brought to This Woman by High Priest." Holding on to the arms of her chair to maintain her composure, Gertrude then admitted to sharing the same bed with Bernard and Zelia on many occasions.

With this, magistrate Breen declared that he had heard enough and closed the preliminary hearing, sending the evidence to the grand jury. Bernard never testified, nor did the defense get to rebut testimony or put on a single witness. Attorney Jordan made another motion to reduce his client's $15,000 bail, but the judge refused and then launched into his summation.

"I find that the charge has been fully sustained," Breen said. "There was not only systematic, but scientific seduction. This girl, Gertrude Leo, of Seattle, one of the two complainants, has been inveigled into a den of iniquity for the purpose of perpetrating a shameless outrage. She has been marked, I say, in every respect save physical murder, and I shall not reduce the bail I fixed when I first read the complaint and before the testimony showed the dangerous character of this man and his practices."

He banged his hand down on the table and repeated, "I shan't!"

The week's events drew the attention of the entire nation. Even postal inspector Anthony Comstock made an appearance, to lend his support to the efforts against white slavery. Comstock held a long conference with assistant district attorney Reynolds and dropped off a bundle of letters purportedly sent to him by persons with knowledge of those trafficking in women (though it was never ascertained whether the letters held any direct connection to Bernard and the Tantriks).

Meanwhile, Bernard was remanded to the Tombs, a notorious prison at the Criminal Courts Building on Centre Street. He shared one of its 406 cells, designed to hold single prisoners but inhabited by two or more on most days. Some fifteen thousand men and women were jailed there every year. There weren't enough beds or blankets, and prisoners had to take turns sleeping in a single cot. Boys and men were thrown together, as were hardened criminals, pickpockets, lunatics, rats, and nations of lice.

Many defendants took a guilty plea rather than spend another day there, preferring to take their chances in the work prison on Blackwell's Island, in the middle of the East River.

Back in Humeston, Iowa, the tiny town where Bernard had spent part of his boyhood, the farmers were celebrating the earliest spring they'd seen in a while. The oats were sown and the pastures green and the corn was going in the ground. On Wednesday, May 11, the farmers and townspeople opening the *Humeston New Era* were treated to a rehashing of the week's events in New York City. The headline was "Omnipotent Oom Held," and at the end the *New Era* added a local angle. "The Pierre Bernard mentioned in the above article is thought by many people here to be the same Bernard who was a resident of Humeston several years ago."

Bernard's disgrace was now complete.

His followers had scattered, hiding from the law, awaiting the outcome of the upcoming trial. The Tantriks' home on West Seventy-fourth Street stood completely empty except for the housekeeper. Zelia, Gertrude, and Jennie, along with several detectives, had returned to the brownstone during the week of hearings looking for more evidence and possible witnesses. While they were there, the telephone rang, and Gertrude answered. Recognizing the voice as that of Ora Ray Baker, Gertrude pretended to be the housekeeper and asked Ora Ray to meet her in ten minutes at the new 110th Street subway stop on Broadway.

Though she appeared to be a Victorian shrinking violet in court, on the street Gertrude showed a grittier side. Ora Ray appeared as she said she would, standing alone at the wide intersection of Broadway and West 110th Street. When she saw that Gertrude was not the housekeeper and deduced that the two men with her were not friends but policemen, Bernard's half sister took off running. Gertrude sprinted after her and caught her by the arm.

"Let me go! Let me go!" Baker screamed. "I don't want to get mixed up in this thing. I'm going away." Since there were no charges against her, the detectives did just that.

On May 23, the New York grand jury returned two indictments against Bernard, for abduction and fraudulently impersonating a doctor, and his trial was added to the slow-moving summer schedule of the Court of

General Sessions. With the Great Oom indicted and locked up, the DA's office stepped up efforts to tie him to the white-slave conspiracy, searching across the country for more witnesses. There *would* be further charges, the public was told; white slavery was undoubtedly involved.

Behind the scenes at the DA's office, however, there seemed to be dwindling faith in these assertions. Bernard's case had been bumped down the prestige chain from the superstar Reynolds to assistant DA De-Ford and now to *deputy* assistant DA John Kirkland Clark, whose job seemed to consist solely of saying no to Bernard's attorneys as they petitioned the court for more reasonable bail and a speedy trial.

Bernard's case quietly disappeared from the front pages as he continued to languish in jail. With unbathed convicts doubled up in shabby bunks and the throng of prisoners packed to the rafters, the Tombs was as unpleasant a summer stay as the law could manage. Though he was given the opportunity, Bernard refused to plead guilty to a lesser charge and maintained his innocence, seeking his day in court.

In June, attorney Jordan brought to Clark's attention the testimony of several eyewitnesses who disputed Gertrude Leo's honesty, her stated age, and her "previously chaste character." She was twenty-one, Jordan said, an experienced adult woman who had, back in Seattle, slept with Winfield Nicholls, and there were plenty of witnesses to this. When Jordan offered to produce these tattletales in court, the DA dropped Leo as a witness *and* as a complainant, but kept the case on the docket. Bail was lowered to $10,000, but the sum was still too high for Bernard to raise and he remained in jail.

Then in early August, the Hopp family decided they no longer wished to be part of the prosecution. Zelia's brother, L. G. Hopp, and her older sister, Mrs. Betts, the woman who had introduced Bernard to the family, told ADA Clark that Zelia had moved out of state and would not appear in court—not ever. The family wanted the charges dropped. Clark told Mrs. Betts that the state of New York would do nothing of the kind; in fact, he informed her it would "do no harm" to keep Bernard in the Tombs for a few more months. She then visited Bernard's attorney, Jordan, telling him that the family had learned that the Seattle girls' stories about Bernard were not true, but designed to get the Hopp family to press charges. Zelia, who was sicker now than ever, was "nearly driven insane" by the experience. Zelia's brother wrote a plaintive letter on behalf of the entire family, informing Jordan and the court that "knowing the true facts concerning P. A. Bernard the defendant in the case concerning us, [we] have decided to forget and bury all knowledge concerning same and would ask you to act as you see fit in disposing of said case." The entire Hopp family, he added, had moved out of the state and had no intention of returning.

On August 25, attorney Jordan again petitioned the court for Bernard's release. His client had been denied a speedy trial, and now all the witnesses, including the sole complainant, had not only left New York but expressed a determination never to return. The application was granted by Judge O'Sullivan, but he still refused to dismiss the charges. Bernard walked out of prison that day, under indictment but a free man for the time being, released on his own recognizance. He had spent 104 days in the Tombs in the summer of 1910, but he never spoke publicly about it.

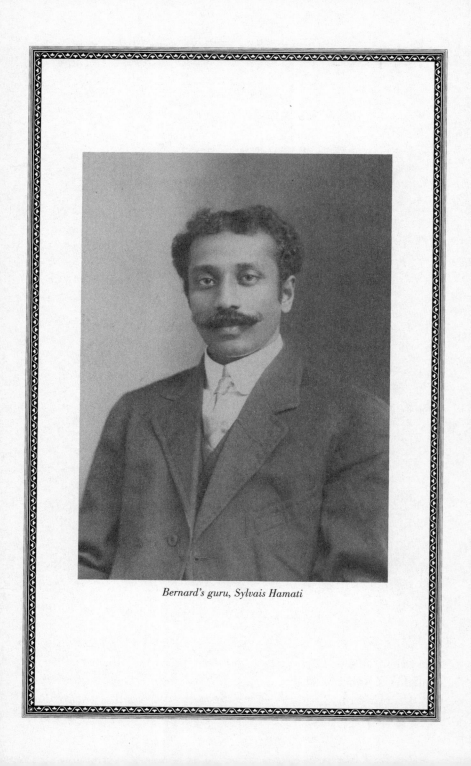

Bernard's guru, Sylvais Hamati

Chapter 6

YOGA AT LARGE

A yogi
Is a sort of holy fogy
That does not wash or shave:
His ways are rather logy
From living in a cave.
He dines off water, dates,
Cheese-parings, plantain-rind,
Then sits and demonstrates
The Universal Mind

–Marguerite Merington, 1906

ierre Bernard was not the only American talking about yoga in 1910, nor was he the first one to take up the practice. The transcendentalists and the Theosophists had begun their initial inquiries before Bernard was born. In fact, word of yoga arrived in the United States nearly a century before his birth—an idea in a cloud of ideas, both sacred and profane, from what was called "the Orient": the vast, unknowable *out there*. In 1805, William Emerson, the father of Ralph Waldo Emerson, published the first English transcription of a Sanskrit text in the United States, a drama titled *Sacuntala*. His son fell under the spell of India's sacred literature, especially the

Bhagavad Gita, the Song of God, which Emerson read in translation for the first time in 1843. "It was as if an empire spake to us," he wrote of the Gita—"nothing small or unworthy, but large, serene, consistent, the voice of an old intelligence."

Yoga is first mentioned in the Rig-Veda, the oldest of the four sacred Hindu scriptures known collectively as the Vedas. These texts date back some 3,500 years, though twentieth-century archaeological evidence indicates that the practice of yoga is even older than that—more than five thousand years old. The idea of yoking human action to the hope of liberation from the cycle of birth and death is explored somewhat more deeply in the Hindu texts known as the Upanishads, the oldest of which were composed circa 800–500 BC. Out of the Upanishads arose the Bhagavad Gita, composed 500–200 BC, in which the path to liberation was broadened to three avenues: karma yoga, or service to others with no expectation of reward; bhakti yoga, the yoga of devotion; and jnana yoga, which seeks wisdom or knowledge. The philosophy of yoga is next explored in the Yoga Sutras, written by a mysterious scribe named Patanjali in the first or second century AD and later called raja or classical yoga.

Around the first century AD there also arose a new religious tradition called Tantrism, a practical philosophy and culture based on the sacred literature known as the Tantras. The unifying principle among the dozens of Tantric sects and schools that sprang up was the worship of the divine feminine creative principle, Shakti, who may be called by hundreds of names but is always the consort of the masculine god Shiva. Out of this tradition of goddess worship, the yoga of the perfected body, hatha yoga, began to be codified around the ninth century AD and grew in popularity in the fourteenth century, when the seminal hatha yoga text, the Hatha Yoga Pradipika, was composed. In the seventeenth century, the two other widely used hatha manuals, the Gheranda Samhita and the Siva Samhita, gained acceptance, the latter containing descriptions of the esoteric beliefs—superhuman powers, the "subtle body," the chakras, and the kundalini awakening—that are to this day associated with the practice of advanced forms of physical yoga.

In 1849, Emerson's friend Henry David Thoreau wrote wistfully that he aspired to become a yogi and succeeded "to some extent and at rare intervals." Thoreau read deeply in the Indian sacred texts, but he and

Emerson and the other Concord intellectuals—earnest, brilliant men and women all—were destined to remain outsiders. At its root, yoga is an experiential practice, its wisdom transmitted master to student, which requires actual masters, who were in quite short supply for most of our nation's early history. It wasn't until 1883 that the first Hindu cleric lectured in the United States, coincidentally or not in the parlor of Emerson's widow in Concord. Six years later Bernard began his apprenticeship with Hamati.

By then, Americans' understanding of yoga was shaped by the views of the Theosophical Society, the previously mentioned spiritualist-reform group founded in New York City in 1875 by Madame Helena Blavatsky and Colonel Henry Steel Olcott. The Theosophists, like the transcendentalists, studied Eastern texts, embraced a variety of Hindu and Buddhist beliefs, and threw in more than a few of their own. By 1901, the Theosophical Society was a worldwide force in Victorian-era spirituality, and more important, an alternative to mainstream worship for millions of highly educated seekers. With five hundred active chapters in forty-two countries, the society was rich and powerful enough to engineer Hindu and Buddhist revivals in India, where it established schools, publishing houses, and libraries to hold copies of ancient religious texts.

Theosophist scholars were among the first translators of Sanskrit texts. They devoted special attention to Patanjali's Yoga Sutras, whose meditative disciplines and ethical teachings have been referred to as raja yoga since the sixteenth century. *Raja* was translated to mean "royal," denoting the high road to liberation, and the Theosophists used the term to distinguish it from hatha yoga—the low road—which they wanted nothing to do with.

In their lectures, Theosophists spoke in hushed tones of Indian yogis who had demonstrated Faustian powers over time and space, "over men and natural phenomena." They believed in the awesome possibilities of the mind—astral projection, telekinesis, clairvoyance, communicating with the dead—but seemed to fear and loathe the human body—"raja, yes; hatha, no" summed up their philosophy.

A slightly more down-to-earth take on yoga came from the followers of Swami Vivekananda, the great Indian religious figure who arrived in the United States in 1893 and met Bernard a few years later in San Francisco.

A follower of the mystic saint Ramakrishna, Vivekananda became a member of the Theosophical Society as well as a Freemason, establishing a place for himself among the emerging Anglophile Indian elite. He was also a celibate who had renounced worldly pursuits as a young man in favor of the wandering ascetic's life. His view—that a meditation-based yoga was a safe, practical, and scientific way for Westerners to dial the human soul into the frequency of the infinite—overlapped with the Theosophists' vision, though he was far less preoccupied with occult powers. Vivekananda expounded at great length on the three paths of devotion mentioned in the Gita (karma, bhakti, jnana) and added a volume of his thoughts on Patanjali's raja yoga—the ultimate calling.

Vivekananda's influence in the United States was immense. Completing two extended speaking tours before his death in 1902, he established a network of outreach centers—called the Vedanta Society—in New York and California and left behind a series of sold-out volumes based on transcriptions of his lectures. The Vedanta Society, whose philosophy is based on the Vedas and whose members believe in the unity of all existence, the divinity of the human soul, and the harmony of all religions, sent its emissaries into the urban boulevards and small-town byways of America. These refined young men in flame-colored robes spoke like kindly parish priests and moved with ease among the matrons and widows of Boston, New York, and Chicago. It was all very polite. The yoga the Vedantists taught was mental exercise—yoga from the neck up—and it went over very well in the hushed parlors of Back Bay, Fifth Avenue, and Lake Shore Drive. Any controversy it provoked derived not from scandals of the flesh, but from the domestic frenzy that ensued when its most fervent American converts followed the trail of incense to its logical end and renounced all worldly desires, in some cases breaking ties with husbands, wives, children, and family fortunes.

Vedantists and Theosophists shared the view that hatha yoga's body-centered practices were queer and dangerous. Blavatsky warned that pranayama, the breath-control practice that may have saved Bernard from drowning in 1895, was "injurious to the health," and useless to those seeking spiritual liberation. Vivekananda, for his part, dismissed hatha yoga's asanas as "nothing but a kind of gymnastics," and later put a finer point on it for curious followers. "We have nothing to do with it . . . because its practices are very difficult, and cannot be learned in a day, and, after all, do not lead to much spiritual growth." Even in the liberal halls of academe, hatha yoga was dismissed as absurd. Oxford University's famed nineteenth-century Indologist Sir Monier Monier-Williams mocked it as "a strange compound of mental and bodily exercises, consisting [of] unnatural restraint, forced and painful postures, twisting and contortions of the limbs, suppression of the breath and utter absence of mind."

In India, hatha yogis were forced to the margins of society, as they had been for centuries, not only by the British colonizers and their Indian sympathizers but also by the Christian missionaries from the West, who saw such practices as the embodiment of heathenism. As a result, the generation of educated monks who came to America around the turn of the century were essentially a coterie of Theosophical-leaning Tantric-deniers and hatha haters.

Sylvais Hamati, on the other hand, represented himself first and foremost as a Tantric, a follower of a revolutionary tradition that had evolved from its first-century origins into an elaborate oppositional philosophy to Vedic asceticism. Tantrism is, above all, of this world. The body is divine and thus the practice of hatha yoga became central to its sanctification. Tantrics believe that enlightenment is most profound when it involves the entire human body. Hamati was a skilled adept in the postures, breathing, and meditation of hatha yoga, and steeped in the subversive beliefs behind them. He molded the young Perry Baker in his image, to delight in the world as it was—a divine manifestation. This was the essential tenet of the belief system Pierre Bernard then passed on to those who came into his circle: to embrace the ferocity of existence and resist the mind-body dualism of the day.

"Body and soul are co-existent," Bernard insisted. "One is but a manifestation of the other. The best way to perfect the soul is through the body and the senses." In his network of Tantrik lodges, he was evolving the architecture of a new, energetic, and dynamic American yoga, combining hatha's postures and breathing with a keen respect for the powers of sex and desire. "The first duty of every initiate," he announced "is to purify his body and through his body improve his spirit." The difficulty of the postures of hatha yoga was precisely the point—Bernard believed in Americans' ability to master them. The rest would follow.

His mission as he saw it was to drag yoga out of the ascetic's cave and into the sunlight. "The ascetics are really the most selfish men," he said. "They have the wrong idea of nature, which leads them astray and to do things which are very harmful." Flying in the face of Victorian propriety, Bernard had been teaching his followers in San Francisco, Seattle, Portland, Chicago, St. Louis, and New York that the body was not evil, that sexual desire was part of a healthy life, that it was wrong and unnecessary to leave your wife or husband to study yoga. "The only way to control nature so far as it is harmful to humanity is not by absolutely killing desires," he said, "but by moderate satisfaction of those desires and carefully considering their usefulness and importance in life."

Yoga was loose in the land of the free, taking its cues from the Theosophists, Vedantists, and Bernard's Tantrikas, who all contributed to a growing awareness of the practice. In their wake appeared an assortment of self-proclaimed gurus claiming knowledge of Eastern philosophy. Some of these freelance teachers were outright con artists, like Yogi Bill Ellis, a grifter who lured women into palm readings and then slipped knockout drops into their tea while he took off with their money and their secrets. Others were sincere, if misguided, healers, like Dr. William Latson, a charismatic silver-haired man in his thirties, who counted among his patients some of New York City's most successful and sophisticated women. In his office on Riverside Drive, he presided over elaborate secret rituals—Hindu dancing included—designed to free his female patients from their libidinal restraints. In the Midwest, Sakharam Ganesh Pandit, a whip-smart young Brahmin, set up his School of Applied Philosophy and Oriental Psychology in Chicago, where he tutored thirty mostly female students. In 1910, Pandit advertised his services for one-off engagements and "parlor talks" on subjects like "the fourth dimension and the teaching of Hindu sages." If students couldn't come to him, he offered correspondence courses in yoga and metaphysics for $2.50 a month. Pandit, like Bernard, taught a form of hatha yoga, but only in private lessons, and his star burned out nearly as soon as it was born, snuffed out in a scandal that sent him looking for a new profession.

Yoga also played into a new medical-spiritual trend known as Mind Cure, which William James called America's "only decidedly original contribution to the systematic philosophy of life." Mind Cure—the power of mental processes to treat and cure disease—was the central tenet of both the Christian Science and New Thought movements of the late nineteenth century, and brought about the popularity of a mysterious author whose pen name was Yogi Ramacharaka. Ramacharaka, a former lawyer from the Midwest named William Walker Atkinson, explained the wisdom of the East through the lens of New Thought in thirteen popular books, including *The Hindu-Yogi Science of Breath, The Yogi Science of Relaxation, Secrets of Yogi Breathing, Hindu Yogi Practical Water Cure,* and *The Science of Psychic Healing.* These books covered the subjects of mind control, mental healing, and Hindu philosophy. There is no evidence that Atkinson (or his pseudonym Ramacharaka) ever taught students, and much about his biography remains unknown to this day. In 1904 he wrote *Hatha Yoga, or The Yogi Philosophy of Physical Well-Being,* a commonsense health manual appended to a few pages of primer on breathing and exercise, having little to do with hatha yoga. Two years later he published *Raja Yoga or Mental Development (A Series of Lessons in Raja Yoga).* Atkinson's readership was immense, but the yoga he imparted in these self-help manuals did not have much to do with the practices Bernard had been teaching—and those we would recognize today.

Hatha . . . raja . . . karma . . . these distinctions were for the most part lost on mainstream observers, who considered all yoga followers to be dupes. For decades yogis had been considered fools and naïfs, but of the harmless, cross-legged, navel-gazing variety. By the time Bernard was arrested, however, a series of highly publicized events had given rise to the notion that something more dangerous was afoot, that these gurus and the morals-loosening effects of yoga might well pose a danger to Americans—American women in particular.

In the spring of 1908, for example, Purdue University president Winthrop Ellsworth Stone confessed to his board of directors that his wife had left him and their children to study yoga. The scandal compelled him to tender his resignation publicly. "I am utterly crushed," he told his fellow parishioners at the Presbyterian Church in Lafayette, Indiana. "I can scarcely bear up under it. I want your sympathy and your prayers. I love my wife; I would welcome her back. She is as dear to me as she ever was, but I am so sorry for her. I hope that in a year or two she will come to her senses and return to me and my boys."

At about the same time, a group of well-known and wealthy American women began to display alarming behavior in the company of their friends and families. In Cambridge, Massachusetts, Mrs. Ole Bull, a devotee of Eastern philosophy, disinherited her daughter, leaving $500,000 instead to the Vedanta Society. A fellow New Englander, Miss Sarah Farnum, bequeathed her entire fortune to a Hindu summer school. Miss Ellis Shaw of Lowell, Massachusetts, was legally restrained by her family from turning over her fortune to a holy man. Back in Indiana, Mrs. May Wright Sewall, a high-ranking Theosophist and advocate for women's rights, was said to have fallen "dangerously ill" under the guidance of her unnamed yogi in Indianapolis.

The controversy became too much for the Theosophical Society, which in September 1909 officially banned even a discussion of yoga as part of its movement. In a series of contentious meetings in Chicago, pro-yoga and anti-yoga factions faced off over what seemed to be the unstated but underlying issue: yoga's adverse relationship to marital stability. The followers of Annie Besant, president of the American Theosophists, called the pro-yoga women "animalistic." One reporter, attempting to decode the group's rhetoric and still make it palatable for a newspaper audience, wrote that the philosophy of the pro-yoga folks "seems to suggest the proposition of setting aside the institution of matrimony on occasion—to cleanse the mind," which sounds very close to a precursor to the philosophy of the 1960s swingers' movement.

At the center of the Chicago controversy was none other than the young Brahmin teacher Sakharam Ganesh Pandit, who was accused of giving a female student a neck rub during a private yoga lesson. Pandit, a member in good standing of the Theosophical Society, withdrew his membership when accused of this "immorality." A spokesman for his school then tried to explain that if any women in Pandit's classes developed "yogaistic tendencies," they would be told to withdraw.

His capitulation was not enough. Death threats were mailed, and Annie Besant, in an attempt at reconciliation, allowed that "it will be best for him" if Pandit took his yoga ways with him back to India.

What was turning out to be an American war on yoga was joined by the white-slave hysteria that had figured in Bernard's arrest. Six months after his unceremonious release from the Tombs, Chicago police raided the home of Evelyn Arthur See, who was branded a guru and cult leader like Bernard. See, a Christian mystic, was actually charged as a white slaver, and his trial was a virtual replay of the Bernard proceedings, drawing standing-room-only crowds in Chicago and millions of newspaper readers across the nation. See was consigned to a fate much worse than Bernard's, however. Tried and convicted of the crime of abduction, he was sentenced to four years of hard labor at Joliet prison.

In May 1911, at the height of the See trial, the gentle Dr. William Latson was found dead in his office on Riverside Drive, "a bullet hole through his brain," according to the *New York Times*. Latson's grisly death was officially ruled a suicide, though several coroners at the inquest disagreed, calling it murder. When a heartbroken female follower made her own attempt at suicide, the combined news sent a jolt through polite society, and on May 28, the *Washington Post* bundled See, Latson, and Pierre Bernard into a massive story headlined "This Soul Destroying Poison of the East: The Tragic Flood of Broken Homes and Hearts, Disgrace and Suicide That Follows the Broadening Stream of Morbidly Alluring Oriental 'Philosophies' into Our Country." This was a Sunday special composed of three separate articles and an assortment of racy photos and illustrations, including one of Ruth St. Denis, the famed performer whose Hindu dance, the author stated, "typifies the sensual allurement of the Orient."

But the main subject of the exposé was Oom and his Tantrik Order. The names of Gertrude Leo and Zelia Hopp were again invoked; black magic powers were again attributed to Bernard. His group was said to be the funneling organization "to which nearly all of the American devotees of Hindu occultism belong." The article was a classic *Reefer Madness* combination of falsehoods, titillation, and fearmongering. All the inflammatory notes were rung: the sexy nautch girls, the degrees of initiation, the sexual rites, the medieval graveyard rituals, the blood, the lust. By June 1911, when the divorce of Mr. and Mrs. Stone of Purdue was finalized, everyone knew the culprit had to have been yoga.

A flurry of feature-length exposés blaming yoga for "domestic infelicity, and insanity and death" followed in newspapers across the country, and the U.S. government soon began an official investigation of "various swamis and Hindu priests" to determine how many American women had been taken abroad or relieved of their wealth. Pierre Bernard had escaped trial and long-term imprisonment, but the world he was released back into in the autumn of 1910 was anything but contrite at his wrongful imprisonment. For any teacher of yoga—not to mention the profane hatha yoga that was Bernard's calling—the public had nothing but contempt.

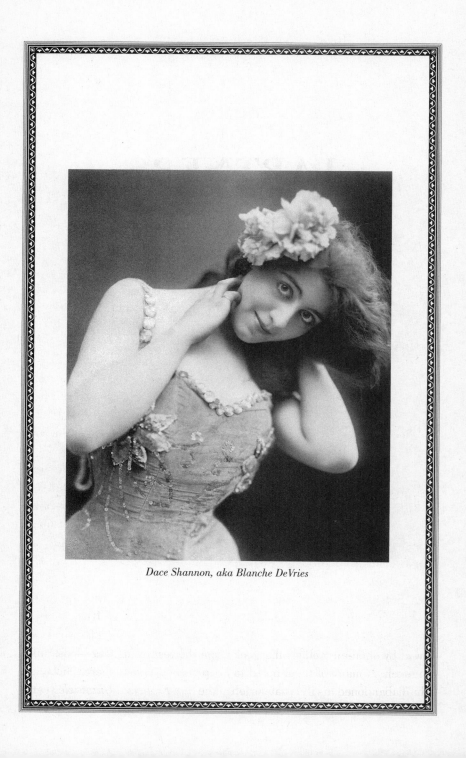

Dace Shannon, aka Blanche DeVries

Chapter 7

PARTNERS

fter five months of pleas from his attorney, the courts dismissed the abduction charges against Bernard on February 10, 1911. About the propriety of his romantic affairs with the two young women, he never offered an opinion. The consequences of his actions, however, were obvious. Tarred with notoriety, branded with a humiliating new nickname, he had become a pariah to the wealthy set who'd funded his ventures. The Tantrik Press had failed to take off, his followers had scattered, and he was flat broke. He needed a refuge, a haven where he could figure out his next move.

The day after the charges were lifted, permitting him to leave Manhattan, he ferried across the Hudson River to the borough of Leonia, New Jersey, where pretty bungalows sat on wide streets atop the cliffs of the Palisades. Bernard's pupils from the West Seventy-fourth Street house followed, including Nicholls, Jones (whose wife had left him), Ora Ray, and the two men from the West Coast, Bradlaw and Sanford.

Leonia was a low-cost, warm-weather hangout for New York City artists, many of them newspaper and magazine illustrators who went there originally to paint the dramatic junction of the Hudson River and the plunging rock face of the Palisades. The commute—a short ferry ride followed by open-air trolleys that took them the rest of the way—cost only a nickel, so many of them opted to keep second homes there. Nicholls, who'd abandoned his illustrator's job at the *San Francisco Chronicle* years earlier, must have felt at home in the liberal art colony. At the least, the

Tantriks' sojourn in Leonia provided them with a restful holiday after the frantic pace of the last two years.

But New Jersey proved too tranquil for Bernard, too far offstage, and he was anxious to return to the cultural capital of the world. In April, he snuck back into New York and began a new enterprise in a far less conspicuous setting than his last Manhattan address. The New York Sanskrit College set up shop at 250 West Eighty-seventh Street, at Broadway. "Comfortable seats, cool place," read the announcement, tucked discreetly into the columns of classified ads in the *New York Times*. Discretion was the watchword of the new undertaking. Bernard opened the college using another alias, Homer Stansbury Leeds (though he is listed by his real name as the dean in the school's literature). He hired a small revolving faculty—credentialed professors from India—to expound on the Bhagavad Gita, the Upanishads, the Vedas, and the Tantras, as well as Sanskrit language and science. Equipment was installed, yoga mats laid down, lectures booked. Swamis and musicians from different regions of the Indian subcontinent came to teach and perform. In his typical spirit of reciprocity, Bernard later explained that he wished "to enable young Brahmin students to perfect themselves in the teaching and coaching of Sanskrit language so that they could secure private pupils and thereby support themselves during their stay in this country." In a few cases, he provided extended room and board to Indian students who had come to the United States to attend college.

How Bernard was able to finance his own institutions always fascinated those who chased after him, and he rarely offered a full explanation, except under duress. When he was forced to talk about his finances in a legal deposition several years later, he offered this: "The money which I put in the libraries and apparatus . . . has come not merely from the fees charged pupils, but also special fees which I have charged for private instruction and outside coaching, exhibitions and exhibitions of special phenomena." It seems Bernard was establishing an altogether different side business from the private lessons he'd been conducting for years. Like Harry Houdini, he'd found a lucrative niche making his knowledge of magic and illusion available for sale to debunkers and scientific skeptics, "giving them instruction which would enable them to unravel supposed phenomena or exhibitions of mysteries"—in other words, to expose frauds and confidence artists among spiritualists and mediums.

And he never stopped giving private yoga lessons, again to many in the theater community, which was still in full thrall to all things Oriental. He tutored the wife of one of the Sire Brothers, well-known Broadway producers, as well as the wife of George Blumenthal, who'd made quite a name for himself as Oscar Hammerstein's publicist. Private clients like these were responsible for the most remunerative form of teaching Bernard undertook.

Back at his fledgling academy, the first season's offerings included free lectures followed by ancient Hindu Vina music daily at 8:15 p.m. and "physiological yoga," as the school called it, which was taught privately and only on the weekend. The schedule looked like this:

SUNDAYS, Vedic Philosophy services.

MONDAYS, Ancient Hindu Vina music.

TUESDAYS, Indian History, Ancient and Modern.

WEDNESDAYS, Teaching Sanskrit language.

THURSDAYS, Ayur Vedic Botany.

FRIDAYS AND SATURDAYS, Physiological yoga.

This setup was a far more academic endeavor than the West Seventy-fourth Street townhouse, and it was housed in a far less glamorous space, too: a run-down set of rooms in an average Upper West Side apartment. Morning sunlight streamed into the main studio from the Broadway windows and a dried-out potted plant sat on the sill. Oversize gilded letters on one wall of a large room spelled out Y-O-G-A, beneath which could be seen a gallery of devotional photos of swamis and gurus, including Hamati. There were rickety folding chairs and a worn Persian rug. The metal emblem of the Tantrik Order in America hung on the wall. On the long blackboard appeared the week's schedule, and there it was noted that Indo-Aryan history would be illustrated by a slide show.

Over the next several months, the college became a hive of activity for visiting Indians, interested students from Columbia University, and others. Throughout the spring and into the summer, new guest speakers arrived, lecturing on subjects ranging from "Mysticism of the Orient" to "Secrets of East Indian Guruship," the latter the specialty of an itinerant scholar named Pandit Prabodhacharanda Shastri, who'd found his way to the Upper West Side of Manhattan from a monastery in India. Hindu religious figures like the renowned mystic Baba Bharati, who was billed to American audiences as the "Henry Ward Beecher of Calcutta," turned up to lecture and teach. Dr. U. L. Desai, who'd roomed with Bernard in New York years earlier, and Dr. P. C. Banerjee of the University of Calcutta joined the faculty and became lifelong friends of Bernard's.

And then there was Hazrat Inayat Khan, an Indian mystic and musician who was in the United States that summer on a self-appointed mission from God to spread the news of Sufism, an Islamic brand of mysticism that stressed love and acceptance. Khan had arrived at Bernard's school with his three musician brothers to perform and raise money, but compared with many of the gentle, unthreatening Indian missionaries who had preceded him, he looked every bit the powerful, handsome guru capable of sweeping women away—"very dark, good looking and wears a short, pointed Van Dyke beard and well waxed mustache," one reporter noted.

After one of Khan's musical performances at the Sanskrit College, Ora Ray Baker experienced a strange and powerful attraction to the handsome newcomer. Now twenty-one, she had been in her half brother's care for more than five years and wanted to find her own path in life. She had grown up to become a graceful woman, Bernard's perfect hostess, who always knew the right thing to say to people to make them feel at home. Ora Ray believed in her dreams as powerful portents, and as Khan's music trailed off into silence, she no doubt recalled the one in which a sage from the East took her into his arms and together they flew away over the oceans. Khan was six years older than Ora, sure of himself, a Muslim prince who had gladly traded his birthright for the chance to cross the seas to make converts to Sufi Islam. He gave her music lessons, and for a few days she kept her feelings to herself out of respect and awe for him.

After meeting Bernard and reading the *Journal of the Tantrik Order*, meanwhile, Khan had nothing but the highest praise for the American's devotion to India's spiritual traditions. "I do not hesitate to say that our people accept your word as final in the canon of Vedic interpretation," he wrote to Bernard in June 1911. "The zeal which you have shown in introducing to the Western world the texts of the Eastern philosophies and religions is most commendable."

Bernard's zeal was not enough to turn the school into a profitable enterprise, however, even with the support of many members of the Indian community. The public's disapproval of yoga and yogis, along with Bernard's own sullied reputation, worked against the academy's success. In the fall it became clear that he could not manage to pay the rent.

In November, in an effort to wring a little extra income from his property, he made the acquaintance of Miss Emma Rosalsky, who'd placed an ad seeking a location to conduct her morning kindergarten. Rosalsky's primary enrollee was the son of a prominent Wall Street lawyer, William Grossman, whose wife had encouraged her to find other pupils so that she might meet her expenses and have a bit left over for her efforts. She agreed to pay Bernard a few dollars a week for morning use of the Sanskrit College building, when the rooms would be empty.

But Rosalsky's associations with both the Grossman family and the scandal-tainted Bernard proved irresistible to the city's journalists, many of whom had never let the Tantriks out of their sights. On the overcast morning of December 14, 1911, Rosalsky had hardly begun the school day when a pack of boisterous reporters confronted her with clippings clutched in hand. She was educating these children in the very lair of . . . "Oom the Omnipotent, the Loving Guru of the Tantricks." Was the young lady aware of that?

Miss Rosalsky threw the intruders out, slammed the door, and tried to go about the rest of her day in a normal fashion. Not content to let things lie, one of the reporters hoofed it ten blocks north to West Ninety-seventh Street and rang the bell of the Grossman residence. Alarmed, Mr. Grossman rushed down to the Sanskrit College and knocked but received no answer; on the other side of the door, his son's teacher was so unnerved by the rabble that she wouldn't answer for anyone.

The reporters camped outside, and after an hour the young teacher rushed past them with her students. Undeterred, the gentlemen of the press proceeded to canvass the neighborhood in the hope of digging up fresh dirt on Bernard. They were quite successful. "What my wife and I have seen through the windows of the college is scandalous," said F. H. Gans, who lived across the street. "The windows of the place were open last Summer. We saw men and women in various stages of dishabille. Women's screams mingled with wild Oriental music. We told the janitor to notify the police, but the orgies have continued." Another neighbor, Thomas Richardson, said that the goings-on at the college kept him up until three or four in the morning. Still another said that "well dressed women were in the habit of coming to the place in taxicabs at midnight and staying there several hours."

The witnesses, led on by the reporters, were embroidering their impressions, projecting suspicion onto unfamiliar practices, interpreting Indian vocal music and chants as screams and yoga togs as dishabille. It was no doubt true, however, that the Tantriks kept late hours, and wealthy women, and even women of the theater, were always welcome at the Sanskrit College, even in the late-evening hours after performances.

This time Bernard confronted his accusers directly. "I am conducting a perfectly respectable Sanskrit school," he told the reporters. "It was true that two women complained to the District Attorney that my West Seventy Fourth Hindu school was a disorderly resort last year. But the women were bribed by the district attorney and the newspapers to do this, and both of them left town with big rolls of greenbacks when the case against me fell through." He introduced the reporters to Prabodhacharanda Shastri, who seemed to impress the man from the *New York Times* with his good breeding. The reporter described the Indian as a "good looking man whose accent is very English and who smokes a very English bulldog briarwood pipe."

Manhattan district attorney Charles Whitman was unmoved by Bernard's high-class company. He assured the citizens of New York that he would be keeping a close eye on Bernard's newest venture. On the evening of December 21, he made good on his promise, sending a team of investigators uptown to finally hunt Bernard down and to arrest him on charges of "violating the educational law" by running a school without the proper diploma or license. The search was fruitless—as usual Bernard had slipped away—but he took the hint. He abandoned New York City for the foreseeable future.

* * *

In 1912 his band of yogis and yoginis regrouped at a large house at 145 Christie Street in Leonia, near a pretty creek that drained into the Hackensack River. Here Bernard set up living quarters with Ora Ray, who helped out with teaching, bookkeeping, and housecleaning. Jones and Nicholls were frequent visitors, though they also maintained New York

City addresses, and several of Bernard's new friends crossed the river to Leonia as well—men like Dr. Banerjee and four or five other Hindu scholars. News of Bernard's teachings had begun to reach far beyond his small circle. Two students from the universities of Edinburgh and Glasgow came to Leonia to sit at his feet, bringing an intellectual component to his allure that Bernard would continue to welcome and encourage over the years.

Lessons continued much as they had in New York, with Bernard guiding his students in mat work, breathing, and lectures on yoga. That August, he gathered his faithful remnant and described his mission for the newcomers: "The Tantrik Order is simply . . . a body of men, Yogis, who for their evolution, for their happiness, follow a certain system, a certain science of Life, which being in accordance with nature is best suited to bring about the consummation which everybody desires, happiness." Pure common sense, Bernard said, naturally led any thinking person to acknowledge the usefulness of hatha yoga. "My definition of the spiritual man therefore is a man who follows nature's laws. Nature's laws have been reduced from time immemorial by intelligent men to practical use. Yoga is the only system in which we get these laws. It is actual knowledge of investigation and practical application of those laws in human life. The purpose of human happiness is the purpose of yoga."

Ensconced in Leonia, Bernard was beginning to formulate a dignified language by which his teachings could be justified. Time and again he would refine and alter this treatise to suit the interests of the times and the temperament of his followers, whose personal lives were as much his concern.

Unbeknownst to Bernard, however, Ora Ray's secret attraction to the Sufi musician-poet Inayat Khan had developed over the past year into full-blown romance, and in 1912 she informed her half brother that *her* human happiness would be possible only as the life partner of Khan. Bernard refused to give his permission and vowed to stop the romance in its tracks. Khan was penniless, he pointed out, an itinerant mystic with no prospects, nor much in the way of earthly ambition. Her beloved holy man lived on handouts, was in fact out of sight even now, traveling and performing for his bread. Even Khan's brothers were politely but firmly against the marriage. Determined to ensure that the man now out of sight was put out of his half sister's mind, Bernard intercepted Khan's subsequent letters to Ora Ray, hiding some of them and destroying the rest. He also made sure that Ora Ray was otherwise occupied when Khan boarded a ship for London later that year. His Sufi friend, whose insights and admiration Bernard had once held dear, was now a man he publicly denigrated.

Ora Ray continued to pine for her mystic, but Bernard was not persuaded, even as he pursued a new romantic interest in his own life. Or perhaps he was preoccupied, blinded by his feelings for a beautiful young dancer named Dace Shannon Charlot.

She was not yet twenty-one when Bernard first laid eyes on her. She had thick, dark hair and lovely, outsize features, the most striking of which were her eyes. Dace was a creature born for the stage, physically and emotionally; haughty and needy in equal parts, she exhibited a distaste for the mundane and talents large enough to take her from the backwaters of Michigan to the variety stages of Broadway. She'd arrived in New York as a teenage soprano with dreams of an opera career, but her attraction for a powerful older man pushed her off course.

When Bernard met her, Dace was living in Leonia with her mother and sister, having fled and filed for divorce from her abusive sixty-year-old husband, a Frenchman named Charlot. Four years earlier, he had spirited her away to Mexico, and she'd managed to escape only through the intervention of her pistol-packing mother. The real-life soap opera of their breakup was playing out in newspapers across America in 1913 as the scandal of the moment. But Dace wasn't scandalized. To the contrary, she reveled in the attention, charming reporters and photographers with her quick wit and showgirl looks.

The date Bernard first met Dace was never recorded, but it's likely they were at least acquainted by the time she secured her divorce in August of 1913. She had taken Hindu dance lessons at the office of the late Dr. Latson on Riverside Drive, then moved on after his tragic death to the Sanskrit College, where she'd befriended Dr. Banerjee. It was Bernard's flamboyant attorney, Clark L. Jordan, in fact, who represented her in the divorce, securing her alimony and court costs as well.

Post-divorce, Dace wasted little time reinventing herself. With her mother and sister, Franci, she had taken rooms at a boardinghouse on Christie Street in Leonia, where she planned her return to New York's stages under a new name: Blanche DeVries. The *Charlot v. Charlot* divorce spectacle had given a boost of notoriety to her performing career, a quality she hoped to capitalize on by perfecting the sinuous writhings of the oh-so-modish nautch girl dances. The classes that she'd taken with Dr. Latson and the Sanskrit College Tantriks would be put to good use.

But it seems that she was fated to employ those talents in another capacity. Her friend Marian Dockerill, a fellow veteran of New York's yoga-and-dance scene, was present at the lunch in a New Jersey boardinghouse at which DeVries threw in her lot with Bernard. In recounting the meeting in her book, *My Life in a Love Cult*, Dockerill insisted it was Blanche DeVries who proposed the partnership, while Bernard sat back uncharacteristically passive during the meal—"quiet, unobtrusive, a rather bald young man."

"Look at our divorces, suicides, murders, other tragedies that follow in the train of mismating!" DeVries said. "That should not be. It's all because American women and men don't know the first thing about love. Not the first thing!" In her excitement DeVries brought her hand down on the table with this ringing endorsement of Bernard's rhetoric. And she knew full well that repeating it in the presence of its creator would have the desired effect. "We can teach the Anglo Saxon how to love," she continued. "At least Pierre can. I'm only a woman. The Hindus don't think so much of women as teachers. Women are only the receptive ones in the love line. Think you could do a lot of loving, Pierre?" she teased.

The flattery had its intended effect. At the end of their lunch together, Dockerill noted, Bernard "nodded solemnly" over the prunes on his plate to DeVries's teasing question. From then on, the two were a team. He was her first great teacher. She became his most devoted student, his lover, and his acolyte, and she proved her usefulness to the Tantrik Order from the earliest days of their relationship.

Their attraction was by all accounts a powerful fusing of two souls. Each had enormous strength and willpower, along with a highly developed libido. Matched in their strengths and complementary in their weaknesses, together they would need but a few years to become the nation's premier occult power couple. Both had fierce ambition and were private to the point of paranoia. Both had burned through several pseudonyms and were veterans of yellow-press exposés (though DeVries seemed to better enjoy her newspaper outings). In letters Bernard addressed her as Sakti, the supreme Tantric goddess, and signed himself Shiva, the name of the prominent Hindu deity—the god of destruction.

In a more meaningful way, they completed each other. Bernard loved the risk and reward of business and possessed an innate ability to transform his pursuits into profits. DeVries was an aesthete who treasured the finer things in life but ignored their cost. She was carefree with her finances and head over heels in love with music and dance and beauty, a polished counterpoint to the occasionally rough finish of her partner's character. Bernard was strong medicine for some: bursting with energy, an alpha male in extremis, first son of a first son, and so preternaturally confident that he chafed as many people as he attracted. Blanche DeVries had developed into a gracious woman, cultured and smooth of manners over a steely core. She was also a talented visual designer, expert in the domestic arts, and a natural flatterer of women with great wealth.

DeVries had come along at an opportune time for the Tantriks. Ora Ray Baker, who had functioned as the group's poised and polished hostess, had plotted her escape. While cleaning out Pierre's desk, Ora Ray had stumbled upon Inayat Khan's home address in Baroda, India, and in 1913, she slipped out of her love-struck brother's sight and boarded a ship for Belgium. She and Khan reunited there and were married—first in a religious ceremony on a boat to England and again in a civil ceremony in London on March 20. She took the veil of a devout Muslim wife, never showing her face in public for the rest of her life. As Pirani Ameena Begum, Ora Ray attained a place of high honor among Sufis, and she never returned to the United States. Bernard, his eyes fixed on his own future, broke all contact with her.

<hr />

In 1914, as Europe descended into war and American newspapers turned their attention there, Bernard was able to go about his business free from the snooping press. Living in New Jersey, visiting private students in New York, he was able to fill his time lecturing and studying, and he encouraged DeVries to deepen the education he was giving her with her own reading in science and philosophy.

In December of that year, he traveled to Haverford, Pennsylvania, to attend the forty-sixth annual meeting of the American Philological

Association. This organization was the principal society for classical studies in North America, and its members were also making strides in the
discovery and translation of "Oriental" manuscripts like the Yoga Sutras
of Patanjali. Of the 150 attendees at Haverford that year, Bernard was one
of only six who listed no university affiliations.

It is doubtful that any of his fellow scholars realized that Dr. Pierre
Arnold Bernard had not completed even a formal grade-school education.
A brilliant autodidact, he held his own in the company of erudite men and
women and considered himself a lifelong student; he valued his connections to groups like the Philologists and the Royal Asiatic Society, and he
eventually became a member or fellow of more than fifty other learned
societies and academies.

Bernard's pride in these connections was genuine, but they also served
to counter the public's perception of him as a fraud and lothario who'd
espoused a dubious philosophy. By keeping prestigious intellectual company in public, he was giving the outside world little reason to scrutinize
his actions in private, where he and DeVries were teaching some extremely
risky concepts: Sex, they told the inner circle of followers, was not just
natural; it had the potential to be sacred. On May 9, 1915, he gathered
together those who had pledged themselves to secrecy and signed their
names in blood. Bernard launched into a rambling lecture on marriage,
orgasm, evolution, yoga, and oral sex, "that marvelous intimacy." The lecture was titled "Sex Perversion, Chemical and Anatomical Values," and
from his surviving notes, it is clear that his views on the primacy of sex in
human relationships were dangerously ahead of his time.

"Ninety-nine percent of divorces are the result of sex perversion," he
said, which he defined as either an insufficiency of sex, "celibacy," or an
"overdose"—not getting it right in quantity or quality. In "mouth congress," as oral sex is called in the Kama Sutra—"there is a great shock,"
he added. "Orgasm is prolonged ten times longer than during sex congress," its intensity so extreme that the subject "has no mind left. . . . The
sensation is so terrible that some say they die. Some cannot endure it."

Oral sex, a crime punishable by as much as twenty years in prison
in the United States, was in India an ancient, sacred practice, Bernard
proclaimed. "Thirty-five hundred years ago this self same thing was done
by the people of India of [the] Brahmanical branches," and it was this

interplay of the erotic and the sacred that formed a major part of the South Asian Tantric culture he had adopted as his own. "If sex is right," he told them, "that is the whole secret."

During this time Bernard continued to slip back and forth across the Hudson, and by 1916, he'd audaciously set up a suite of offices in Manhattan at 662 West End Avenue, where he rented rooms to medical doctors, including Dr. William Jenkins, a former health commissioner of the Port of New York. With the talented DeVries on board, Bernard was finally able to expand his vision. He opened new yoga studios that were beautifully decorated, again thanks to DeVries—one on Riverside Drive for women and another on Park Avenue for men—and he restarted his outreach program, deploying the lady-killer Nicholls and the saintly Florin Jones, to places where like-minded people might be found. At least once during the war years, Jones ventured as far as London to drum up new clients and teach hatha yoga, but he aroused the suspicions of the British authorities and was quickly deported. No matter, the most fertile ground for new recruits was, they discovered, right in their own backyard, at Carnegie Hall. During these war years, the annex to the great auditorium was on Sunday nights a honeycomb of hip, youthful activity, with simultaneous competing parties thrown by the artists who lived and worked there. From all over the city came actors, dancers, sculptors, photographers, singers, and painters, who drifted from studio to studio as the evening wore on: dancing, drinking, playing music, eyeing one another's work, and all the while hoping for a connection that might lead to a commission or possibly a romance—a happy hunting ground for Nicholls and Jones.

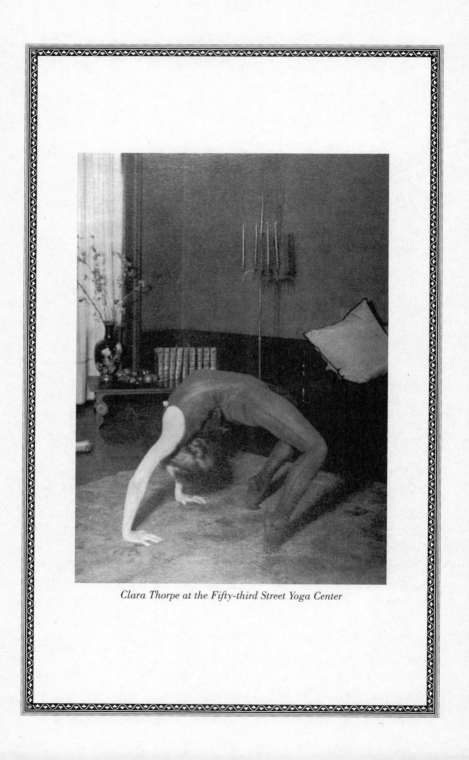

Clara Thorpe at the Fifty-third Street Yoga Center

Chapter 8

EXPANSION

n one of those Sunday nights at the Carnegie Hall studios, Florin Jones made quite a first impression on a pretty ballet dancer named Llellwyn Delores Smith. A native of Portland, Oregon, she had been dancing on Broadway in Florenz Ziegfeld's spectacle *Miss 1917*, but her aspirations to classical dance had led her here to the studios, where she had studied with Isadora Duncan's adopted daughters, Anna and Liesel. Llellwyn was also taking private lessons in Hindu dancing with a famous performer named Roshanara, one of Ruth St. Denis's vaudeville followers.

Like an emissary from another universe, Jones was standing patiently before a dozen or so artists and actors assembled in Helen Jacobs's painting studio, just as he had stood before other crowds in Seattle and Portland in his long years of service to Bernard. He spoke of the benefits of yoga, the path to nirvana, and other marvelous things he'd learned and wished to share. His voice was nearly hypnotic in its power. "I didn't understand much of the philosophy," Llellwyn later wrote, "but I enjoyed his almost musical way of speaking. . . . Unlike anyone I had ever met before, [he was] mysterious, with an air of self composure and authority. . . . He spoke of a knowledge hidden in Yoga, beyond human comprehension, available only to those willing to take the sacred path."

Jones was physically attracted to Llellwyn from their first meeting, but he kept his distance. Because this young dancer was probably seventeen years old and looked even younger, he wisely refused to take her anywhere near Bernard's yoga studios. "The papers might blow up a story because you are a dancer in the Follies," he told her. "With a little imagination, they could have a headline like this: 'Yoga Cult Hypnotizes Young Follies Dancer.'"

Instead he took her for rides in Central Park in the little Ford coupe he kept in the city. On these trips he shared his dreams for the next chapter of his life, which included opening his own yoga school in Leonia. He owned a bit of property out there, he said, with a tumbledown house on the cliffs overlooking the Hudson River. In his quirky and self-deprecating manner, he had named his home Dinky Dump. He also confessed to her that he and Bernard did not always get along, that they clashed over their different ways of teaching.

As time passed, Llellwyn convinced him of her seriousness and he began to teach her yoga—in private, of course. She was the perfect student in many ways, a typical member of this new Lost Generation—disoriented by the war and the pace of the times, bewitched by the possibility of glimpsing the mysteries of life. And she was physically gifted, too, a very charming blonde with a sweet, trusting face and a dancer's lithe body.

The forlorn Jones nicknamed her Cheerie, a name she kept and used happily for years. Gentle and bookish and tending toward depression, he confided in her about his terrible heartbreak over another woman— presumably his ex-wife, Duval—which only endeared him to her. While Cheerie vacillated between feelings of worship and love, Jones made no secret of his place in the Tantrik Order: his function in these matters was to find and groom students and pass them along to his guru, Bernard— but only when he deemed them ready and trustworthy, not to mention of legal age. "He warned me that when I progressed, P. A. Bernard might accept me as his pupil," she wrote, "and my loyalty to him [Jones] might not survive the test."

Jones kept his worries in check; after all, he had a job to do. And then, after months of preparation, he dutifully took his young charge up to visit Bernard's yoga school for women at Riverside Drive. Cheerie later recalled her first impression of the corps of young female yoga teachers. "Their natural beauty impressed me," she wrote. "Their radiance and healthful glow, without a trace of makeup, I thought far surpassed the most renowned of Ziegfeld's beauties." She told Jones that she was now even more anxious to meet Bernard, but he insisted the time was not yet right. In his desperation to retain her affection, he blurted out that they ought to be married.

Cheerie was bewildered by Jones and his proposal, but for reasons she could never explain, she agreed. His ardor simply bowled her over, she later said. She'd passed up an offer for a five-year contract at the fledgling MGM Pictures on the West Coast—and with it the chance for the performing career she'd always wanted—and in 1917, the two were wed at his little house on the Palisades. The marriage, which went unconsummated, was "a strange mistake" in Cheerie's words, though she never lost her affection for Jones.

She continued to live at home with her parents, keeping her marriage and her interest in yoga a secret from her family. She worked when she could, took classes and lessons, and began a lifelong friendship with Clara Thorpe, another talented but underage dancer, who had found her way into the fold at Riverside Drive. Eventually Cheerie's parents discovered the depth of her devotion to Jones and his yoga teachings, and they demanded that she stop immediately. She refused outright, convinced that her elders could never understand this new world—her world—so influenced were they by the newspaper scandals linking yoga to hypnotism and black magic.

During this family turmoil, Jones finally took her to meet P.A., as Bernard was called by close associates. They knocked on the door of his study on Riverside Drive and entered. Cheerie was shocked by Bernard's appearance. She had pictured "a saint in yellow robes seated in meditation. To my disbelief, I met a vigorous man of about 40 in a white sport sweater and wearing baseball pants, smoking a big cigar." When she looked into his eyes, Cheerie made a life-altering decision on the spot. "I saw a leader, self-assured and untouched by all outside influences. I trusted him[,] feeling that whatever path he chose for me I would follow."

By then Bernard was able to boast that he operated eight studios, keeping thirteen teachers busy with fifteen students per class. Classes were segregated by gender (for the most part), and the schools were operated more or less like business franchises, financed and run by his teachers.

DeVries's theatrical decorating style began to assert itself in these eight studios, which were located in townhouses and apartments in good

Manhattan neighborhoods. At the women's townhouse at 662 West End Avenue, she chose a color scheme of deep, fiery red. Heavy crimson draperies covered the windows. On the floor were giant red carpets that sat atop gym mats, upon which DeVries and Clara and the others demonstrated postures and trained their students. The elegant bathrooms had attached lounges, which were furnished with luxuriously upholstered chairs and chaises and decorated with tapestries. The gentlemen's studio at 330 Park Avenue consisted of three rooms that opened to the street and was decorated in a harmonious palette of blues. At Fifty-fourth Street and Fifth Avenue, blue draperies shielded the windows, and the teachers and clients wore green tights and bathing suits. Some of these quarters were large enough to maintain rooms to rent for boarders and private rooms for the yoga staff. The Riverside Drive mansion, where DeVries resided as leader of the female staff, was also spacious enough to devote a room to Bernard's growing library.

After a few years' respite from the baying hounds of the press, the Tantriks' expansion again caught the attention of reporters for William Randolph Hearst's *New York American*. They began digging for dirt in earnest. But rather than run with the exposé on its own, the paper turned over its files and leads to the DA's office in exchange for exclusive access to the ensuing investigation. Manhattan district attorney Edward Swann welcomed the collaboration of the press in bringing down Bernard, who piqued the special enmity he reserved for spiritual fakers.

To lead the sting, Swann called upon one of his best undercover officers, Mrs. Ada Brady, commanding her to gain the confidence of a member of Bernard's inner circle—no small feat, since each of these members had taken a blood oath not to reveal the slightest bit of information to outsiders. Brady summoned her legendary poise, turning herself into "Mrs. Shaw," a bored young society woman looking for attractive men and new kicks. Soon enough, one of Bernard's wealthy female followers unwittingly fell for the policewoman's blandishments and arranged an introduction with the Great Oom.

"Dr. Bernard shook hands after I had introduced myself," Brady told a reporter. "I told him I was Mrs. Shaw and was sent by a Mrs. Burgess. He said: 'Oh yes, I know about it.' I told him what I wanted. He said there would be certain exercises taken, lying for example on an operating table, which he indicated right at hand, and moving the body about in such positions that every muscle was educated to move at will and in any way that you desire. He said the treatment was wonderful. He said many actresses of note were his patrons and they were wonderfully enthusiastic about it. He named one noted in vaudeville and one in motion pictures."

Bernard tried, politely, to interest his visitor in yoga lessons, playing on her modesty. "He said there were some people who do not like to appear in tights and go through the exercises in front of other people. But if we were not averse to doing it, we could take our treatments in class with perhaps fifteen other people."

Brady attended her first hatha yoga class at the 662 West End Avenue townhouse, where she took detailed notes that were later published in the *American*. A young girl, described by Officer Brady as very blonde, came in and gave a demonstration of what the policewoman called the "nautch girl" dances. Convinced that what she was seeing was an all-too-innocent front, Brady complained to Mrs. Burgess, her unwitting informant, that the classes weren't enough. She wanted to be initiated into the inner circle. She also wanted to know, specifically, "Will I meet men?"

If the policewoman received an answer to her last question, there is no evidence of it. But she reported back to DA Swann that "male and female classes in rejuvenation were held in that house on Tuesday night. And that the 'Lectures Upon Imagination' were [to be] delivered by Bernard in person to the initiated. Some of these dress in tights." This last detail was enough evidence to warrant another raid.

On Tuesday evening, April 30, 1918, an assistant district attorney, an inspector, and five deputies stormed the West End Avenue address. Bernard was not there at the time—as usual—but the police took into custody Winfield Nicholls and four others, moving everyone downtown for questioning. The investigators listed the occupations of those who rented rooms in the house: "psychics, soothsayers, cryptic name purveyors, spiritualists and trance mediums," some of whom, they informed the paper, were preying on the wives and girlfriends of soldiers and sailors overseas.

The next day the *New York American* ran a long page-one story that proudly proclaimed its role in hunting down Bernard: "Twelve Cult Worshippers Taken in a Raid upon Home of the Great Oom," read the headline. "The disciples of the cult, whose practices continue all night, include both men and women. An admitted disciple of Bernard and an initiate into the practices of the Inner Mysteries and Sex Worship, is expected to supply valuable information. Well-known names have already declared to be members."

Bernard lay low once again—nobody knew how he always managed to avoid the police—expecting worse to come, and come it did. The next day, investigators descended on three more of his yoga schools. Police questioned DeVries and others, including a woman identified as Sister Beatrix, a former Episcopal nun who ran a private school for girls in Rockland County. The cops harassed staff and students, leaked names to the press, and described their efforts to reporters as a "round-up." The accusations against the group, trumped up to begin with, were then escalated to something close to treason. The United States was at war and rife with fear that German undercover agents were infiltrating its citizenry. So when the DA's office leaked to the public that German aliens living in the Riverside Drive house could view the movement of American battleships in the north Hudson, suddenly Bernard wasn't merely a salacious cult leader; he was a traitor, harboring enemy spies during wartime. The DA also let it be known that this bit of intelligence had been forwarded to the Justice Department, which was already investigating swamis at the New York Vedanta Society for conspiring with the Germans against the Allies. Of course, Bernard had nothing to do with any of this, and neither the New York Police Department nor the U.S. Justice Department ever produced evidence to bring a single charge against him. One of Oom's renters, a séance medium, was indicted in New York, according to press reports, but no other arrests followed, and none were ever made. The point, however, had been made yet again that in the name of "purity" this kind of harassment, sanctioned by the city government and aided by the press baron Hearst, was not about to stop.

Then again, Bernard was a stubborn man, and he had recently hit a geographical gold mine with his latest yoga school for women at Fifty-fourth Street and Fifth Avenue, right in the heart of Millionaires' Row. This time, the depredations of the establishment were not powerful enough to change his course or even slow him down.

In the closing years of the nineteenth century, many of the great American families had built their homes along this stretch of Fifth Avenue, where the Vanderbilts alone had nine mansions. One of these, at 660 Fifth Avenue, was located just a few blocks from Bernard's Fifty-fourth

Street yoga studio, and it had symbolized Vanderbilt wealth and excess for decades. Six-sixty Fifth had been built in 1883 by Alva Smith Vanderbilt, the ambitious first wife of William Kissam Vanderbilt, to gain entry for her in-laws into Mrs. Astor's Four Hundred, the social elect of New York City. The Tantriks' entrée to this world arrived via Margaret Rutherfurd, the daughter of the second Mrs. William K. Vanderbilt.

Tall and good-looking, Margaret was the progeny of Anne Harriman Sands and the legendarily handsome (and now deceased) Lewis Rutherfurd. When her mother married Willie K. in 1903, Margaret became a member of the richest family in the world. As a teenager, she was wooed in Paris by Kermit Roosevelt, the big-game-hunting son of the president, but she eventually married an ambitious young suitor named Ogden Mills, a politician with substantial wealth and social connections to more than match the Vanderbilts'.

By the time she ran into Florin Jones in 1917, Margaret had been struggling for more than a year—including a stint in a sanitarium in Maine for a nervous breakdown—to reconcile herself to an unhappy marriage and her birdcage existence. Her life was freed by unimaginable wealth and bound by the strictest social codes, a plight shared by all the Gilded Age heiresses. "You don't know what the position of an heiress is," wrote her cousin Gertrude Vanderbilt in her journal. "You can't imagine. There is no one in all the world who loves her for herself. No one. She cannot do this, that and the other simply because she is known by sight and will be talked about."

With her husband off fighting in France, Margaret had been spending less time at the Washington, D.C., home they shared and more time with her friends and family in Manhattan. She'd also undertaken a personal spiritual quest that led her in the direction of metaphysics and yoga— and into the recruiter's sights of Florin Jones. Jones set her up in yoga classes with Blanche DeVries, who as a natural teacher and born confidante worked brilliantly with Margaret. The two women became close companions—they were roughly the same age—and soon enough the heiress had declared herself a committed student of yoga and its philosophy. When the time was right, she was told, if she proved herself worthy and ready, she would meet a master of these things.

Wealthy and connected at the highest levels of high society, Margaret was a prize catch. DeVries took the young heiress in hand and smoothed the path for her, surely hoping her friends and family would follow. But that would all come later. As the Great War entered its final year, Bernard had plenty of money coming in, even without access to the Vanderbilt coffers. He was charging new students $100–$150 for a series of classes—as much as $2,000 in twenty-first-century dollars—and demand for his services was still growing. Always a good businessman, Bernard had invested in real estate and put a portion of his profits into the stock market. "Made quite a little money in International Mercantile Marine," he said later. "Bought it at $30 . . . and sold some of it at $70 a share."

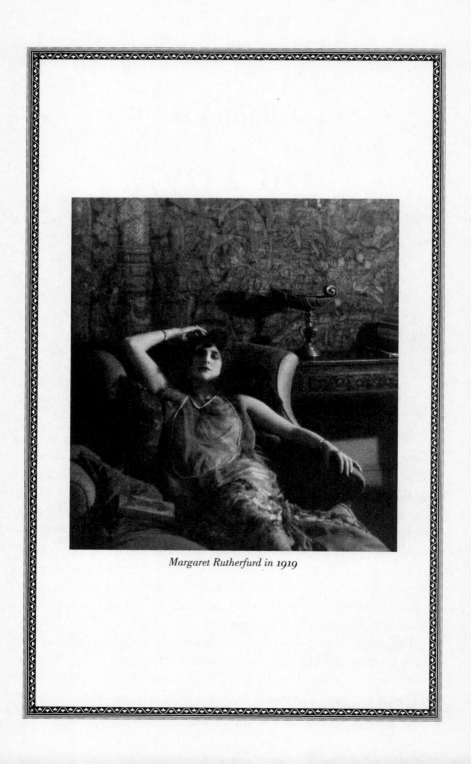

Margaret Rutherfurd in 1919

Chapter 9

FOR LOVE
AND MONEY

he Great Oom himself met Margaret Rutherfurd Mills in 1918, not long after the DA's failed raid on his operation—"introduced by Miss DeVries at somebody's house in New York," he later recalled. The Tantriks were about to leave the city to set up their first—and it turned out only—summer camp on Long Island's East End, and it took only two or three private lessons with her teacher to compel Margaret to ask to come along.

That summer their school and resort in the Hamptons attracted about thirty pupils, who took open-air classes in hatha yoga followed by lectures and socializing. As usual, this gathering of eccentrics lived and worked side-by-side in a group of houses they leased to be near their guru. Margaret and DeVries roomed together, and in their spacious bungalow they entertained friends and family visitors—prospective clients in DeVries's eyes. Her wealth and connections aside, Margaret turned out to be a devoted student. She kept up her reading, which no doubt included the *International Journal of the Tantrik Order,* the primer Bernard pressed on all his initiates. And she faithfully attended his lectures, given three or four times a week in the afternoons.

Though the Tantriks left no further footprints in the sand that summer, it is clear from what transpired afterward that Margaret had developed an intense attraction to Bernard. Was it love? She clearly thought so. Though she was still married to Ogden Mills, who was by this time a

New York State senator, the marriage was all but ended in her mind. The young heiress, heretofore constrained by society's rules, was emboldened by Bernard's message of transformation through love and his reverence for the power of women.

"Through the lips of a woman the breath of divinity passes," Bernard wrote in the *International Journal of the Tantrik Order*. "There exists nothing that the true love of her cannot cause a man to achieve. In that sweet bosom is to be found more pure and sacred emotions than in all the churches, pagodas and mosques that stand." In Margaret's bosom there was swelling an attraction for her guru more powerful than even her heiress's inhibitions could withstand.

Unbeknownst to Margaret, however, on August 27, 1918, Bernard married Blanche DeVries in a civil ceremony in Richmond, Virginia. It was an impetuous act, by all indications, with no planning or announcements, and with little regard for the legal niceties of matrimony. In front of a judge and witnesses, the newlyweds placed their signatures next to outrageous falsehoods on their certificate, claiming bogus residences and fictitious parents. DeVries even allowed herself a French father named Jean. In the months that followed, the newlyweds proceeded to keep the marriage a secret, even from their closest associates.

In September, the group moved back to New York. Margaret took the oath, became an initiate of the Tantrik Order, and was given her club name, Durand. By the fall, she had introduced her entire family to yoga, and it seems this new exercise regimen, with its strange philosophy, had become part of the Vanderbilt family's table talk. Margaret's stepfather, Willie K., now in his late sixties and suffering from degenerative heart disease, took physical exercise with one of Bernard's teachers, Harry Sanderson, at the Park Avenue studios, as well as privately at 660 Fifth Avenue. Harold Stirling Vanderbilt, Willie K.'s son by his first marriage, was a natural yogi; years later he recalled that the headstands and postures he performed every day had been taught to him by Oom himself. Margaret's mother, Anne Vanderbilt, observed first with bemusement, then with admiring conviction, that even her younger daughter, Barbara, had become somewhat interested.

In November, while the world celebrated the Armistice, Margaret poured out her feelings to Bernard in a letter, bubbling over with her new passion and struggling to prove herself worthy of her guru, after an evening they'd evidently spent together.

> I want to tell you (& please believe me!) that the love in me for you is not a barometer or changeable as it seems to you & as you thought last night but is deep & true growing day by day [. . .] A love really big should develop the very opposite characteristics in an individual, infinite patience & understanding. I *know* darling it is in me to be the most patient & understanding person in the world, but at present I am still like a child that has been knocked & bruised. I have been longing & longing for you so long & even when you did finally come I kept on blindly knocking not realizing that finally you had heard & that you were the one.
>
> But I resent the fact so that I can't come to you simply & be yours & that we can't be happy in every way now instead of letting more time elapse & settling such superficial conventionalities[.] It seems so wrong to have to cow tow [*sic*] to a lot of fools whose lives hang together by a set of man made laws[.] Every drop of blood in me cries out against it [—] why should one have to sacrifice 5 minutes of one's happiness to that. . . . I want to be all yours monkey in every way, conventionally & unconventionally in all ways conceivable & you sweet have chosen me for your own out of this foolish old world so why should we wait any longer so far as settling those obstacles, there is nothing to be gained by waiting now—
>
> I wish you were here now in my arms darling & I would kiss you & contemplate your beautiful face, sweet. I could gaze on your face for hours[.] It is worship I feel for your whole being. To breathe you in to feel & be near you is all I ask for, & to some day be worthy of you & your love. I kiss your dear dear eyes sweet.

There is no record of Bernard's response to this letter, but perhaps he didn't need to put it on paper. Obviously, he had Margaret's complete submission already—achieved partly by his own magnetic charms and partly by shattering her upper-class assumptions. Bernard had given her a glimpse of a bigger universe than the one laid out for her by wealth and station, and she desperately wanted to be part of it.

Wisely, she didn't share these revelations with her mother. Anne Vanderbilt saw only the splendid results of Bernard's work with Margaret, Harold, and Willie, and she approved. She was especially pleased with the dispositions of the young women of Bernard's academy—notably Cheerie Smith and Clara Thorpe—whose exemplary charm, fitness, and balance made them fine role models for her two daughters. Yoga was now taking its place alongside the traditional Vanderbilt pastimes of yachts, Thoroughbreds, and entertaining. Anne's friend and fellow socialite Mrs. Charles C. Goodrich, wife of the Goodrich tire heir, joined her in her newfound passion. And they spread the news of this healing philosophy to their social circles in Paris, Newport, Bermuda, and Hot Springs, Virginia. Even one of the Vanderbilt family doctors, Guy Otis Brewster, endorsed yoga's beneficial effects.

✦✦✦✦✦

All who knew Anne Vanderbilt said there was a depth to her, a softness and empathy that opened her soul to the pain of others. She turned out to assist at every tragedy of her time, large or small. She organized transportation for the stunned survivors of the *Titanic* when they spilled onto the docks of New York's West Side. She enlisted Mark Twain to raise funds for San Francisco's earthquake victims, donated $1 million to build housing for TB sufferers in New York, founded the Big Sisters organization, and created safe and secure dance halls for working women in the city. Her only weaknesses, according to those who knew her well, were Paris couture and men with spiritual power. By early 1919, she had thrown herself fully into the role of sponsor to the Tantriks, who were getting ready to open yet another enterprise, the Fifty-third Street Yoga Center for Women. In January, she signed over checks in the amount of $10,000 to Bernard and DeVries to help them get it going. Then in February, just a block south of where Margaret had first studied yoga, the beautiful new yoga school for women opened. On March 14, Anne invited the Bernards to her home at 660 Fifth Avenue and donated another $10,000 toward their efforts. With her husband ill and her daughter Barbara increasingly prone to fits of moodiness, Anne had begun to lean on the sisterly strength of DeVries and the fatherly wisdom of Bernard for emotional guidance.

The Fifty-third Street Yoga Center itself was a welcome diversion for Anne. It's likely she even picked out the location, and if so, it was a testament to her good taste. Sixteen East Fifty-third Street was a distinguished five-story townhouse with an elaborate wrought-iron portal and Juliet balconies, nestled between Fifth and Madison avenues. This school was to be Bernard's first true joint venture with his wife, as well as a significant upgrade from the smaller space on East Fifty-fourth, which had been shut down (though the West Side schools and men's studios continued to operate). DeVries leased the Fifty-third Street property in her name and conducted the academy according to Bernard's principles. She hired and outfitted the staff, who wore starched white aprons over black leotards. She trained the teachers in hatha yoga and offered private instruction herself to a few select clients. And with her usual alacrity she made the place sumptuous and inviting for wealthy and educated women who were accustomed to fine surroundings. In the airy, light-filled marble lobby, she installed expensive Italian furniture and gold-framed mirrors. Clients were greeted by a hostess and escorted to the rear of the building, to an open-cage, French-style elevator, which lifted them to the upper-floor studios, steam baths, and irrigation rooms. With the proper recommendations in hand, along with an advance fee, the female clients were given a physical examination by one of two physicians affiliated with the center. "Then they were led to private rooms," according to *Town & Country*, "handed Annette Kellermann [*sic*] bathing costumes and told to disrobe."

Even the ladies' workout wear was chosen with care. Annette Kellerman, the Australian swimmer and diver who'd made the tight, one-piece sleeveless unitard with formfitting short shorts famous—or infamous to some—was also a women's rights advocate. The decision was undoubtedly DeVries's doing, and it telegraphed a message in keeping with the spirit of the establishment. This was the twentieth-century suffragist's workout wear of choice, a fitting uniform, if the slightest bit risqué, for the forward-looking American women who would be drawn to yoga. Each studio room was painted and outfitted according to its own color scheme. On the walls were posters bearing friendly reminders that "Cleanliness Is Next to Godliness" and "A Clean Colon Insures a Clean Mind." New students started with simple yoga exercises of rolling the stomach muscles and touching the toes.

But what was really going on in the Tantriks' inner circle? According to the notebooks left behind by Cheerie Smith, she and the others were as busy as students in any other private academy. There were classes in anatomy, psychology, English literature, and Sanskrit, with lectures on Vedic philosophy and comparative religion. Hatha yoga—postures, movement, and breathing exercises—shared equal billing with healthy living, and nothing was the least bit untoward.

In this new iteration, the Bernard-DeVries team stressed balance and moderation in all things. Alcohol and smoking were forbidden—except for Bernard's cigars—and fresh, healthful meals were served to clients and staff. Taking responsibility for one's actions, especially maintaining one's health, was a cardinal rule. Illness was avoidable, DeVries repeated over and again, something that smart, highly evolved women could learn to prevent. It was a timely message that would resonate powerfully with the worried wives and mothers who heard it, as the Spanish influenza had the previous year broken out into a full-fledged pandemic, infecting a third of the world's population and killing 30 million, most of them young.

The message *and* the method caught fire. The Yoga Center was bustling from early morning to late at night. With the exception of Bernard, it was staffed solely by young women. Some of these teachers and staffers went home after work, but a core group of eight or so lived on the premises as an extended family, with Bernard and DeVries in the role of surrogate parents. Bernard bounced around from East Side to West, keeping an eye on the operations of his other, less glamorous franchises. He kept living quarters in a few of them, including the upper floors of the Fifty-third Street townhouse, where he maintained an office for private sessions with clients. And on designated lecture nights he gathered everyone together for his renowned talks.

<hr />

Cheerie Smith gave him her rapt attention as she transcribed his words into her notebooks and later typed them for further study. His language "affected me deeply," she wrote. His practical and pragmatic approach to the subject of yoga was quite different from that of her first teacher, Jones. Bernard, she said, "used no ponderous phraseology, but graphically, and even ruthlessly, unveiled the weaknesses and stupidity of human behavior. I had always thought that developing one's talents was so important. Now I changed my ideas; developing the best in one's character was of greater value."

After one final blowout with her parents, who refused to come around to her new way of life, Cheerie packed her belongings and moved to Fifty-third Street. Changing not only her address but her very identity, she now went strictly by her nickname and worked at the center full-time as a housekeeper and occasional teacher. She labored hard and happily, she said, behind the scenes from 5 a.m. to late in the night in return for room and board and a free education. "[We] gathered like a family around 'Our Father' Bernard," she wrote. "I was the youngest among the women who lived there and the last to join the 'Inner Circle.' I knew nothing of housework or cooking, but I was both willing and eager to learn." She recalled her new boss, DeVries, as a "woman who had the strength and will of a tiger. She was determined to carry out P.A.'s ideals, no matter what. She was completely dedicated."

Committing herself to the Yoga Center also brought Cheerie the unforeseen privilege of hanging out with its main sponsor. Anne Vanderbilt liked to drop in behind the scenes and socialize with the "girls," as she called them. After hours, she often sent her chauffeur to pick up Cheerie and the other members of the inner circle, and together they'd meet at Anne's box at the Metropolitan Opera or attend Broadway shows in a group.

In her interactions with Cheerie and the other Tantrikas, Anne must have wondered how these young women might be drawn into her efforts to mentor her flighty younger daughter, Barbara Rutherfurd Hatch. Barbara's marriage to Cyril Hatch, a society dilettante seventeen years her senior, was even more stilted and unsatisfying than Margaret's. Barbara had given birth to a son, Rutherfurd, just as her husband suffered financial reverses, forcing the young woman back into her parents' home, baby in arms. But Barbara's troubles ran deeper than money, her mother knew.

Visited by fits of indolence and outbursts of temper, Barbara was ill-equipped to be a responsible parent to Rutherfurd, who ultimately grew up under Anne's care. The young mother was besieged by jealousy of her prettier older sister, yet she refused to divulge any interests or desires of her own, despite her mother's tireless encouragement.

Finally, at her wit's end, Anne turned to Bernard's teachers to lend a hand. She asked if Cheerie wouldn't mind coming by the house to give her daughter dance lessons, as Barbara had recently returned from a Hawaiian vacation and had shown a spark of curiosity about the hula.

Cheerie happily obliged, walking the block and a half from Fifty-third Street to 660 Fifth Avenue. She rang the bell and entered another realm of earthly existence. Noting the white marble entry, the medieval tapestries, the luxury she spied in every corner of the main floor, she made her way up the staircase to Barbara's bedroom. A maid hung freshly pressed laundry in Barbara's enormous closet, while servants moved silently through the corridors, delivering breakfast trays, placing flowers in vases, going about the brisk business of readying the great house for a new day.

Barbara sat at her dressing table, yawning, while a maid finished the morning routine of brushing the young woman's hair. She was dressed in a white cotton batiste nightgown beneath a blue dressing robe, which, Cheerie noticed, was trimmed in ermine. The furnishings on the dressing table were gold French antiques, decorated with carved Cupids. While the maid finished with Barbara's hair, the heiress toyed idly with her jewelry. Cheerie, whose own upbringing was quite well-to-do, was bowled over by this opulence, but there was one detail that caused her to gasp. Folded at the foot of Barbara's magnificent canopied bed lay a comforter made entirely of mink.

Barbara had returned from the Hawaiian Islands with a trunk full of hula costumes and puka shell necklaces. She'd also brought back recordings of Hawaiian music to play on the Victrola. On this sunny morning, however, no holiday exuberance was in evidence. She sat uninterested as Cheerie demonstrated the dance, Barbara's body "so listless, [it] didn't respond as I wished," Cheerie said.

It took several more visits for Cheerie to cajole Barbara into progress, but on the day of the last lesson, the heiress rewarded her teacher with a hand-me-down velvet dress and a short mink jacket. These clothes probably meant little to Barbara, but Cheerie kept and treasured the gifts for decades.

It didn't take long for Barbara to fall back into her funk, as if the hula dance had been performed by an impostor. Exasperated, Anne tried a more rigorous approach, ordering her daughter to submit to Bernard's idea of work therapy.

"Some folk like to spout a lot of Sanskrit terms like *Prana*, *Pranayama*, and *Karma* and whatnot, as if there were some virtue in foreign words," Bernard told his followers, "but it would do their souls a power more good to be on a course of household drudgery, scrubbing floors and so forth." With this advice ringing in her ears, Anne summoned Cheerie's services once again. "Since my job was scullery maid of the kitchen," she recalled, Anne "required me to teach Barbara how to clean the back stairs, top to bottom." Early on a Monday morning, Barbara walked the block and a half from 660 Fifth to the backstairs kitchen at the Yoga Center to learn firsthand the pleasures and terror of domestic labor. To her credit she arrived early, Cheerie noted, sleep still in her eyes, wearing a dainty white organdy dress and a lace apron.

The two women trudged up to the fourth floor. The heiress took the scrub brush, dipped her hands into the bucket of hot, soapy water, and immediately burst into tears. But then she quickly gathered herself together, and three hours later had worked her way down the stairs and polished the last step. In the end, she was reported to be pleased with her efforts.

Barbara, it turned out, was not the only society woman scouring the floors at the Fifty-third Street studio. Several women of social prominence, noted *Town & Country*, were "sometimes seen by milkmen and late-night revelers scrubbing down the marble front steps at the crack of dawn." It was a good way to tamp down the egos of pampered ladies, and like the Betty Ford Center fifty years later, Bernard's Yoga Center considered the upkeep of the facility another component of healing and therapy.

With its nuanced methods for healthy living, tailored specifically for women, the center attracted luminaries such as business entrepreneur Helena Rubinstein, actress Ethel Barrymore, and Frances Payne Bolton, who would later be one of the first women elected to the U.S. Congress. They came because Bernard's down-to-earth advice worked, Cheerie said. "He understood how to Westernize this ancient philosophy, making it more useful and practical." The center stood for "beauty, cleanliness, and efficiency," Cheerie noted, "more proof to show visitors that yoga succeeded materially as well as spiritually. Unlike the swamis of India, our guru believed in material success as well as spiritual enlightenment."

One had to admire these women, who possessed enough backbone (or faith) to publicly associate with Pierre Bernard at this time. Despite the chaste practices taking place inside the walls of the Fifty-third Street Yoga Center, to outsiders his reputation remained anything but sterling. By the time Anne Vanderbilt was sending Barbara to scrub Bernard's floors, his yellow-press nickname, the Omnipotent Oom, had so thoroughly worked its way into American culture that it had become shorthand for any spiritual charlatan with a taste for the good life. In the nascent film industry the "evil swami" as seducer of women had become something of a stock character—a trope that in 1917 made its way into the Sunday comics, where an episode of the immensely popular syndicated strip *Hairbreadth Harry* featured a villain who hypnotized suckers and pocketed their jewels before ushering them into a secret chamber with a trapdoor. The title of the episode made its point precisely: "The Omnipotent Oom Gets Two Customers."

Evil . . . charlatan . . . villain. There was never a scrap of evidence to sustain these charges, but the police continued to track Bernard like a criminal. One morning, as Cheerie and Clara were working the front desk at Fifty-third Street (they happened to be checking in Margaret and Barbara Rutherfurd), the doorbell rang. Two young policemen, looking somewhat abashed as they entered the fancy lobby, held out a search warrant for the premises and pronounced the names of the two eighteen-year-old females they wished to question—who, as luck would have it, were the receptionists themselves. The policemen explained that their precinct had been informed of the girls' presence there and wanted to make sure they weren't being held against their will. Cheerie burst into laughter and assured them that she was fine. To stall them, she looked the policemen over with the feigned brazenness of a seasoned flirt while Clara quietly rang upstairs. DeVries was aware of the kind of ruinous publicity her own appearance could provoke, so after a hushed exchange with Clara on the house intercom, she sent down an assistant to shoo the cops away.

The ruse worked. After the police left, having barely set foot in the building, Margaret and Barbara Rutherfurd reappeared in the lobby like apparitions. They had shrewdly melted away into a nearby coat closet at the first appearance of the law. The sisters were, it turned out, seasoned pros at shying away from unwanted publicity, and for the moment at least, a crisis had been averted.

But the Yoga Center went into a quiet uproar anyway. To DeVries the timing of the police visit couldn't have been worse—while Anne Vanderbilt's daughters were right there! Bernard, too, became concerned at the law's renewed interest in his operations. "He thought this [was] only the beginning of future police encounters," Cheerie later wrote. "He worried about me especially as the youngest and most gullible of the girls at Fifty-third Street. A young former Follies dancer might be dramatized into another newspaper story, hurting his efforts to establish his good name as a guru."

Cheerie regarded Bernard as father and protector, the commonsense mentor who would guide her life. But his genuine concern for her well-being encompassed self-interest too. Bernard considered himself an expert at divining the deepest needs of the human heart, and he knew how to convince his subjects to see in him precisely what suited those needs. Cheerie was clearly a young woman in search of a father figure. Her vaudeville past made her inviolable purity an absolute necessity to the Tantriks; otherwise, her visibility at the reception desk could mar the Yoga Center's legitimacy. So if Cheerie considered Bernard her protector, it was a role that he was more than willing to play.

Margaret Rutherfurd, on the other hand, was clearly being encouraged to behold the same man as a lover and an idol. The language of her letters escalated from admiration and affection to out-and-out worship as she wrote to him from the cold limestone glory of her family's French château on Vanderbilt Row.

Beloved! My love for thee has grown till it now absorbs my entire being. In thee + through thee I see + feel the whole of life. In me there is ever a longing to worship thee, thy form, to contemplate thy face of surpassing beauty. I have gazed deep in those eyes I love so much + seen all (which before was unrevealed) the depth of love & the highest bliss[—]love for thee has opened my heart to a life immense. A life all concentrated in thee who art the universe embodied. Beloved I worship at thy shrine with my life & for all eternity.

Not only was Margaret falling more deeply in love with Bernard, she was thinking of rewriting her will and leaving everything she owned to him. She'd been in attendance at the center throughout these first months of its inception, but whatever had transpired to prompt such epistolary passion had gone on behind closed doors and remained a mystery to those around her.

Bernard read her letters and kept them safe for the rest of his life, but he, too, kept his true intentions close by. Certainly he must have considered the life that might await him if Margaret divorced Ogden Mills and married him. A privileged world of mansions and yachts and private railroad cars must have beckoned like a mirage on the horizon, but if it did he didn't let on to anyone—except maybe to Margaret herself.

Anne Vanderbilt was too busy with other matters to be anything but oblivious to her daughter's dalliances. There were plenty of details to arrange, as Anne prepared to take her ailing husband abroad. April for the Vanderbilts meant a return to France, which in 1919 was gearing up for the first postwar racing season. The prospect of seeing his Thoroughbreds return to the winner's circle revived Willie K.'s spirits when little else could. His health was poor and deteriorating, and his decline was devastating for Anne, who'd worn widow's black twice before. She had come to depend on DeVries and the young women of the Fifty-third Street Yoga Center for companionship and peace of mind, and her profound gratitude was evident in a hastily written note she sent to DeVries on the morning of her departure in late March.

660 FIFTH AVENUE

SATURDAY 7 A.M.

Good bye dear DeVries please forgive me for not seeing you out[.] I feel strained to the breaking point[.] My stay here has been a little journey into hell. I do not ask for sympathy—or understanding as no one can enter into another's heart and soul and see the conflict going on—Only one thing I want for you to believe and that is that nothing can or will ever make me forget your great kindness and patience with me under all circumstances, nothing can repay for what you have done for me & Willie[.] Think of me as kindly as you can and I will do all in my power to apply what you have taught me. . . . Please thank & say good bye to all 53 St.

On Friday, April 4, Anne wrote to DeVries again, this time from London, stressed and much in need of the comfort her teachers had imparted. Foreseeing this, DeVries had obliged the older woman by sending along a cache of thoughtful travel gifts and advice.

Ritz Hotel
Piccadilly London

Dear de Vries how I miss you and what would I not give to have you here just now, I am trying so hard to be philosophical and to put into action all that I learned from you and the Doctor; as far as the outside world goes I feel sure that they see nothing but calm and poise, but inside I am full of seething[.] Sometimes, it is all so much harder than I thought it was going to be, traveling even for robust people is strenuous, and for an invalid more so. Mr. Vanderbilt is so patient, but it is very hard to sit by and see him suffering, racked by a dreadful bronchial cough and to me growing weaker every day, I don't feel as if he could possibly stand the journey tomorrow but I shall not breathe freely until we are safely settled once more in his own house, it is a terrible responsibility—You poor dear I have done nothing but grumble so far, and I meant only to write a line to thank you for the wonderful basket full of surprises, it was so dear and thoughtful of you in your busy life to think of me; and I more than appreciated it I assure you. Neck brace was most appreciated and I kept well in every way all the way over, but so far no exercises which I sadly miss, and shall start early Sunday morning. . . . We are having winter weather and London is living under war conditions the climate is most depressing . . . here nothing but fog and . . . I don't see how they stand it.

My brain is not working this morning I need a good walk but don't dare go out so forgive this stupid letter, thanks for the line you sent with the basket. I only wish I lived up to it.

The Divine Mother [—] if I could only attain that. . . .

While Anne was far from home and burdened with concern for her husband, her attention drifted from her daughters, who were alone in New York for a time, free to pursue whatever their hearts desired. In any case, they'd have to weigh their allegiance to the Tantriks in haste: Bernard and his people were once again on the move, this time to the bucolic Hudson Valley.

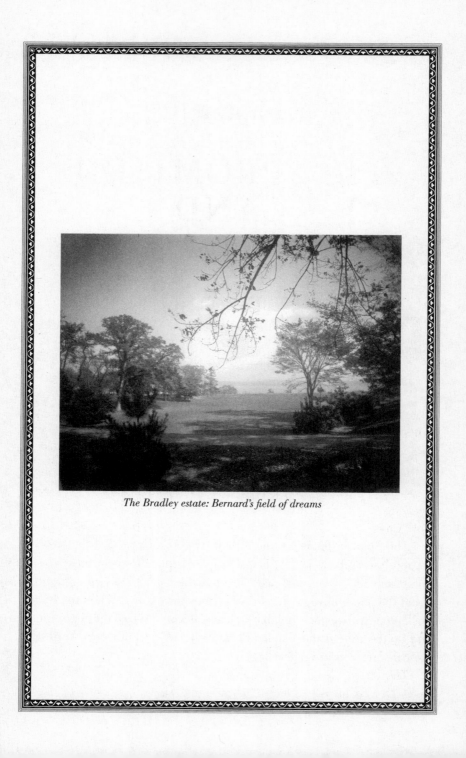

The Bradley estate: Bernard's field of dreams

Chapter 10

THE PROMISED LAND

ack in the fall of 1918, while Margaret was composing her love letters to Bernard, DeVries was making regular trips to an old upstate village called Nyack-on-Hudson. She had been brought there by Sister Beatrix—the former Episcopal nun who'd been caught up in the Manhattan DA's raid that spring—to teach feminine deportment at the ex-sister's Riverhook Select School for Young Women. DeVries fell in love with this charming hamlet twenty-five miles north of Manhattan, and when she learned that the school was running short of the funds it needed to continue operating, she brought Bernard up to have a look at the property. There was an abundance of acreage, hills and valleys for privacy, and a good number of buildings, and the two began to consider its prospects as a new venue a safe distance from New York City.

The Spanish flu killed more than 675,000 Americans that year—37,000 New Yorkers in October alone—so it must have seemed like an opportune time to consider an escape from the city, DeVries's protestations about the power of yoga over sickness notwithstanding. When the Riverhook property became available for lease, Bernard seized the opportunity, and by the time Anne Vanderbilt had set sail for France in April, the Tantriks were packing their bags.

They began leaving the city in shifts, in a small fleet of automobiles. "It took us less than two hours to reach the countryside," Cheerie

Smith recalled. An urban girl at heart, she described their home-to-be as "bypassed and ignored, tucked away, green and lush in the Hudson Valley."

Nyack in those days was surrounded by spacious, rolling countryside divided into dozens of small farms and a growing number of sprawling estates, a few of which ran a half mile or more from the wooded uplands down to the water. Land was cheap and virtually tax free. In downtown Nyack, brick-and-stone commercial buildings dominated the intersection of Main and Broadway. To the south, Broadway quickly turned residential, with gas lamps and towering elms; to the north, in Upper Nyack, old-growth oaks and maples mingled with evergreens to produce leafy riverfront vistas reminiscent of coastal New England. "On account of the salubrity of the climate, beautiful and romantic scenery, and good society, it is a very delightful place for a summer residence," a popular historian had written in 1866. It was an even better deal fifty years later, when it was convenient to reach by train, car, or ferry. Judges, doctors, state assemblymen, lawyers, and Tammany politicians had found it a perfect weekend retreat.

Nyack ferries carried shoppers to and from Westchester on the hour, and dozens of passenger trains stopped there daily. The locals—descendants of shoemakers, boatbuilders, fishermen, and farmers—were proud of their Carnegie Library and private schools, and they boasted to newcomers that their town had been a busy stop on the Underground Railroad as late as 1855. Religious communities nestled in the hills around town, and of these the largest was the Missionary Training Institute in South Nyack, a fundamentalist Christian institution that sent its graduates to make converts in India, China, and Tibet. In nearby New City, Paramount Pictures president Adolph Zukor had purchased three hundred acres for his own summer estate, where he entertained his stable of silent-film stars.

In short, it was an ideal destination for Bernard's vision: a country club–academy that would combine yoga, deluxe accommodations, and homegrown entertainment with his own style of Eastern education—a truly American ashram. Here, he hoped, he could relax and spread out, free to go about his esoteric teaching with a minimum of interference from the police and the press, a matter that became more important than ever now that the publicity-shy Vanderbilt women were fully committed.

Locals called Bernard's new home the Maxwell estate, after its original owner, Hugh Maxwell. This rectangular parcel of seventy-six parklike acres contained two mansions—one on the east boundary of the property and another on the west. In between were seven additional residential buildings. The grandest structure was the Braeburn House, an eighteenth-century redbrick mansion near the Hudson. Formerly the casino and clubhouse of the Nyack Country Club, it came to be known as the Brick House by its new owners. According to legend, it was once the home of a French pirate who dug an underground tunnel to the banks of the Hudson to secretly offload his booty.

The Brick House was three stories tall, with thirty rooms, lovely verandas, and wraparound balconies. There was a large ballroom for social functions and a seventy-foot-long gymnasium with a stage at one end, where classes in breathing and posture and acrobatics were held, along with amateur shows and lectures on Tantric philosophy. Bernard moved his library to a big room at the house and placed a billiard table in the middle of it. Guests who booked themselves into the residential quarters there had access to all of these amenities, as well as professional-level tennis courts just outside.

A quarter mile away, at the far west side of the estate, was a slightly smaller mansion: a three-story, eighteen-room stone-and-stucco Tudor that had been the country getaway of Van Wyck Rossiter, an executive for the Vanderbilt family's New York Central Railroad. Rossiter had leased the property to Sister Beatrix for several years, and it was she who'd transferred the lease to Bernard and DeVries. Once the club was up and running, the Rossiter House would also function as guest quarters, with Bernard and DeVries bedding down in a small cottage nearby.

This enormous estate required more than a bit of visionary thinking before it would be transformed into the empire of physical culture and learning Bernard had in mind. Parts of it were completely run-down, and some of its buildings had been abandoned for years. The Tantriks pitched in cheerfully, however, working in teams. DeVries, Cheerie, Clara, and other women cleaned the houses and made curtains, while Bernard set Nicholls, Jones, and the rest of the menfolk to planting fruit trees and working in the gardens. "For our labors we were told that ours was a cooperative effort where we all shared equally in the ownership of these estates," wrote Cheerie.

As usual, the press had taken to snooping around. According to a *Los Angeles Times* stringer, Sister Beatrix "renounced her Episcopalian vows, embraced the Yogi cult of the Hindus, leased the clubhouse in South Nyack in which she had conducted a boarding school for girls—and disappeared." The paper then mused about "the strange things that have been taking place about the old clubhouse since she surrendered possession."

Actually, there was little strangeness going on in those days. That spring saw nothing more than a good deal of sweat equity. The young crew moved from one building to the next, working long days and into the nights. Bernard employed a few local workmen for heavy labor, but the staff and students of his yoga schools did just about everything else. The plan, according to Cheerie's recollection, was to embark upon a huge expansion of the efforts they'd begun in New York City. The cottages and rooms would then be rented out to wealthy visitors and serious students keen to study yoga in a country setting.

DeVries took aside "her girls"—Cheerie's words—for monthly lemon sessions, in which she ruthlessly picked apart their failings and faults. She instructed the young women in what she and Bernard had termed "suggestive values." This meant that they were to keep up their general appearance, cleanliness, posture, and smiles, ever mindful of their roles as walking advertisements for the positive effects of yoga. DeVries reminded each one of them, time and again, "You can be a success, an outstanding personality, a star."

Bernard's advice sounded slightly more portentous: "Live dangerously, carefully," he told them.

<hr />

With Anne and Willie K. in Europe, Margaret continued the family's active support of Bernard's work, writing a series of checks for close to $2,000 in April alone. In May, when she and Barbara reluctantly set sail for Europe to join their family, Margaret left Bernard fully in charge of her finances, giving him power of attorney to write checks on her accounts. She'd also rewritten her will, turning over her entire fortune to Bernard upon her death.

In France, she traveled from one Vanderbilt estate to the next with minimal interest, her heart fixed on the man she'd left behind. She was forced to spend languid, stifling days on the family yacht, which was docked in the Mediterranean. *Valiant* was the largest private pleasure boat in the world at the time, the closest thing to a floating New York City mansion that money could buy: twenty staterooms, grand piano, library, salon, Chippendale chairs fitted with brass for maritime use, and all the furniture upholstered in crimson velvet.

For Margaret, it was a floating prison. She felt certain that she was being spied upon in these close quarters, that her stepfather was opening her mail, and the constant scrutiny made her disagreeable. But she read her Bhagavad Gita and wrote to Bernard about their plans for the future. It was proving difficult to keep her heart's deepest longings to herself.

Finally she was asked to accompany her mother on an automobile trip across France to survey the damages of the war. "Things are very bad," she wrote to Bernard, "the roads abominable & my poor old womb had the hell of a time. . . . After reading Krishna it is all so different . . . everything explains itself clearly."

The worst part of this trip was not the devastation of the battlefields, or the new restlessness of the lower classes, but her painful separation from her lover. By June, though she had not received a letter from him in over a month, she decided she must tell her mother what was in her heart. In the French countryside, Anne and Margaret found a few hours of uninterrupted quiet by themselves, providing "the propitious moment," as Margaret later described it, to tell Anne about her love for Bernard, about their plans to be together forever and her desire to divorce Ogden Mills. "Needless to say it was no surprise to her, as I well knew it would not be," Margaret wrote to Bernard.

> She is very happy about it now, though at first there were many questions in her mind[,] but have put her at rest about all of these. She seemed to worry chiefly about the effect of our action upon the work & people concerned, their resentment & lack of understanding thinking it would do the work a great deal of harm. All natural objections, ones I have thought of & you also probably thousands of times. I explained all to her as best I could & have left her with great peace of mind & confidence about it all. She sees well what a marvelous & wonderful thing it is for me Sweet & is only anxious

that I should live up to the situation which she also realizes is not an easy one. Darling it is very difficult to put all down on paper but rest assured that she is happy[,] very happy about it all which is what I so much wanted her to be. Oh, Sweet, if I ever see you again nothing in god's earth will ever separate us.

As she signed off this letter—postmarked June 17, 1919, and sent discreetly to Bernard's post office box at Pennsylvania Station—Margaret mentioned as if in passing that she had informed the unsuspecting Ogden Mills about her plans. He was of course bewildered and furious, but Margaret seemed to care very little. Another young woman contemplating a public society divorce and the revelation of a relationship with one of America's most infamous figures might well have sought to shelter herself from the storms of controversy that were certain to follow. Not Margaret. In the grip of her obsession with Bernard, she didn't seem to give it an iota of serious thought.

Am now going to get all dressed up as am going to pose for a very talented young French artist for a sketch I hope it will be good & will give it to you if you want. Good bye Precious one take care of yourself.

What was Bernard thinking as he read this? That in a cruel twist of fate he had met his heiress a few months too late? He had been married to DeVries for less than a year. Then again, they'd continued to keep their union a secret, even from their followers and closest associates—no doubt from Margaret. Bernard's natural disdain for authority, combined with his and DeVries's cavalier treatment of their marriage certificate, suggests neither felt fully bound by their legal vows. If Margaret was quite ready to change her entire life for Bernard, what remained unclear at this point was to what extent Bernard had led her on. Was he deliberately stringing her along to keep her family's financial support coming? Or was Margaret perhaps a little delusional, their bond a one-sided infatuation that presented itself to Bernard as merely a problem to be settled in the most financially advantageous fashion. His thoughts, his motives, his plans for their future together or apart—these he kept to himself. He did not write back to Margaret.

After four anxious days of waiting for a response, Margaret could wait no longer. On June 21, she cabled from Paris.

CANNOT UNDERSTAND WHY I HAVE NOT HEARD FROM YOU IN OVER A MONTH [STOP] AM TERRIBLY MISERABLE . . . [STOP] IS THIS ENGAGEMENT BETWEEN US AS IT WAS WHEN I LEFT [STOP] CABLE ME AT ONCE AS IT MEANS MY WHOLE LIFE [STOP]

Though there is no remaining record of Bernard's telegraph response to Margaret, whatever communication he sent contained the necessary reassurances. For in late July 1919, making her final preparations to leave Paris, she cabled him again.

TANTRIKAM, THANKS FOR CABLE [STOP] FORGIVE ANXIETY [STOP] VERY HAPPY [STOP] AM SAILING SAVOIE JULY TWENTY SIXTH [STOP] ADDRESS ME PERSONALLY RECEIPT OF THIS [STOP]

Margaret returned to Nyack with the expectations of marriage and a life with Bernard, whose effect on her was, as she'd written to him, an "overpowering force . . . a magnet attracting me, sucking me in." What she found was a busy man preoccupied with rehabbing the huge estate he'd just leased. Work was still under way, even while guests from Margaret's social set began arriving. The tennis courts had been refurbished, a baseball diamond laid out, buildings made ready for the winter. None of this interested Margaret, of course, who wanted only one thing: to be married to her guru as soon as a divorce from Ogden Mills could be arranged.

Bernard later said he'd curtailed Margaret's ardor by confiding an essential fact to her mother: "I assured Mrs. Vanderbilt that [marriage] was impossible; that I was already married and without mentioning names or dates I explained to her the circumstances of my marriage."

From the start this was an affair mired in ambiguities. Did Bernard and Anne withhold this information from Margaret, or did he lead her to believe that they would indeed be married down the road, though it might take more time and his own divorce, too? It seems undeniable Bernard and DeVries conspired to do whatever it took to keep Margaret happily in the fold—for financial reasons, certainly, for romantic and possibly sexual ones, too. Margaret, who prided herself on her rebellious ways, may even have welcomed the idea of sharing her lover with DeVries, whom she had come to admire as well. In letters to Bernard, after all, she had promised herself to him "in every way, conventionally & unconventionally . . . in all ways conceivable."

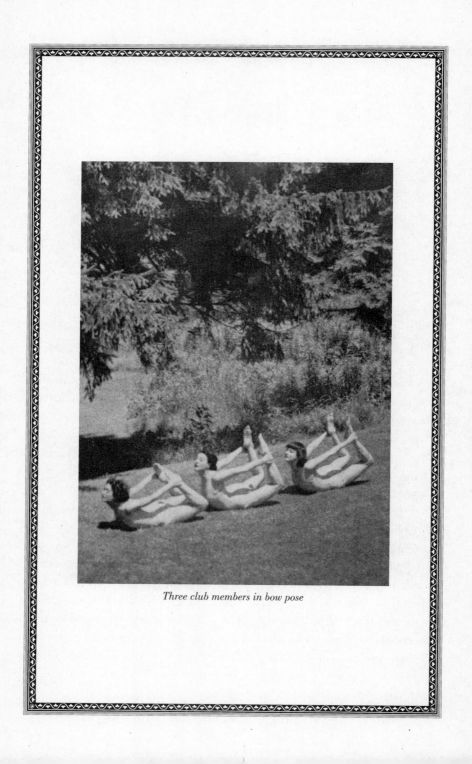

Three club members in bow pose

Chapter 11

WELCOME
TO NYACK

he summer in Nyack had passed in a blaze of work and progress. In just a few months, the club was 150 members strong, and the place filled up with fifty or sixty guests each weekend, even into the fall, as the locals had noticed. On a gorgeous Indian summer morning in October, the villagers were out in numbers, shopping and socializing in the sixty-degree weather—comparing notes about the glamorous newcomers who'd descended upon them. The natives maintained their distance, but kept their eyes trained on the comings and goings at the old Maxwell estate, now called the Braeburn Country Club. Most of these visitors motored up from New York City; some were even driven by chauffeurs and accompanied by servants who toted their linen-lined gladstone bags. Out on the lawn, wives of prominent attorneys and stockbrokers mingled with doctors, professors, writers, dancers, artists, and entertainers. Some guests arrived with reputations and prodigious talent, others with nothing but youth and physical beauty. It was a mixed crowd of the rich, the young, the bohemian, the blue bloods—all of them drawn to this retreat for the country air, the activities, and the man who ran it. The members, men and women alike, played outdoor sports like tennis and badminton. At night, there were large communal dinners and do-it-yourself entertainment: amateur theatricals and vaudeville shows, in which everyone was encouraged to sing and dance along with the talented professionals of the club.

Blanche DeVries patrolled the grounds and kept a watchful eye on everyone, including Margaret and Barbara Rutherfurd, who'd become weekend regulars since their return from France. Cheerie and Clara and the corps of young yogini dancers helped the guests with their exercise and otherwise paraded about in their glowing youth, looking like pretty walking billboards for yoga.

Bernard had assumed the humble title of general manager of the club, dressing as he pleased in baseball pants and loose sweaters. Visitors noticed that he walked these grounds as if he possessed the sweetest of life's secrets, talking as easily with landscapers, mechanics, and merchants as he did with linguists and theologians.

The village of Nyack had been buzzing with rumors and sightings ever since Sister Beatrix closed down Riverhook in June. The newcomers, striking young women and handsome, athletic men, brazenly took their exercise outdoors and in plain sight, the matronly Nyackers murmured.

A few well-off townspeople had politely applied for membership and been turned down flat, so the general opinion gathered credulity that this was the exclusive domain of a snooty coterie of urban weekenders. A sign with stern warnings not to trespass was posted at the entrance to the Braeburn. Indignant at these rebuffs, the citizens of the village had mobilized into an army of spies. Mailmen, telephone operators, milkmen, and others with access to the grounds registered their impressions. Curious villagers lined up at the borders of the property with binoculars or opera glasses, duly reporting everything they saw to their pastors and policemen.

What did they see? Men and women wearing athletic clothes, bloomers, and sandals, and going about hatless in the sun. Near the public roads they spied adults playing tennis and badminton, sometimes with children. Still, the rumors persisted that these daytime frolickers were also involved in the "queer antics" of a godless cult. The rectors of St. Ann's Catholic Church and Grace Episcopal had both inquired at the club about the alleged presence of a "yoga colony." They, too, were rebuffed.

But on this pleasant Saturday in October, an ambitious reporter from Hearst's *New York American* passed through the hive of Nyack's suspicion and ambled onto the grounds of the Braeburn, no permission asked or given. He noted the identities of the socialites, the brazen casual dress and comportment of these young rebels, observed the games, the exercises. At the Brick House, he finally came upon the man he wanted to see.

Slouched across a chaise on one of the building's shaded verandas, Bernard appeared to be napping. He refused to stir or even to acknowledge the reporter's existence; he didn't even turn his head until the first question was asked. "A cult here?" he said dismissively, waving the reporter off. "The only cult we know anything about is that of health and the great outdoors. If there be any religion in that, we embrace it. Health! Exercise! Life! Those are the things we want here."

Taken aback by Bernard's decidedly "Occidental" bearing, the man from the *American* pressed on. He had questions about Sister Beatrix, about rich society ladies, about sex, and, of course, about yoga. "If there is a yoga cult here, I never heard of it," Bernard repeated. "The nearest religious element to the club is the little church across the way. We are purely a recreational club, a sort of Summer colony. When the Autumn gives us such fine weather, we keep open house through October and November.

"As for Sister Beatrix, I know absolutely nothing about her. She is not here."

"And about your membership?" the reporter asked.

"That depends on who wants to join us," Bernard answered, providing a string of details regarding necessary introductions and recommendations. Contact the club secretary, Mr. Edmund Trowbridge Dana, he advised.

"Do you admit men as well as women to the club?"

"Oh yes," Bernard said. "It is just like any country club that goes in for outdoor recreation."

Just then, two female members walked past in their stocking feet. These were city women, casually dressed in white blouses over bloomers, wearing neither shoes *nor* hats. One of them had draped a red opera cloak across her shoulders as if to accessorize her disdain for proper daytime attire. The reporter registered his shock at the women's lack of manners, Bernard's intransigence, and the generally shabby condition of the house. The floors were unwaxed and dusty, he noted, and these girls, unskirted and unashamed, were walking contraventions of traditional feminine decorum. In this state of dishabille, the two women sauntered off to the tennis courts.

If the sight of these women in such provocative attire distracted the reporter, Bernard's stonewalling rekindled his curiosity. He returned to the

Braeburn the next evening with additional questions. Unable to find Bernard, he interrogated others. Chalmers Wood Jr., a debonair Wall Street stockbroker and man-about-town, listened while the reporter repeated allegations, whispered in social circles, that he, Mr. Wood, was not quite happy about his wife's course of exercise at the club. Absolutely wrong, said Wood. He was completely satisfied, and no, there was no connection here to what the reporter called the "yoga ritual."

On Monday the *American* broke this story with a front-page dissection of the "women devotees of Oom." Twenty-four-year-old Barbara Rutherfurd Hatch appeared in a photo, beautifully dressed in fur, gloves, walking stick, and beret. Margaret, twenty-eight, was pictured as well, identified as "one of the pupils of 'Oom the Omnipotent.'" The story boldly proclaimed—and falsely, it turned out—that Mrs. William K. Vanderbilt was on her way home from Europe to rescue Barbara.

<hr />

The yellow press had followed Bernard upriver. When Pulitzer's *New York World* realized it had been scooped, the paper sent a reporter speeding north to Nyack to dig for more—or at least different—dirt. Loyal fellow that he was, Chalmers Wood stood up once again for Bernard and the Braeburn, insisting there was "nothing queer about the exercises." The women wore tights and bloomers, he said—"the costumes are the same worn in gymnasiums."

The *World* spun the story with a new angle and a few more facts, reporting accurately that E. T. Dana, the secretary and treasurer of the Braeburn, was the grandson of Henry Wadsworth Longfellow. Dana, a Harvard graduate, was a disciple of George Bernard Shaw and also a free-thinking socialist. And yes, the Vanderbilt heiresses were indeed members of the club; they were patients of Dr. Brewster, who testified that he had sent them there to take the rest cure. In his newly appointed role as club physician, Dr. Brewster added that Bernard was "a great man doing a wonderful work for humanity, and that his philosophy was based on physical exercise and fresh air."

The reporters were undeterred. They had picked up the commingled scents of sex (yoga), society (the Vanderbilts), and scandal (the Great Oom himself)—a newsroom trifecta if there ever was one. Now they contacted law enforcement sources to inquire about the police response—or lack of it—to the idea of a yoga cult setting up shop in Nyack. Sheriff Alexander Merritt of Rockland County said he would personally investigate if the rumors turned out to be true, and that he had already contacted the county's district attorney, the Honorable Morton Lexow, who was himself ready to act.

The local papers finally picked up the story: "Bernard in Seclusion; Society Women Vanish," read the headline in Tuesday's *Nyack Evening Journal.* This new report not only promised investigations by Sheriff Merritt's office; it warned that the New York State troopers were standing by, waiting for an invitation to pounce on the Braeburners.

The invitation had, in fact, come that morning. The troopers in those days were called out to enforce blue laws, inspect buildings, maintain quarantines, and bust unlicensed dentists, doctors, and other violators of state law and moral decree. When a formal complaint about the Braeburn yoga cult arrived Tuesday morning, Sergeant Faber and his officers mounted up and rode the ten miles or so into Nyack, then spread themselves out across the seventy-six acres of Braeburn grounds. Leaving nothing to chance, the sergeant searched each of the buildings himself. What exactly they were looking for was never spelled out; anything out of the ordinary could be construed to be hidden or discarded evidence of yoga practices. The *New York American* reported on the paucity of their findings.

> The women and children and the few men who were present were attired in bloomers and sandals, but instead of the grotesque Yoga muscle dances, gyrations and writhings that had shocked the community of Nyack, the troopers were treated to only the simplest of physical culture drills.

Jockeying for position in the unfolding controversy, the state constabulary and the Rockland County authorities then announced their intention to conduct their own investigations of the affairs of the club. DA Morton Lexow attested that if occult practices were going on in his jurisdiction, the matter would be laid before a grand jury. Sheriff Merritt, meanwhile, dismayed at the troopers' disappointing performance (and subsequent monopoly of the headlines), insisted on leading his own search party around the Braeburn's grounds on Wednesday. The sheriff announced that he was hunting for Vanderbilt heiresses, and that social rank would provide them no shield from the law. What law they might have broken he didn't mention.

Having tasted the thrill of big-time publicity, Merritt became unstoppable. He befriended most every reporter who showed up in Nyack, and after reviewing the records from Bernard's 1910 arrest, he declared he was convinced that female captives might be held at the Braeburn. Then, pay dirt: a secret tunnel discovered by his men under the Brick House. The passageway, Merritt surmised, was of recent construction and could have been used by Bernard as a prison.

Anxious to play their part, three Nyack clergymen from the prominent Episcopal and Catholic churches said they were planning a trip to New York City to furnish information to the city's district attorney and to plead for the cooperation of both jurisdictions to drive Bernard and his yoga cult from Nyack once and for all.

At a Thursday night meeting at Nyack's Hotel St. George, local politicians decided it was high time to go public. One state assemblyman rose up to inveigh against the Braeburn and urged the rest of the meeting room authorities to "find some way of taking action." A legal expert from the area suggested that "a committing magistrate be empowered to subpoena witnesses"—a way to force Margaret and Barbara to testify. DA Lexow added that Nyack was "not the place" for such a man as Bernard. That same night, local residents took matters into their own hands and defaced the Braeburn's sign.

It had taken less than a week for this small town to work itself into a moral panic, though nobody was quite sure about the nature of the immorality. No matter: Bernard and his guests were alleged to be in hiding by week's end, perhaps even driven from the peaceful streets of Nyack. The anti-yoga forces declared victory. "Oom's Flock Flies Before Sheriff," read the *American*'s headline.

But Bernard gave little evidence that the week's hysteria had fazed him. "The greatest possession is self-possession," he told his followers time and again, and he lived by those words. That weekend he let it slip to the *Nyack Evening Journal* that he was thinking about *buying* the Maxwell estate, all seventy-six acres of it—just as soon as the seller named his price. He also let it slip that his club and its members had been dropping $6,000 a month (equivalent to $73,000 today) in the village since early summer.

Well, of course, that changed matters substantially. So, eight days after the first newspaper story re-besmirched Bernard's reputation, slandered his society guests, and targeted him as the object of a witch hunt literally designed to run him out of town, certain clear-minded citizens of the small town of Nyack began to see things in a different light. The *Nyack Evening Journal* reported on the sudden U-turn: "Chief of Police of Upper Nyack Gives 'Oom the Omnipotent' Clean Bill."

Thus absolved, Bernard spoke freely about the big turnout he now expected for his Halloween celebration the coming weekend, his forty-third birthday. After all, he couldn't help gloating, the local and New York press had combined to make him the beneficiary of "about $50,000 worth of free advertising." Chief Wannamaker, a son of one of the oldest families in Nyack, and a man who chose his words wisely, suddenly spoke up for Nyack's newest citizen. "They didn't get anything on him," said the chief. "He's all right."

Bernard had learned a valuable lesson in the matter of village politics. At the end of the month, he threw his birthday party for a bigger crowd than had ever been to the Braeburn. He then offered to lease out his ballrooms to interested parties. He made donations to the local volunteer fire departments and even joined one for a time. He made sure that all of his purchases were made through local dealers. He attended Little League games and joined the local Masonic Temple, where he courted the friendship of the eminent justice Arthur S. Tompkins, who would soon be elected Grand Master of the Free and Accepted Masons of the State of New York. Judge Tompkins said of the Braeburn Country Club that "he and the Chamber of Commerce, to which he belonged, were all for it."

With the prominent locals won over, Bernard turned his attention to the New York City operations. Together with DeVries, who'd managed to elude the press and police throughout the October madness, he closed down the Riverside Drive studio to better concentrate their efforts on Fifty-third Street. This location was thriving beyond expectations. On most days a stream of limousines and taxis could be observed dropping off and picking up well-to-do female yoga students in front of the prim gray townhouse. After completing several beginning and intermediate courses, promising students were informed about the opportunities for advanced study up in Nyack. And then, if these students were willing, they could seek Bernard's personal approval and join the Braeburn Country Club.

The New York–Nyack pipeline had an auspicious start. One of the Yoga Center transferees, Frances Payne Bolton, would become one of the Braeburn's most crucial and loyal sponsors. An heiress to the Payne family fortune, she'd married into one of the oldest and most politically connected families in Ohio. Her pockets were deep, and she idolized Blanche DeVries—her style, her discipline, her grace and elegance. Bolton commissioned DeVries to decorate her family home in Cleveland, as well as the dormitories for a new nursing college at Western Reserve University, setting up DeVries in a sideline business that she continued throughout her life. Despite her conservative background, Bolton was an enthusiastic yoga student who came to the club often, even against her husband's wishes. "After each visit we lived more affluently," Cheerie remembered. "Rooms redecorated, another car for P.A. and more jewelry for DeVries." It was generous women like Bolton who would become the backbone of the club in the years to come.

***

In January 1920, Bernard made good on his promise to the *Evening Journal* and purchased the Maxwell estate for more than $100,000. The sale was front-page news in Nyack, where it was described by the local press as "one of the largest real estate transactions ever made" in the area. He paid in cash.

Anne Vanderbilt had returned from Europe in November, and that winter she and Bernard talked finances and the future of "the work." On March 15, she gave him $75,000, which he used to help finance a new real estate holding company he named the Biophile Club Company, Inc. He issued her stock in the corporation and insisted she accept interest payments of 6 percent a year on the money. Two days later, as Anne prepared to return to Europe, she appointed Bernard her attorney and agent in the Biophile—with power to vote for her in all corporate matters—the appointment to last until her projected return to the States on October 1. With a cash-infused real estate fund and total control of its use, Bernard began surveying the surrounding land with the eye of an acquisitive monarch. He next set his sights on a showpiece estate located one and a half miles south of the Braeburn. Owned by S. R. Bradley, a local utilities executive, this gentleman's farm—complete with a huge home, a barn, stables, and other buildings—spread out over thirty-nine acres of fields, farmland, orchards, and uplands with unbounded views: a panorama of the blue-gray Hudson River with the Westchester hills in the distance and the little town of Nyack below. When he purchased the Bradley estate in May, Bernard became the biggest landholder in the area, his holdings now totaling 115 acres, and thus one of the area's most important citizens.

While the Tantriks began the long process of refurbishing yet another huge property, Margaret split her time between France and New York. There were no more love letters, but a series of checks she wrote in 1920 indicated her ongoing support of the club. On April 4 she signed a check to Bernard for $1,000; another on May 8 for $1,371; $617 on May 17; $1,500 on May 24; $1,000 on July 31 and again on September 1. Moreover, she gave Bernard power of attorney on her Nyack bank accounts in her absence. Any talk of marriage, however, remained on the back burner.

The money poured in and the Tantriks matched it in their efforts to fix up the property. When they weren't hanging tapestries and painting walls, they studied and played, partied and performed. In February and again in April, they put on bazaars featuring cuisine and entertainment from around the world. Margaret and Barbara were active participants in both benefits, serving on the planning committees and joining in the fun. Barbara even took the stage for the second benefit, performing a dance pantomime of Scheherazade, after which Winfield Nicholls starred in a skit called *The Fakir of Thebet,* juggling and showing off the sleight-of-hand magic he'd picked up over the years.

That summer the club grew by leaps and bounds. There was the opening of the summer music school, and to spice things up just a little bit more, Bernard added coed baseball—hardball, no less—to the club's menu of sporting activities. Though the games drew the ire of a local resident named Frank Crumbie over the immorality of playing on Sunday, baseball at the club continued uninterrupted for years to come, and Bernard ingeniously worked the national pastime into his Tantrik philosophy.

At the Brick House, formal classes in Sanskrit, Imagination, and Breath Work continued. Nicholls, who'd mastered the kind of body control Bernard had exhibited—he, too, could endure repeated piercing of his skin and still his breathing and heartbeat—taught many of these classes, under his official billing as calisthenics instructor.

The members were treated to the occasional lecture from a visiting Brahmin, the most memorable of whom—to Cheerie, at least—was an ambitious young monk named Parahamansa Yogananda, who would later become renowned as the founder of the Self-Realization Fellowship on the West Coast. "He stood out dramatically in his yellow robe," she wrote of his visit in 1920, "his very large brown eyes with long black lashes, his long raven-colored curls resting on his shoulders[,] touching the yellow silken robe. . . . He lectured on yoga, ending the talk with a song, accompanied with an Indian instrument which he played. The song, 'Oh, God, Beautiful' . . . he sang over and over, rolling his lustrous eyes lovingly and generously in the direction of the pretty girls watching him."

Yogananda and Bernard respectfully parted ways after this visit for good reason: the Indian swami was uninterested in hatha yoga—disdained it, actually—and never taught it; Bernard placed hatha yoga at the center of a rapidly growing enterprise that was becoming more varied by the day. Bernard was his own man and the Braeburn a one-guru club. In 1920, another Indian swami named Yogananda tried for a year to build a hatha yoga institute in Harriman, New York—less than an hour's drive from Nyack—but there is no record of friendship or even interaction between Bernard and this newcomer, who eventually returned to India.

Mystics are driven to go their own way. And like the freelance metaphysicians flourishing in postwar Europe that very year—G. I. Gurdjieff and Aleister Crowley—Bernard was constructing, piece by piece, a self-contained spiritual biosphere that would sustain its own growth. By attracting devotees from the literary and artistic worlds, he and DeVries also drew the requisite roster of rich benefactors to keep things going—not just heiresses like Anne Vanderbilt and Frances Payne Bolton, but men and women from across the country who'd distinguished themselves in their careers and had come to Nyack to relax, learn yoga, and mingle with the artistic elite: E. Warren Everett, a fiery red-haired attorney from Chicago; Lester Wilson, a professor of education at the International Institute of Teachers College at Columbia; Morris "Whit" Whitaker, a retired naval architect and Yalie; Percival W. Whittlesey, a Connecticut Yankee and blue blood who'd served as an undercover spy during World War I; and Charles Ezra Scribner, chief engineer at Western Electric, a visionary who held more patents than any other inventor in his field.

The summer music school, another draw for prominent and cultured people, was administered by a longtime devotee named Harriet Seymour. A piano teacher of well-to-do children in Manhattan, Seymour had achieved national renown with several instructional books that emphasized the enjoyment of music over by-rote études. She was a true believer in Bernard's hatha yoga, and she encouraged many of her own students and friends to come study with her at the club. But what really gave the school and the club marquee credibility was the arrival of three world-class musical luminaries—the conductor Leopold Stokowski, the British composer Cyril Scott, and the Danish soprano Povla Frijsh. Each musician came to Nyack separately, but together they formed a troika of accomplishment that not only boosted the reputation of the club but also drew even more wealthy followers willing to pay extravagantly to partake in such a cultured scene. All three mingled with the club members, helped with the school and the performances, and flirted with abandon—causing a few Tantrikas to be overcome by mad crushes.

Harriet Seymour's greatest contribution to the Braeburn turned out to come in the form of three young recruits—friends of *her* friend Elizabeth Newman, all of whom were in their early twenties and ready for a little adventure. Marie Louise Schreiner, Ruth Bartholomew, and Mildred Ryder were so immediately enamored of the Tantrik community that they never left, and their talents and enthusiasm were so pronounced that Bernard and DeVries decided to personally train all three of them. The trio put in long hours on the weekends and in the case of Marie Louise paid for the privilege of living and working there. Every morning they were up and ready for the 6 a.m. asana class, having started the day with a cup of hot water and an enema. DeVries, the taskmaster, ran the day-to-day activities of the club and gave out the orders to these young women, just as she did with Cheerie and Clara. Since Marie Louise had grown up with servants, DeVries made sure the younger woman learned how to prepare food for others.

The point of their training, they were told, was not to bliss out by themselves in Nyack, but to teach others. "Get a knowledge of yourself, know your weaknesses, organize [your] yoga teachings," Bernard told them in January 1920. On another occasion, he put it this way: "The pleasure, peace, happiness you get out of all that composes life may be termed *Moksha*." And the highest calling was to spread it around. "We can't all go through life with *Moksha* on our faces," he said to them. "We've got to produce the conditions that put *Moksha* on the other guy's face." Bernard gave them their marching orders: "We get yoga and then we sell it. . . . It should be our philosophy, our religion, our art of life, our idea of life lived."

Eventually, Bernard and DeVries would send the three women out on the road. When his favored clients couldn't get to Nyack in the off-season, they would head off to the east and west to teach private yoga lessons at the salons and private homes in Chicago, Cleveland, Philadelphia, Pittsburgh, and even Europe, spreading moksha and in the process picking up hefty fees for Bernard.

Back at the Braeburn the pursuit of enlightenment was folded into the club's everyday activities, even in mundane chores. All of the members cleaned their own rooms, cooked and served meals to one another, kept up the property, and entertained themselves. Some even worked in the fields alongside hired men from the village, cleaned up for dinner, and then attended philosophy lectures, arguing late into the night about life and love.

Cyril Scott, who'd first come to Nyack to calm his nerves during a long string of American performance dates in 1920–1921, delighted in the company of his fellow Tantriks. "I can truthfully say that they were sane, balanced and tolerant-minded persons, with whom it was a pleasure to associate," he wrote. "For Dr. Bernard would brook no cranks and emotional personality-worshippers among his chelas."

By summer's end, the entire Braeburn community was immersed in preparations for what would be the club's first annual circus, the epitome of Bernard's theory that communal activity could be used as therapy and education. Everyone was expected to get into the circus spirit, creating their own acts or pitching in behind the scenes with costumes, props, and lighting. Lawyers and teachers and heiresses would be transformed into clowns, tumblers, high-wire artists, magicians, trapezists, animal trainers, barkers, and prop masters. Cheerie recalled summer days bent over vats of boiling dye for the curtains, while in her head she planned her solo in the spotlight.

"For some time I had observed how many people of wealth were miserably bored," she mused. "They had everything, they thought, except a motive and a need to work. During our rehearsals, no one had a chance for boredom. Talents were discovered, there were jobs to be done and a frenzy of activity prevailed."

There was never a word in the country club's brochures or a sign at the front door promising cures or rehabilitation—no advertising save word of mouth. But even in these August days ending his first full year in Nyack, Bernard's club was gaining a separate distinction as a sanitarium for men and women troubled with depression, alcoholism, drug addiction, and other maladies of the mind. While the Braeburn's stunningly original artistic-recreational-philosophical scene was still the primary draw, Bernard was quickly gaining renown as an expert who worked wonders with difficult family members and treated his clients with dignity and discretion. Combining the principles of yoga, his innate approach to behavioral psychology, and an almost constant round of physical and social activities, he helped people get their lives back. It was a winning strategy of serious fun, and there was no limit in sight for the endless demand for the club and its services.

Supplying the idle wealthy with recreation, parties, and celebrity buzz had proved just the ticket Bernard needed to advance the hatha yoga cause. Anne Vanderbilt's assistance had been instrumental to his success at the start, but Bernard knew better than to take her generosity—and her daughter Margaret's affections—for granted. With the energy of a man half his age—he was forty-four—he was continually searching for the latest hook, the untried angle, and he would transform the Nyack club and its mission many times in the years to come. Still, he had found his home, and for the rest of his life he would rarely leave it, never venturing overseas and only occasionally traveling away from it at all.

Q ᵢt is stated that you have taught that one of the first
things that people must do to involve themselves in
this theory of religion is to divorce entirely what you
might call the Anglo-Saxon or Christian idea of right and
wrong, that those practices and beliefs present everything
of that sort. Have you ever taught anything of that sort?

A I hardly think so.

Q Well, have you?

A No, sir. That is a scream.

Q They say that you advocate or sanction sexual intercourse
between people who are not husband and wife?

A Never on God's green earth. No living soul ever
heard me say such a thing. There are men who do those
things but they do not say it; so I am informed by the
public press.

Q I am asking you what you advocate and what you do not
advocate. Do you teach any religious theory or any
religious rites?

A No rites on earth, no ritualism.

Q No religious theory or philosophy or school?

A My idea is this; the spirit of all the work I am doing
is this: to inculcate the principle of comparative and
analytical studies of anything which we take up. Now the
leading or basis principle of the whole thing is the

A page from the deposition

Chapter 12

INTERROGATION

ernard had played his cards brilliantly. In a matter of months he'd transformed himself from a pariah to a metaphysically minded country gentleman of the lower Hudson Valley. The expansion funded by Anne Vanderbilt was well under way, accommodating a steady stream of new clients who came to Nyack through the Fifty-third Street Yoga Center and other points of introduction. His followers seemed willing to do whatever he commanded to build his yoga empire. But as the dog days of summer 1920 rolled on, a new saboteur was hard at work to depose the Braeburn king.

Private investigators had been dispatched to Iowa, California, and Oregon to sift old rumors and comb the Tantriks' haunts. They put in long hours at the morgues at leading newspapers, digging through yellowed clippings for damaging information. They contacted Bernard's former associates and acquaintances and questioned them with the intensity of federal agents in pursuit of a public enemy. But this latest inquiry was not the work of the U.S. Department of Justice or the first or fourth estates but rather of a small group of powerful secular agents long established in their role as the guardians of the ruling class.

Henry B. Anderson, Esq., was the archetype of such protectors. He was not the man you would wish to find digging through your past, especially if the party he was paid to protect was a young woman of impeccable virtue, the issue of the best families on two continents, who had declared rather too publicly that she wanted to marry you and begift you her inheritance, too . . . and perhaps more especially *again* if that young woman was the suddenly estranged wife of Ogden Mills, H. B. Anderson's very good friend, and the stepdaughter of Anderson's former client William Kissam Vanderbilt.

After a long, slow decline, Willie K. had died in Paris on July 22, 1920. The significance of this event for his heirs couldn't have been made more publicly clear by the *New York Times* the next day: "Was Eldest Male Survivor of Family That Built Fortune in New York Central: Estate Near $100,000,000: $300,000,000 Left by His Father in Eight Shares Believed to Be Over Billion Total Now."

Both daughters of Willie K.'s widow were that very summer in the midst of pursuing divorces—a procedure that in France was kept secret from the press by law, but obviously not from the husbands of Barbara Rutherfurd Hatch and Margaret Rutherfurd Mills. No doubt these men—or at the very least, Ogden Mills—wanted to know what, exactly, their wives had been up to. Who was this man Pierre Bernard, who'd so inveigled his way into Margaret's heart that she'd rewritten her will, leaving everything to him?

The Vanderbilts had retained Anderson family attorneys for generations: for wills, taxes, family matters, and business disputes, some of which had reached the echelons of the Supreme Court. H.B., who ran the firm with his brother, Chandler, was the Vanderbilts' fixer, the man who could be called when gentlemanly torque needed to be applied.

His investigation into Bernard's life began in the late summer of 1920, after Willie K.'s death, and he let his clients know that he intended to spend plenty of time—and money—putting together this dossier. Anne Vanderbilt was made aware of Anderson's efforts, which were most likely bankrolled by Willie K.'s sons and Margaret's soon-to-be former in-laws, the Mills family. At least one curious newcomer to the club, Chalmers Wood, seemed to have a hand in these machinations as well.

In September, Bernard was summoned to a preliminary conference at 660 Fifth Avenue and informed of the inquest that had been made into his personal life. Questioned by H.B. about his marital status, Bernard refused to answer. Anderson next questioned Bernard about the power of attorney Margaret had granted him, to which Bernard countered that, yes, he supervised her purchases in Nyack, helped her set up a local bank account, and prevented chauffeurs and tradesmen from taking advantage of her. But when the lawyer suggested he had abused his access to Margaret's account, Bernard denied that he ever used it.

Without further ado he was dismissed, but the message from Anderson was clear: he and his men were investigating Bernard's background because of his intimate relationship with Anne, Barbara, and especially Margaret. Understandably vexed, Bernard hired an attorney to help him contend with Anderson, but he also prevailed upon Margaret and her sister to get their mother to step in and stop the investigation.

But Anne Vanderbilt, now a widow for the third time, had greater concerns than the hurt pride of her daughter's new beneficiary. She was in the midst of negotiations to sell the mansion at 660 Fifth—a house she'd never liked—and she still hadn't completed arrangements for the transatlantic passage of Willie K.'s body, which remained locked away in a Paris morgue. In a telegram from Paris, she chastised Bernard for interfering with Anderson's work. Referring to her daughters' pleas to intercede on his behalf, she characterized his effort as "unfair at this distance." She also wrote:

UNDERSTAND YOU HAD RETAINED LAW[Y]ER. . . . RESPONSIBILITY
SHOULD NOT FALL UPON US. . . . YOU ARE THE PERSON TO DEFEND
THE WORK.

A week later, she dispatched a similar telegram to Barbara, who was spending a great deal of time in Nyack:

ANDERSON CABLES INVESTIGATION PROCEEDING BERNARD REPRE-
SENTED [B]Y WISE. YOU MUST LET THINGS TAKE THEIR COURSE AND
NOT INTERFERE. MIGHT INVOLVE GRAVE CONSEQUENCES. MOTHER.

Evidently, Anne's regard for Bernard and "the work" was not subject to the blinding passion of her eldest daughter. She and her two daughters and their many social friends were the leading financial sponsors of the club. If he could not clear his name sufficiently with the Andersons, the entire operation at Nyack could be brought down.

In early 1921, Bernard was summoned to a second meeting with H.B. and another member of the family firm, E. O. Anderson. He arrived with his attorney, Mr. Wise, and the official Braeburn club attorney, one Mr. Staton. They were joined by the Andersons' chief private detective, Lawrence Richey, who had incidentally just signed on with Warren Harding's Secretary of Commerce, Herbert Hoover. The months-long investigation was complete, and he had been paid well for his efforts.

The results had been disclosed to the Andersons, and now Bernard would be called to account for them. The questioning began with a lawyerly probing of Bernard's teachings and beliefs. He responded like the noncooperating witness that he was, seeking to outmaneuver and outflank his interrogators. And when that didn't work, he simply denied or refused to answer.

QUESTION: It is stated that under this word *Tantrik* or at any rate under the suggestion of your religion or your teachings there are several theories or doctrines. One of them is the doctrine of intercourse between a man and a woman as representing the ultimate divine ecstatic condition, the highest ecstasy possible. Do you teach that in any way?

BERNARD: Not unless I was crazy or lost my mind.

Q: You never taught that?

BERNARD: No, never in my life.

Q: It is stated that you have taught that one of the first things that people must do to involve themselves in this theory of religion is to divorce entirely what you might call the Anglo-Saxon or Christian idea of right and wrong. . . . Have you ever taught anything of that sort?

BERNARD: I hardly think so.

Q: Well, have you?

BERNARD: No, sir. That is a scream.

Q: They say that you advocate or sanction sexual intercourse between people who are not husband and wife?

BERNARD: Never on God's green earth. No living soul ever heard me say such a thing. There are men who do those things but they do not say it; so I am informed by the public press. . . . Truth is what we want. What we care for most is pure intelligence. We are not interested in any particular doctrine or dogma or any religion or anything of the kind. . . .

Q: Is there a Tantrik philosophy?

BERNARD: In this sense there is. There are 165 volumes of Tantras, they say. They are indexed and are to be found in the British Museum in Bombay and at Oxford. These individual works which go to make up the whole, treat of different subjects. At different times different people from B.C. times to the fourteenth century . . . have gotten hold of some of these particular works and did not have access to others. They would form a little sect and study out what was in these books and attempt to practice it. That gave rise to about twelve different sects that call themselves Tantriks, each one having different principles, different practices and different beliefs. Different schemes of . . . what? Of culturing or controlling ourselves or increasing our evolution mentally, morally, physically and spiritually; as they believe, a better human being and a shortcut path to it. It is very practical and comes right down to doing things rather than theorizing. . . .

Q: In your teachings up there [in Nyack] your statement is that you *discourage*, not only do not preach, but discourage any sort of sexual informality outside of the marriage state?

BERNARD: Not only that, but I cannot conceive in my comparative study along those lines of an ideal on earth higher. . . .

Q: To get back to my question, you preach that any indiscriminate association, sexual association, outside of marriage is wrong, do you?

Your preaching is on the square of the Christian religion in that respect?

BERNARD: Yes, and further than that—I do not take objection, but I think Mr. Staton could tell you or anybody else that we take great offense at the word *preaching.* Any time a question is put up following these talks we have, I say to them, "You must ask your family minister. I do not preach. I do not settle problems of morals. I know nothing of casuistry. That belongs to your minister. Go to him. I could only give you an opinion. That is out of our jurisdiction."

The discussion then moved to Bernard's views on exercise and medicine, and the nature of the schools he was running. With this he expanded on the intricate franchise structure of his teachers' work, as well as the sophisticated corporate structures he'd put in place to buy and manage the real estate of the Nyack club. It was a feint that managed to confuse four intelligent lawyers, who were much less interested in his finances than in his views on sex and morals. Bernard then waxed philosophical, claiming that recent advances in physics had made it inevitable that the world should accept the Tantric philosophy of monism, the philosophy that states that matter—the universe and humans included—is made of godlike stuff, what the physicists were calling energy. We are all reflections of divinity, akin to the spider spinning its web world from the stuff of its own body.

Enough! Flabbergasted, H. B. Anderson broke in and announced that the real purpose of the meeting was to obtain answers to questions they had yet to ask. Bernard was about to slide into the Anderson X-ray machine, to go on trial for his life before a self-selected jury of wealthy, connected, Protestant power brokers.

Henry B. began.

ANDERSON: Now I will start right in and then we can discuss it generally afterwards. If I make it terse, it is not that I want to be disagreeable but to save time. I have you down as born in Leon, Iowa, October 31st, 1877, is that correct?

BERNARD: I do not know where this report is going. To me it is not a matter of much interest why, where or when I was born. It seems to me unessential.

Q: Is there any harm in telling where you were born?

BERNARD: No harm, excepting this. . . . I do not think it is absolutely fair to have a person's bowels dissected. I do not know where this is going. If it involves anything that is of interest to you here—

Q: It does very much.

BERNARD: What is it?

Q: I want to know if the information I have secured as to when and where you were born is correct.

BERNARD: Who would want such information?

Q: I just asked you the question. I am informed that you were born at Leon, Iowa, October 31st, 1877. I ask you if that is true and you say you do not want to say.

BERNARD: I do not think it is material.

Q: Very well. We will leave it at that. . . .

Then H.B. began drilling into Bernard's background, seeking answers to other basic questions about his family and upbringing. This drove Bernard to angry stonewalling—perhaps to keep his family out of his troubles— and he refused to answer, except to correct Anderson's inaccurate birth date.

Q: I promised you when I get through with this investigation I would let you know the result of it. Now I am giving it to you. You can make or not make any comment you want on it. . . . Dr. Bernard, this is a very damaging record as it stands.

BERNARD: What has where I was born got to do with it?

Q: I have not gotten through with it. It is stated that you never went to high school, never completed a high school education.

BERNARD: No.

Q: It is stated that for several years before they moved to California, you worked in your stepfather's barber shop and later in California in a cannery and then in the barber trade with your father.

BERNARD: In a what?

Q: A cannery, picking fruit.

BERNARD: Where was that?

Q: Oakland, California[,] and Riverside.

BERNARD: I think I was there about two weeks and lost a ruby ring.

Q: We are also informed that your father was a man by the name of E. W. Baker, that he deserted his wife and went to Denver and then to Yates Center and then obtained a divorce on the grounds of desertion.

BERNARD: No, he did not.

Q: In 1881, when you were three and a half years old, your mother married John C. Bernard.

BERNARD: In the first place, your date is incorrect about the birth.

Q: When were you born?

BERNARD: The 31st of October, 15 to 11 o'clock, 1876.

Q: Soon after that marriage[,] in a few weeks they moved to Humeston, Iowa, where their four sons were born, Glenn, Clyde, Ray and Irwin [*sic*]. Is that all correct?

BERNARD: No comment.

Q: . . . Bernard[,] your stepfather, died in an insane asylum in 1903 or thereabouts and then your mother married Robert D. Martin and since about 1910 Mr. and Mrs. Martin lived in Fillmore[,] California.

BERNARD: No comment.

Q: It is stated that you went to San Francisco at about nineteen years of age, or about 1896 or 1897.

BERNARD: I do not remember those dates.

The Anderson team changed tactics and began a roll call of Bernard's alleged crimes: They had it all in a large document in front of them: names, addresses, aliases; Nicholls, Jones, Harriman; Alma Sylvester, opium smoking, forced marriages; charges of fraud, theft, abduction, impersonating a physician. . . . "And we are told you never had any medical diploma in California," said Richey.

BERNARD: You were correctly told, but you were incorrectly told— . . . I was working in connection with different doctors.

E. O. ANDERSON: Did you ever know of a man named Hamati?

BERNARD: Hamati is a fellow that as far back—well not absolutely as far back as my memory will go, but away back in the early days of boyhood I met him in Lincoln, Nebraska[,] and from that time on, except such times as I was on a visit home I was with him continually up until the time I was, oh, I don't know, some place in the twenties, twenty-three or twenty-four, something like that.

Q: Well, you were started in on this method of thought and evolution through him, were you not?

BERNARD: I was. Well, in the sense of being taught by anyone who knows anything. . . . His occupation was that of a teacher of these things, or especially of the eastern philosophies and such and what you men in western language would call the occult, such ideas as some people get nowadays. I recall as soon as I was able to read I was delving into these occult novels.

On and on the interrogation went, the Andersons reprising every scandal and legal scrape that dogged the Tantriks in San Francisco, Seattle, Portland, and beyond. To Bernard's discomfort and rising anger, the lawyers seemed to have discovered quite a bit about his extended family. They produced details about his half sisters Ora Ray, Lula Fay, and Merl Baker. They knew, of course, about the abduction charges made by Gertrude Leo and Zelia Hopp in New York City in 1910; the failure of his publishing company; his brief refuge in the pseudonym "Homer Stansbury Leeds" following his release from prison; the exile to Leonia, New Jersey; the appearance of Blanche DeVries in his life; his stock market victories.

The Andersons' mission was clearly to ruin him, or at the very least to make sure that the daughters of Mrs. William K. Vanderbilt were safely removed from his inner circle for good. Suddenly aware that he could not simply run from this mountain of allegations sliding down on him, Bernard began to change his tune.

E. O. ANDERSON: Well, leaving out the sex stuff, that is all.

BERNARD: Do not leave that out. My personal desires—

Q: We would have to have another session for that. What I mean by sex stuff is this: I have these written statements of three or four girls of varying types. One or two of them I know all about. I regard them as I would a member of my own family as far as their statements to me are concerned as to what has taken place and so forth. I do not feel disposed to go into that.

BERNARD: Don't you want it cleaned up?

Q: I do not see how you can clean it up.

BERNARD: Maybe there is a chance.

Q: What is your idea as to how it could be cleaned up?

BERNARD: Suppose a person has a grievance and they say, here is a crime committed. Now all right, if you prefer to have them start something or go into court with something, that is one way.

Q: How otherwise would you clean it up?

BERNARD: You're just as competent to judge evidence as any trial. Suppose these girls make an accusation. It is up to me to answer.

Q: In the court we would have a jury.

BERNARD: You are good enough jury to suit me.

Q: If a jury did not believe you, you would go to jail. That would be clearing it up. Short of that I do not see how you can clear it up.

BERNARD: I would like to clear it up no matter what grievance they have.

Q: I do not care about hearing anything further. It seems to me that the thing is fairly clear, what it all pictures, I do not know how much more you want. I should advise you to take pains and get a little more adequate answer to some of that. That would be my judgment.

BERNARD: Adequate what?

Q: I would not acquit you on what you said as to that.

BERNARD: Acquit on what?

Q: I should consider after this examination that your whole method and manner of living and associates and connection with people is of a kind that would not justify any man to let his wife or daughter or anybody interested in you to have anything to do with your institution as it stands.

BERNARD: On what ground?

Q: Just on the face of it. I am perfectly willing to stand on that.

BERNARD: What is wrong? . . . Is there anything those people would like to know? What showing can we make that would interest them?

Bernard read through the depositions, but he was helpless to imagine what statement of his own they could possibly be after. His attorney, Mr. Wise, advised him to respond to "the general impression" the women's allegations imparted. "The morality?" Bernard asked.

H. B. Anderson interrupted again at the mention of the word *morality*, which was really his point all along and the heart of the matter. "Doctor," Anderson interjected, "there isn't a prosecuting attorney in the country that would not describe that thing in exactly the same words."

"Let us see what is the nature of the immorality," Bernard answered. "Is it loose living?"

"I will guarantee I could put you in jail in three months on this," Anderson warned, "on the result of this investigation. All I have to do is to go on with it, if you want me to, if you force me to. You go to your lawyers, both of whom are respectable members of the Bar, and talk to them about it and then we will talk again. I have spent three or four thousand dollars to trace up your history and you grant me I have done it fairly. There is nothing in here that was unfairly gotten."

Bernard, at a loss to say anything else, blurted out, "I do not see what is wrong."

"I am not your moral preceptor or your legal advisor," Anderson replied calmly, and with that, the inquisition was finished.

After this day of rather rough treatment, Bernard and his lawyers left the meeting and set about producing a document answering the allegations against him. The resulting words are a masterpiece of fabrication and embellishment that in its way conveys the true story of Bernard's life: he would always be a man no one could truly know, let alone pin down.

"My name is Pierre Bernard," it began. "I was born October 31, 1876, in Chicago, County of Cook and State of Illinois. I lived in Chicago until I was 4 or 5 years of age. I went from there to Bloomington, Ill., for about five years. From Bloomington I went to Des Moines, Iowa, for about two years. From Des Moines I resided in Lincoln, Neb., for about four years. From there I went to Los Angeles, where I remained for about 5 or 6 years."

Except for his name and the date of his birth, the remainder of the opening lines and indeed the rest of the document appear to be truth, half-truths, obfuscation, and outright lies. Why he engaged in this kind of distortion in the face of a professional investigation is not known, though it was part of his Tantrik philosophy to never reveal the truth to outsiders. In retrospect, Bernard seemed to be intent on protecting what was left of the reputation not only of his immediate family but of those who had joined him along the way. He referred to DeVries not as his wife but as "a former pupil of mine," and as for Margaret's expectation of marriage, Bernard dismissed it out of hand as impossible.

The Andersons then upped the ante. On September 17, 1921, a full year after he'd first summoned Bernard for questioning, Henry B. contacted the New York office of the U.S. Justice Department's Bureau of Investigation—the forerunner of the FBI—seeking an audience with its chief, William J. Burns.

I should very much like to get in touch personally with Mr. William J. Burns and furnish him with important data collected by Mr. Richey, who is now connected with Mr. [Herbert] Hoover—data that cost me $10,000.00, but saved my clients and obtained the return of the money that they were blackmailed out of by a dangerous and despicable blackmailer known as Pierre Bernard, who claims he is a Hindu, and teaches young girls immoral practices at a so called school of physical culture at Nyack, New York, as I had a thorough investigation made of this man's criminal activities and have the data and knowing that through Mr. Burns the man can be reached under the Federal statutes, and know that Mr. Burns would be performing a great public service. The man operated first in San Francisco, then here at Nyack, and I think [is] getting ready to pull up stakes and go to Chicago.

Anderson, like the Manhattan DA and others before him, appears to be overstating his case out of a blind fury toward all that Bernard stood for. No evidence was ever uncovered to support Anderson's wild claim that Bernard blackmailed the Vanderbilt heiresses—or anyone else, for that matter—and no evidence exists of any funds returned except for debts paid. There was no plan afoot for the Tantriks to abandon Nyack and relocate to Chicago. In fact, the opposite was undoubtedly true—thanks to the support of a growing number of students, Bernard's Nyack yoga colony was in the midst of a sizable expansion.

On September 27, 1921, Chief Burns of the Bureau of Investigation wrote back to H.B. to say that he would be delighted to review the dossier of charges against Bernard. In the end, however, Burns never found any use for its contents except to add to the bureau's voluminous files on private citizens. Nor did he ever attempt to bring federal charges against Bernard. The bureau's case ends as of that date.

Bernard, meanwhile, had long ago returned to Nyack and gotten back to business. His first annual circus the previous September had gone off without a hitch, undisturbed by the trouble Anderson was trying to brew for him in New York, and its success gave rise to a flurry of activity that made 1921 the first of the greatest run of years in Pierre Bernard's lifetime. There were yoga classes, dances, and baseball games to arrange—Sunday night poker parties, Greek literature classes, even a mock courtroom trial, starring the prominent Chicago attorney Edward Warren Everett—quite the fitting end to Bernard's tribulations at Anderson's hands. On August 27, Everett put on a costume and took up the bullhorn as a barker for the Braeburn Country Club's second annual circus, which this time took place under Bernard's latest acquisition, the largest canvas tent in private hands.

His gamble on a country ashram was in fact paying off more abundantly than any of his previous ventures, including the Fifty-third Street Yoga Center. In April he and DeVries had closed this last of his Manhattan schools, placing all of his chips on success in Nyack.

While new and distinguished members were pouring in, Anne Vanderbilt and her daughters had kept a notable distance from Bernard in the months following the inquest in 1921. But it seems that separation from the Tantriks was far more detrimental to their well-being than any scandal their association with him might bring upon them.

In September, while the Braeburn members basked in their circus afterglow, Barbara returned to New York from Europe in the aftermath of "a complete mental breakdown," in the words of Anne Vanderbilt's biographer. After her Paris divorce, she had taken to drinking heavily, ignoring her young son and lashing out at those who tried to take away her anesthesia. She began an intimate—and to her mother's eyes destructive—relationship with fellow club member Povla Frijsh. Anne had brought her daughter to all the leading lights of French psychiatry, including the famous Emile Coué, but she'd shown no improvement.

Finally, at the advice of Margaret, Anne brought her youngest daughter back to Nyack. Despite all of H. B. Anderson's efforts, the Vanderbilt women could not stay away. Barbara would now be under the care of Bernard and DeVries—their special project.

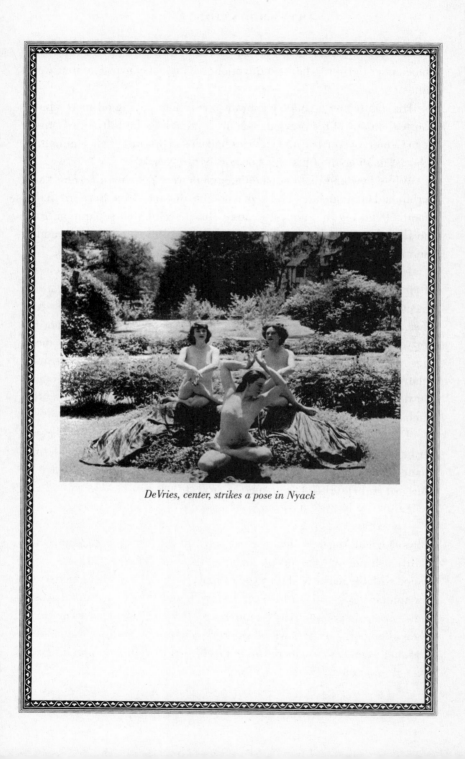

DeVries, center, strikes a pose in Nyack

Chapter 13

BODY AND MIND

hat was Bernard teaching up there on his hilltop that appealed to such a motley assembly of followers? On most Saturday nights sixty to seventy people could be counted on to spread themselves around his easy chair, waiting for his wisdom. As he looked out, he saw some sitting cross-legged on couches and rugs: others, including DeVries and Cheerie Smith, were literally at his feet, emanating great love and reverence. Though Bernard had built his early popularity on occult fireworks and feats of endurance (which he often said he could reprise whenever he wished), he had long ago moved away from yoga's ancient emphasis on superpowers and mind control. Instead, he taught yoga as the proven road to health and balance in life, as long as it was built on a bedrock of character.

Cyril Scott called it "Tantrik Yoga, a combination of Monism and Physiological Yoga," which is a fair start. In fact, the curriculum at Bernard's ashram on the Hudson included the study of Sanskrit texts, combined with the mastery of physical asanas, breath-control, and meditation techniques. What made his approach uniquely American was its insistence upon vigorous activity—students hit the mats at 7:30 every morning, then filled out their days with hard work, exercise, and fun. What made it twentieth-century was its devotion to self-expression, diet, and an attention to inner cleanliness.

All of these parts were brought together under the philosophical tent of monism, the view that—simply put—all is one. Bernard took it a step further: he believed that the human body, as part of this divine universe, was worthy of worship. The body is the sole vessel of our consciousness, he said, which in turn is the only earthly path to enlightenment and freedom. These are goals toward which we should be constantly evolving. In fact, as Bernard put it, the material world is lit to its atoms by the spark of God. The key to the mystery of life—if you care to know—is this unrealized unity. Our tragedy is that we fall for the illusion of separateness—*maya*, in Sanskrit. In this view Bernard echoed Emerson, who a half century before had written, "God re-appears with all His parts in every moss and cobweb."

The mystic's claim—the ability to contact the divine and teach others how to do it—lay at the heart of Bernard's authority. He told his followers that he had experienced the essential unity of existence and that the enlightenment brought about by this experience informed every moment of his life. This mystical state, even the aspiration to achieve it in some form, was the truest and fullest expression of self. He would show them the way.

Bernard was absolutely certain of his vision, and the strength of his convictions drew people to him and kept them at his side. One night, he began a lecture with a series of leading questions, supplying the answers as well.

What are we here for?

To live . . .

To live for what?

Happiness . . .

How are we going to get it?

Fullest expression of self.

For those who were searching for a purpose in life, here it was, take it or leave it. Our mission in life is to realize the divine within us and without. How to do that may take years of training, but Bernard was willing to transmit the techniques used by yogis for centuries to prepare the human body for spiritual liftoff. He taught them what he knew of the mental concentration and autonomic mastery that enabled him to still his breathing and soar off into what was called samadhi, the cosmic connection. "God consciousness," Bernard called it and later described what it felt like.

"Consciousness of names and forms leaves you. . . . The first effect is peacefulness—no feelings of fear, trials and troubles—an un-clutching, letting go—a feeling of trust and faith."

What Bernard described was the holy grail of yoga practice, the rainbow's end. Beginners might be content to take away from their training better physiques and successful sales careers, he said, but that was not the final destination. For Bernard, whose real business was the training of the next generation of teachers, every journey started with the cornerstone texts of Hindu theology—the Vedas, the Tantras, Patanjali's Yoga Sutras, and the Yoga Samhita.

But the mind could properly comprehend these texts only if the body was properly prepared—and that meant physical exercise. All exercise, he said on several occasions, is composed of three parts. "The idea or brain action; the impulse following down the nerve and muscular contraction and relaxation. All muscles when used should be considered as being filled to its limit with all life forces, held and emptied of its lifeless debris. That is the process of Nature. He who knows the philosophy of exercise knows all about Life."

<hr>

Bernard read deeply on the body-mind connection. His library was stocked with hundreds of health volumes and medical texts, some arcane (*Surgery of the Brain and Spinal Cord*, volumes 1–3; *The Ileo-Caecal Valve* by Rutherford), many by popular physical fitness and wellness buffs like Bernarr Macfadden and J. H. Kellogg. There were six texts alone on the biology and art of breathing, over one hundred on the sexual health of women. Bernard also admired the work of R. Tait McKenzie, director of the Department of Physical Education at the University of Pennsylvania, and he often cited him in his lectures.

Effort and sweat! Dismiss the servants! Get down on your knees and scrub the floor yourself. Bernard insisted that "character," the single great requisite for a good life, can actually be installed into the cells of the body by the constant repetition of beneficial acts, acts that subjugate the ego and open the soul to universal potentialities. That belief is hatha all the way and Tantric to the core. The human body—purified, toned, and tuned properly—can then receive the message of God-consciousness. This grace is available to us if we ask.

And we ask through our breathing, he insisted, our most intimate connection to the universe. Exercise is fine for developing muscles, Bernard said, but its chief value is in tricking us into more respiration. In Nyack, Bernard taught the necessity and value of deep yogic breathing: slow, rolling, lobe-parting, chest-swelling breaths that opened capillaries, lifted ribs, lit up the medulla, and brightened the pink, tender skin beneath our toenails. In each of our metabolisms, he believed, there was a continuous epic battle for life and against death and entropy—good versus evil in a molecular sense. Bernard explained this Manichaean standoff in chemical terms as carbon versus oxygen, the dross versus the prana—the Sanskrit term for the divine purifier of blood and brain and sinew.

"Most people use only one-fifth of their total lung capacity," he said. "Breathe more deeply and more slowly. Hold air in longer, and out longer. You will get interesting results in circulatory control." He then tied these results to the highest forms of mysticism, which can be found, he said, in ancient respiratory practices. "The Yogis have an elaborate science of breath," he explained. "There is meaning to them in the length of breath, the distance away from one that is disturbed by the exhalation of breath."

In short: "All the divinity we can ever know is in our carcasses."

But there was one more ingredient in Bernard's recipe. None of this mystical divinity can be attained without the desire provoked by a fundamental aspect of the mind he called "imagination." "Our formal study here has been Yoga," he said one Saturday night. "Aside from a few cross-legged postures and a little sniffing of air, it is entirely a study of *imagination*. . . . There is no desire without imagination. No cognition without imagination. There is no *will* without an action on the part of the imagination. These three states are therefore just three operations on the part of the imagination. Yoga gives us the necessary exercise for a rounded-out schooling of the imagination, which is what we all need."

Imagination, one of the grand themes of Bernard's life's work, stands like an idée fixe in his thirty years of lectures. It is Bernard's term for a well-developed action-oriented consciousness, which motivates meaning-ful human activity. Without a study of it, he insisted, yoga devolves into a series of postures and puffs. Without it, the human mind cannot begin its necessary journey inward; for advanced students of yoga, there is no concentration without it, no meditation without it, certainly no experience of samadhi, the mystical unity that beckons all true seekers like a pot of gold. All of it has to be imagined first, and Bernard said he would teach his students how to do that. The word that this rather unlikely American possessed the road map to samadhi had been spreading far and wide, and an even greater assortment of seekers would make their way to Nyack in the years to come.

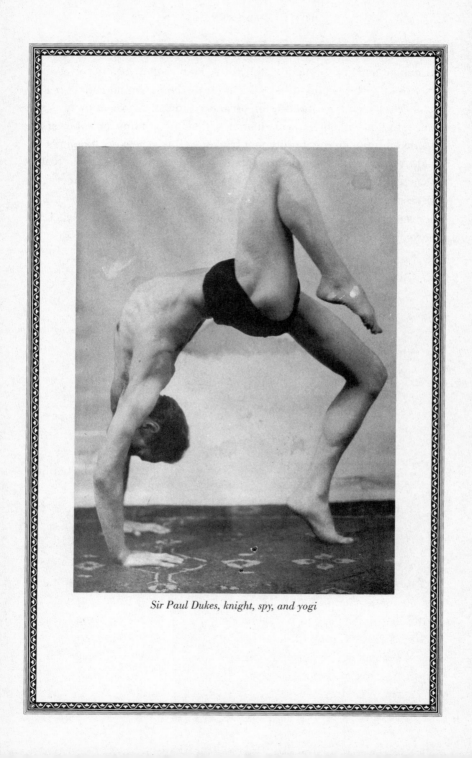

Sir Paul Dukes, knight, spy, and yogi

Chapter 14

ENTER SIR PAUL

hile the Great Oom was building his following, answering their questions, and revealing the philosophy of his American yoga, Barbara Rutherfurd Hatch was making progress on her recovery from her nervous breakdown. In fact, she appeared to be a shining example of Bernard's curative powers. She hit the yoga mat at 7:30 every morning, pitched in on household chores, took music lessons, and socialized with the other Tantriks—a far cry from the indolent young woman Cheerie had encountered in her Fifth Avenue bedroom. To keep Barbara's demons at bay, Bernard and DeVries made certain her days were packed with activities, including meditation and pranayama, and devoid of booze.

As for her sister, Margaret, her obsession with Bernard was about to be transferred to another man, the celebrated British spy Sir Paul Dukes.

As an undercover agent in Soviet Russia during the Great War, Paul Dukes had assumed as many as eight separate identities, evaded capture for years, and transferred vital information to the Allies—at mortal danger to himself. For his bravery he'd been made a KBE (Knight Commander of the British Empire) in 1920 and was publicly lauded by King George V and Winston Churchill. On his first lecture tour in the United States the following year, he played to packed houses in Boston, Chicago, Pittsburgh, Cincinnati, and a dozen other smaller American cities. Introduced to adoring American crowds as "the man of a thousand faces," Dukes spellbound his audiences with a mix of informed commentary on Russian culture and tales of derring-do and great escapes. And he had plenty to talk about. During his years in Russia he had managed to infiltrate the Communist Party at the highest levels.

Dukes had first learned about the Braeburn in the summer of 1921, when he'd been invited to the old-line conservative Nyack Club to lecture on Bolshevik Russia. Despite having won most of the town over, Pierre Bernard continued to provoke the ire of certain upstanding citizens of Nyack, and these grandees made their opinions of the Braeburners and their fascination with yoga known to their guest after his talk.

"You don't have to go as far as Chicago to find charlatans preaching yogi stuff. We've got them right here in Nyack."

"Awful people," said another.

"Monstrous," said a third.

"Absolutely indecent. . . . Why, the women wear slacks."

"They stand on their heads, men and women together."

"The fellow who runs it is a notorious rascal."

Dukes listened attentively to the negative sentiments expressed by his stuffy hosts and made a mental note: I must meet this man.

From the time the Englishman was a small boy, he had been an unrepentant, energetic seeker, determined to collect the wisdom of the world's most celebrated mystics. While studying music at the Saint Petersburg Conservatory in 1913, he had explored Theosophy and hypnotism, befriended the philosopher P. D. Ouspensky, and become the first English student of the mystic G. I. Gurdjieff. Gurdjieff told him about yoga's power; now Dukes was determined to see it demonstrated by an American master.

On his U.S. tour he'd already made several side trips in his quest for esoteric knowledge, including one to the Chicago suburbs to try to meet the elusive Yogi Ramacharaka. But instead of a best-selling yogi *auteur*, he found only a warehouse full of badly written yoga books, presided over by a tough, gum-chewing young lady who laughed at his polite inquiry and waved him off. This and other thwarted efforts merely whetted Dukes's longing to meet a real teacher and bona fide mystic.

The pious Nyack clubmen, in their disdainful murmurings, had just given Paul Dukes the key to his search. He went to the Braeburn the next day, introduced himself to Bernard, and applied for membership, only to be summarily turned down. Bernard had been "curt and uncommunicative," Dukes later recalled. He asked permission to attend a lecture that evening and was turned down a second time. The Tantriks were a suspicious lot, he was learning. The Englishman returned by train to New York City but immediately set about communicating his credentials to Bernard's lieutenants, hoping his good intentions and recommendations would guarantee a warmer reception on a future visit.

Several weeks later, he was on his way. His battered thirty-foot motor launch, playfully named the *Ark*, pushed its way west through the waters of Long Island Sound, moving in the chop past the mansions of Sands Point, Great Neck, and Little Neck that would inspire the setting for Fitzgerald's *Gatsby*. In sight of the skyline of Manhattan, the little boat crossed Flushing Bay, slid into the treacherous watery crossroads known as Hell Gate, and turned north into the Harlem River, heading for the Hudson River and its final destination: Nyack.

Paul Dukes kept a leisurely watch with the October sun on his back. He was in an exultant mood. The *Ark* represented his only permanent address in America and served as the repository for everything he owned in the world. He'd bought the boat in Huntington, Long Island, bargaining an old salt down to $500, placed a Union Jack at the stern and a Stars and Stripes on the prow, and called her home.

It was a full day's sail to Nyack—sixty miles by his reckoning—and late at night Dukes dropped anchor in the snug harbor of the Nyack Yacht Club. The next day, a Saturday, he rolled back the tarps on his boat and climbed the steep hills up from the Hudson's banks to the Braeburn, confident that this time he would find what he was seeking.

He found Bernard dressed in dirty overalls, bent over the engine of an old Stanley Steamer automobile, cussing enthusiastically. Bernard looked up at Dukes and squinted. "We met before, I think," he said. "Would you like a look around?"

The men toured the grounds, passing by a baseball game in progress, with players of both sexes in full uniform. They went into the Brick House and entered Bernard's impressive library, which housed several thousand books, many of which were works about yoga and philosophy and religion, encircling a billiard table in the middle of the room. "Good many books on health, too," Bernard added. "Folks here crazy about health. Believe in keeping fit. Good citizenship."

The distinctive noises of human exertion could be heard coming from another room. Bernard pulled back a sliding door, revealing a long hall with a platform at one end, and on the floor mats about a dozen people taking yoga instructions, learning to stand on their heads. The walls were decorated with anatomical charts of the human body, along with those of horses, cows, and rabbits.

Dukes, impatient to know everything at once, asked why they considered this inverted posture so important. "If you stick around here a bit, you'll see," Bernard answered. "That isn't the only thing that's important. Lots of things are important."

Then the doctor, as Dukes began to call him, excused himself and went back to the Stanley Steamer, leaving the Englishman to the wiles of the enthusiastic yoginis. They petitioned him to join them on the mats, and he obliged them—"to their delight," he later said. As the women in Bernard's circle no doubt noticed, the young spy carried himself with the grace of a dancer. He possessed a pleasing face and a lean, strong body, long legs, and remarkable flexibility. They were as excited to have him in their midst as he was to be permitted to attend his first lecture that very night.

<hr />

Later in the day, Dukes made his way back to Bernard's library and billiard room. It had grown chilly outside, and flames popped and crackled in the fireplace. Bernard, pool cue in hand, finished his game while the late arrivals drifted in. He'd changed into expensive flannels and an open shirt, and once everyone was present, he took his place in his designated armchair. The lights were turned low. As always, Cheerie took notes in the dark in her good schoolgirl script, but this time she was joined by Dukes, who recorded his notes in a spy's tiny shorthand.

Dukes was impressed with the clarity and force of Bernard's arguments for yoga. In the fuzzy world of metaphysics, he had learned, clarity is the rarest of qualities. "The background of true yoga," Bernard insisted, "is not booklore or metaphysics, but character. Without character all the booklore or metaphysics are as sounding brass or tinkling cymbals."

It was settled that October night. Dukes had found his teacher. Bernard, in turn, had finally found a Tantrik soul brother—a man at home in the world of secrets and illusion, but whose faculties represented everything Bernard was not: educated, sophisticated, *dashing*. Sir Paul possessed the kind of refined good looks that opened doors in social circles. He spoke

Russian and French fluently, had dexterity with German, and conversed in several other languages tolerably well. He was a musician and composer who displayed an easy and capacious empathy for his fellow man. He had many times in Russia demonstrated the ability to befriend peasants as well as commissars. Women and men alike were drawn to him.

Dukes asked to join the club and was accepted; his club name would be Sabin.

"I understood of course that it was not an ordinary country club," Dukes wrote. "Candidates were not proposed, seconded or elected by ballot; they were vetted by 'P.A.' and by him alone. The qualifications were not primarily wealth, station or class, but the genuineness of the applicant's desire for knowledge." Dukes could not help noticing, however, that along with lovers of knowledge a great many of the club members were indeed wealthy, famous, or both. He recognized many of the names: Scott, Stokowski, Frijsh, Vanderbilt, Rutherfurd, Goodrich, and others from the Social Register and the newspapers.

But it was Bernard himself who made the deepest impression. "He was the idol of sportsmen for miles around," wrote Dukes, and "there was hardly any sphere of activity into which he had not delved, no religious or philosophical system upon which he was not conversant."

So Sir Paul was aware of Bernard's past career as a fame-seeking occultist—Bernard himself was known to trot out pictures of his younger self tranced-out and wearing Dr. McMillan's hat pins and needles at the San Francisco College of Suggestive Therapeutics. But the American had a different story to tell now, and Sir Paul became a convert. Twenty-three years later, Bernard's main agenda centered on a single theme: how to use the tools of yoga to live a better, fuller life.

Dukes was especially interested in Bernard's expertise on the technology of good health. He looked around at his attractive, fit followers and surmised that the club's health education was responsible for "a salutary revolution in the outlook of many on life and thought."

Epiphany after epiphany ensued, and the ex-spy got a good, strong dose of what he later called "Americanized yoga." He admired the no-nonsense, slang-slinging approach chosen by its guru as the best method to impart Vedic wisdom to twentieth-century moderns. And he agreed with Bernard's insistence on cleanliness—his preference for Lysol and Listerine, as well as the benefits of a regularly irrigated colon, which also happened to be the latest obsession of many health-conscious Americans of the time.

Dukes heartily embraced the teachings and came to consider Bernard a close friend. His devotion turned out to be so absolute, in fact, that he put his boat in dry dock and moved to the club full-time until his speaking tour resumed after the start of 1922.

Invited to the White House in January, he doffed his bowler to President Harding and delivered the street-level news about life behind the closed borders of Red Russia. He wrote articles for the *Chicago Tribune* and the *New York Times* on the demoralizing effects of the new regime on Russian children. He kept an audience in Chicago spellbound for three hours without a single interruption. In March, his book-length account of his wartime adventures as an undercover agent, *Red Dusk and the Morrow*, was published to great acclaim, hailed by the *New York Times* as "one of the most entertaining, most informing and most illuminating of all the many books that have been written during the last four years about Russia." Sir Paul Dukes had become an American celebrity.

But he returned every weekend to Nyack, where in the off-season Bernard and DeVries completed their refurbishment of the Bradley estate, relocated their headquarters to the main house there, and renamed the entire operation the Clarkstown Country Club. Moreover, they installed Sir Paul Dukes as the CCC's first president, a nominal role except to insiders, but one that signified how vital Dukes had become to the club's affairs.

By the spring, it was also evident that his affinity for the place was augmented by affairs of the heart: Margaret Rutherfurd Mills, to be exact. Sir Paul does not record whether his initial meeting with the young divorcée was at an evening lecture or on the baseball diamond. Perhaps they met while rehearsing on the club's new indoor stage in the old Bradley carriage house; rumors held that the romance took off as they practiced trapeze holds for the circus, the spy guiding the heiress's body with his strong hands. Whatever the occasion, Sir Paul later noted, "We immediately fell in love."

The courtship picked up steam through the summer of 1922 and culminated on October 3 in a civil marriage ceremony conducted in high secrecy at the Bernards' residence. Only the master of the house, his wife, and justice of the peace Benjamin Haas were in attendance. Sir

Paul's pocket diary for that day read simply "Married Durand," which was Margaret's club name. None of the couple's friends had been advised of the details of the impending nuptials. The bride and groom spent their wedding night at the club and a few days later drove quietly down to New York to board an ocean liner for Paris. Sir Paul threw the press off their trail like an old spy: he let it slip to friends that they planned to marry in Greenwich, Connecticut; then he changed their reservations on the ocean liner *Olympic* at the last minute to the *Berengaria*. Their real names were never added to the passenger list. Satisfied their secret was safe, the newlyweds boarded the liner.

They took their meals in their rooms for the most part and kept to themselves above decks. Nobody on board recognized them. When they disembarked at Cherbourg, however, they encountered a throng of reporters and photographers waiting in ambush, demanding a statement of confirmation. Margaret hid her face and ran down the gangplank; her husband stood and faced the press.

Back in Nyack, New York City reporters descended on the Clarkstown Country Club in search of a marriage license, but to no avail—Justice Haas had kept it under wraps. Still, the *New York Times* and newspapers across the country saw fit to run unconfirmed reports of the marriage on the front page. The chance to revive an old scandal had proved too irresistible: "Sir Paul has made his home as a member of the Braeburn Club, established by Dr. Pierre Bernard, better known as Oom the Omnipotent and Loving Guru of the Tantriks, who found New York too uncomfortable for him nearly five years ago when the police descended on his temple of mystic cults in this city."

Dogged again by all the old accusations, this time Bernard seized the opportunity to establish himself as spokesman for the Vanderbilt family. He told the assembled reporters who had scurried up to Nyack that "any move Mrs. Mills may have made is known and approved by her mother, Mrs. W. K. Vanderbilt, now in Paris, despite any reports to the contrary." Bernard added that Margaret's sister, Barbara, "has known Sir Paul for a long time and most heartily approves of what is contained in the report and she is the only blood relative of Mrs. Mills in this country."

The ex-husband, Ogden L. Mills, was dragged before the press, too. Mills was by this time a U.S. congressman from New York State as well as the chairman of the New York County Republican Committee. Like everyone else, he knew not a thing about his ex-wife's new marriage, but he let it be known that he had no use for the likes of Bernard and his club. Referring to Mills, Bernard, in turn, joked that "Sir Paul may have neglected to have consulted him."

At Anne Vanderbilt's home in Paris, Sir Paul stood by his guru, confirming his status as a Clarkstown Country Club member to a reporter from the *International Herald Tribune*. Adverse criticism of the club, he said, came mostly from members of New York society who had never visited. He attested that he considered his own membership an "inestimable privilege" and that "the hostility manifested in some quarters against Pierre Bernard and the founders of the club is based entirely upon jealousy and ignorance." He gamely dismissed allegations of a secret sexual elite at the core of Bernard's organization. "It is not unnatural that gossip repeatedly refuted falls back as a last resort to some such folly as this," he explained. "For my part I am satisfied that there is no such inner circle and that there is no mystery whatsoever in the club. I am not a person likely to be fooled, as anybody knowing me or my record will concede."

With this verbal flourish, Sir Paul had granted Bernard and his club a newfound legitimacy. The entire world knew the ex-spy as a reliable, discerning witness, so by hounding Dukes the press essentially undermined the veracity of its own allegations. Bernard must have found the irony worth savoring. Not only had he managed to keep Margaret's fortune under his club's control through Dukes; he and his estimable adherent had become the sought-after experts for the affairs of the family of William K. Vanderbilt. And now Bernard was being glorified as a saint in newspapers on two continents by his own urbane representative, a KBE and a genuine hero of the Great War.

Undeterred by the frenzy in the papers, Dukes and Margaret enjoyed a leisurely autumn honeymoon in Europe. In early winter, they returned to Sir Paul's lecture schedule, traveling first to the United Kingdom and then back to the United States. Margaret, now known as Lady Dukes, stayed out on the circuit with her husband, returning with him to Nyack only occasionally over the next few years.

The halo effect of Sir Paul's connection to the club—and his marriage to its greatest benefactor—persisted in Nyack even in the couple's absence. For this and for the press's hand in bringing these connections to light, Bernard couldn't keep from gloating. "All I fear is that some day they are going to stop granting me the thousands of dollars worth of free advertising about my club," he said. "Every time they rehash the old junk about the club, its membership increases from one to two dozen members. Clippings from all the papers of these wonderful stories are posted on the bulletin board at the club, and they afford the greatest laugh ever for the members, who in all their experience with me have never seen or heard of the stuff printed."

To cement the club's attachment to the celebrated couple, Bernard kept his eye on a piece of land adjacent to the Bradley, and as soon as it became available, arranged for its sale to Sir Paul and Lady Dukes for $125,000. The Farm House, as it would be called, would serve as home for Margaret and her husband whenever they returned from touring the world.

Everything, it seemed, had fallen into place. Margaret was married off but still tethered to the club. Barbara had found a new home and continued to make enough progress in her recovery for Anne to keep her in Nyack. And so Bernard was free to turn his attention to his club's expansion, which was about to jump into high gear. The Clarkstown Country Club—with its expanded acreage and refurbished home base—was to be the site of new vistas of creativity combining the spiritual and the temporal in ways the nation had never seen. This new mission would require great imagination, but when put to that purpose, Bernard's had no match.

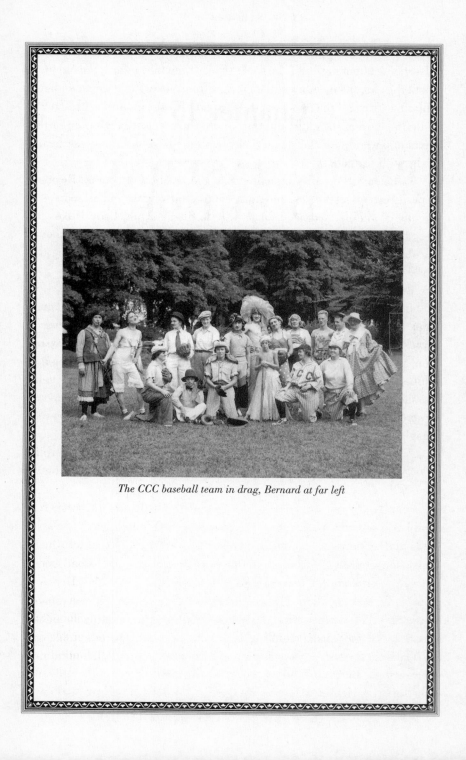

The CCC baseball team in drag, Bernard at far left

Chapter 15

BACH, BASEBALL, AND BUDDHA

he CCC's new headquarters at the Bradley estate were even grander than the Upper Nyack properties. Back in February 1922, Bernard and DeVries had moved into the master suite on the upper floors of a rambling white Victorian mansion with gables and dormers, wraparound porches, and a graceful porte cochere. The main-floor assembly rooms of the Bradley House would be reserved for parties, balls, dining, and other functions of the rapidly growing organization. Bernard nicknamed his new place the Eagle's Nest, as a kind of homage to Margaret's stepbrother, William K. Vanderbilt Jr., who kept a bachelor resort of the same name out in Suffolk County, Long Island.

Compared to the Braeburn's bucolic charm, the Bradley grounds resembled a feudal estate, set on a prominent hill, surrounded by farm fields and orchards and a dozen cottages and outbuildings, all of which were connected by long, winding drives. The carriage house had been renovated, enlarged, and converted into an auditorium, which DeVries proudly named the Inner Circle Theatre—her pride and joy—a venue that featured a forty-foot-wide, thirty-foot-deep stage and seating for eight hundred, the floor space doubling as a banquet room. The other side of the building, the stables, was reborn as a library, lecture hall, and mini-clubhouse for Bernard, who moved his books and billiard table up there from the Brick House. Rooms were added on the second floor for students, and the estate's cottages were leased to club members, who were expected to rent rooms to guests (as had been the case with the Upper Nyack cottages). Finally, one small outbuilding was turned into an informal café named the Cat's Whiskers.

The original operation was not abandoned by any means—the Brick House, which contained the main indoor gymnasium and featured the tennis courts, functioned chiefly as elaborate guest quarters, as did the Rossiter House. Most of the group activities had been moved to the Bradley estate. So, in essence, the Clarkstown Country Club was now composed of two separate campuses—a mile and a half apart—in Upper and South Nyack, which together formed a thriving community of entertainment, commerce, and education.

Doc Bernard, lord of the manor, continued to hold forth every Saturday night in his new lecture hall, speaking into the wee hours in his distinctive oratory, looping far from his starting point to thoughts on medicine, economics, history, philology, and history before circling back to yoga, health, the good life. The lights were dimmed during these lengthy talks, and after a full day of exercise and activity, it was not unusual for a few tired students to drift off to sleep. Bernard pretended to mind but didn't really care; he believed his message was potent enough to get through to the nappers subconsciously, so strong were his powers as a guru.

There in the dark listening to his wisdom were some of his longest-standing associates, like Nicholls and Jones, as well as his most devoted, like DeVries and Dukes. Barbara Rutherfurd, thriving under Bernard and DeVries's care, was also present, as was Margaret, who was then just turning her attention from her guru to Sir Paul. The three young yoga teachers, Marie Louise Schreiner, Ruth Bartholomew, and Mildred Ryder, were also frequent attendees, while Cheerie Smith continued to take down Bernard's thoughts as best she could, filing them away for study later on.

Bernard did not merely teach, however, and there was nothing passive about his pedagogical approach. He issued each listener a call to act, to change, to find happiness and take life by the horns. *Life is action*, he said, in many ways over and again. Club members were taught to learn how to play like children and work until they collapsed in laughter. With their quirky club names and mantras, new skills and garb, new ways to interact with one another, they were given the tools to transform their lives.

Outside the lecture room, however, the changes at the club did not sit so well with the small group of women who had helped make the Fifty-third Street Yoga Center a success years before. "With no warning, a profound change took place," Cheerie Smith wrote. The "yoga cult," as she and Clara Thorpe and others gleefully called themselves—half in irony, half in pride—had suddenly grown into something more public. Not only had Bernard renamed his operation, he'd offered an "open invitation for anyone to join without the commitment," according to Cheerie. "The club now attracted those who found life boring, with too much time and money and those who lacked motivation." Perhaps the worst insult was that the news of the name change had been kept from her; she and Clara and the other young women learned about it from the newspapers. "This hurt me especially," wrote Cheerie later. "It didn't seem fair that money should count more than devotion or dedication. Since P.A. chose not to tell us the reason for this drastic change, I could only speculate on the cause of his decision. He had reached his [forties] and may have decided to conserve his energy. Thousands had listened to his advice. . . . Now it was time for his students to act on their own."

Blanche DeVries, too, was spending more time with newcomers and with new enterprises, including her beloved Inner Circle Theatre. Leopold Stokowski, the famous conductor who rivaled Paul Dukes in the celebrity cachet he brought to the club, organized music and theater classes and lectured on performance techniques. Late into the night, he socialized in the Cat's Whiskers, the hangout he affectionately renamed "the Swiskas." A true Renaissance man, he gave cooking lessons, including one in how to whip up crêpes suzette, as Cheerie recalled. Another time, he set the Swiskas' curtains afire cooking a flambé—a mishap DeVries always recalled with humor.

The summer music program also moved to the Bradley estate, where it continued to be administered by Harriet Seymour. Her talented recruits— Schreiner, Bartholomew, and Ryder—helped out, and this year Ruth brought along her brother Marshall, the director of the Yale Glee Club and the New York City Junior League Choir. Barty, as he came to be known, was handsome, gifted, and ambitious—a thirty-something heartbreaker who drew the attention of the young women at the club. Something of an iconoclast, musically and otherwise, he collected folk songs and Negro spirituals—avant-garde activities for the day—and once gave an open-air recital in the streets of Hell's Kitchen that drew thousands of people out of the tenements and into the streets. At the music school and the CCC itself, Barty was an enthusiastic participant—fully in tune with Bernard's agenda—and he was known to jump in whenever he could, whether leading the orchestra and chorus for Inner Circle musicals or jamming on the banjo at the summer music school.

Another of Seymour's bright piano students, Diana Wertheim, entered the Nyack fold that summer as well. Diana's father, Jacob Wertheim, had died in 1920, leaving his family an estate of nearly $9 million, worth more than $100 million today. She'd grown up in one of the best apartment houses in Manhattan—two floors at the newly opened Alwyn Court on West Fifty-eighth Street—with a coterie of nurses, butlers, maids, cooks, and serving staff to stand attentively behind her when she ate. She'd mastered dressage riding at the Wertheim summer homes in upstate New York and New Jersey, toured the great cities of Europe, and just as readily thrown her hat in for the requisite society entertaining.

Bernard and DeVries would have been aware of how well-off this new heiress was. The entire nation had some idea. In May and June of 1922, a string of newspaper stories detailed Diana's $750,000 trust fund—$8 million in today's dollars—and a request by her mother to increase her allowance to $50,000 a year, the equivalent of $579,000.

A pretty, smiling extrovert, Diana was twenty, tall and carefree, with wavy bobbed hair that sprang from under the caps she liked to wear with her raccoon coat. As a sophomore at Smith College in Massachusetts, she had been recently turned on to the sweet music of monism, as William James called this philosophy of cosmic unity. So when Harriet Seymour enticed her into Bernard's sphere of influence, Diana found herself among like-minded seekers—her favorite being Barty Bartholomew.

Diana moved into a simple cottage on the Bradley estate grounds with Cheerie and Clara, where she took to learning yoga with gusto and living down her trust fund background. Her adoring thirteen-year-old sister, Viola, soon trailed her to Nyack whenever she wasn't at school in the city, happily serving as Diana's wing man, keeping the news of her sister's obsession with yoga—and her fledgling affair with Barty—from their mother. "The girls were enthralled with the club," says Joan Wofford, Diana's daughter. "They were mavericks, they were bright, they were rebels; they did not approve of their parents' lifestyle; they thought it was much too ostentatious and wealthy and uninvolved with important things." At the club they were known as Di and Vi—Diana Hunt and Viola White—and under those pseudonyms they wrote poetry about their early days in Nyack. "I owe the very Breath of Life / Not to the accidental woman / Who bore me, as the price of passing passion / But to him who taught me how to breathe," Diana wrote in "The Twice-Born," which concludes with her asking her guru to "save me from my inheritance—and from myself."

Save me from my inheritance indeed! Not the type to throw herself at anyone or anything, Viola, like Margaret Rutherfurd before her, had also offered to donate her entire financial legacy to Bernard. He did not accept her offer, but did begin to accept regular infusions of cash donations and fees from both Wertheim girls.

There were many more, of course, who'd joined the little colony. A pair of sisters, always referred to as the Misses Jeanne and Martha Powell, became full-time teachers and administrators. An amiable ex-newspaperman named Hamish McLaurin, a close pal of the legendary Damon Runyon, had been coming around for years, but in 1922 he signed on officially with his wife, Amie. In March a Nicaraguan-born physician named Anibel Zelaya put his signature to the roster, joining Dr. Guy Otis Brewster as a legitimizing medical presence at the club. The medical men, who were trusted colleagues and devotees of Bernard's Tantric philosophy, helped out when needed. In this gathering of freethinking young men and women, there were inevitably affairs and trysts. When called upon, the doctors arranged for birth control, treatment of venereal diseases, and other very private matters.

In the years to come, all of these figures would assume major roles in the life of the CCC, but for now they were Jazz Age avatars of the hippies, young and ready for adventure. Many of them had left their straight lives and hitched their fates to Bernard's, pursuing yoga, folk music, and alternative theater in a community that resembled in some ways the communal experiments of the 1960s. Bernard, in turn, offered them a never-ending succession of new and novel entertainments to enhance the appeal of his establishment.

That summer Bernard ramped up his commitment to his favorite non-yoga pastime—baseball—with renewed vigor, scheduling games as often as time allowed, even when there weren't enough hardball-minded members to field two teams. When he needed extra players, Bernard drafted his employees and their families. These he dubbed, with Shakespearean panache, the Mechanicals, pitting them against the club members' team, the Aristocrats. "The Mechanicals seldom lost a game," wrote Dennis Prindle, whose father took part in those contests.

Naturally, Doc Bernard led the Aristocrats from the mound. His money pitch was thrown "with a submarine delivery that could be intimidating," Dennis wrote, adding that "Sir Paul Dukes batted cricket-style, looking for a ball somewhere around his ankles that he could really tee off on." Diana Wertheim, tall enough to cover first base, took to the CCC's brand of hardball—few dispensations granted—with the same aplomb as any of the men.

If the club members were in a creative mood, they might sauce up the game with theatrical antics. On one afternoon, Bernard's team showed up in drag; on another occasion they played dressed in green-dyed costumes and hair.

The playing field, Bernard said, was a classroom and a proving ground on which better human beings could evolve. The national pastime, as valuable as any yoga asana, was "the enemy of death, disease and dirt," he said, if it was played with full attention and concentration. To be a better shortstop, visualize the ball slapping into your glove. "Insipid playing and thinking" drew his disdain, and he commanded his followers to stay conscious on the ball field. "If you do it there, you will do it in life."

Always on the prowl to profit from his passions, Bernard had also set about organizing a semipro team for the 1922 season. To elude Frank R. Crumbie's crusade to expand Rockland County's blue laws to baseball, Bernard built a new field on the South Nyack Bradley estate, where the local jurisdiction was less picky about weekend sports. He hired talented athletes from Tarrytown to Haverstraw and the Bronx, too, picking up a midget second baseman named "Butts" Thompson and a pitcher named James Leddy. He kicked in funds to build bleachers and a grandstand, charging 50 cents admission to cover payroll, which ranged from $250 to $300 a game. He had to sell five hundred to six hundred tickets just to break even, and while it was hard work, he often didn't get his investment back. But his team, the Nyack club (as they were known), won twenty-five out of their thirty games against barnstorming teams like the

House of David, the Brooklyn Blue Sox, the East New York Howards, and the Haverstraw Cuban Giants. At season's end the Nyack papers crowned them world champions, and hailing Bernard as the local baseball czar, the board of governors of the Nyack Athletic Association elected him their president.

While the Nyack ball club trounced its competition, the CCC members stepped up their preparations for their third annual circus. In July a dozen men rolled the big tent out over the lawns of the Bradley estate. This time the club added a fifty-by-fifty-foot stage, with eighteen-foot sidewalls and professional lighting designed by the president of the Architectural League of New York. A full set of trapeze apparatus, high wire, slack wire, rings, trampolines, tumbling platforms, and mats, was installed under the tent, and a crew of stunt trainers from Ringling Bros. arrived to make sure it was all safe and professional. The Wertheim sisters took to the acrobatics like naturals, as did Cheerie and Ruth and the others. Barty organized the choral numbers; Marie Louise Schreiner—affectionately nicknamed Shiny—coached the musical laggards. Margaret and Barbara rehearsed a dance number they were to perform together, but by the summer of 1922 Margaret's attention was fixed on her husband-to-be, Sir Paul Dukes, who wrote the music to accompany their choreography.

The week before opening night, a reporter from the *Nyack Evening Journal* caught up with Bernard as he was attempting to hook up a calliope to one of his new Stanley Steamer automobiles. "It will be one gala day," he announced. "I can make a lofty tumbler out of any hard-shelled dyspeptic old crab." There would be twenty-six different acts, with clowns and magic and exotic animals. He was bringing up an orchestra from New York City to accompany the performers, while everything else, from the costumes to the decorations, was designed and produced on-site. "The scenery, props, lyrics and dances and much of the music have all been done by our members," Bernard boasted, "simply because they enjoy doing it and get a heap of satisfaction out of all the hard work which it takes to make the thing a success."

But all of this excitement would be off-limits to everyone but those lucky enough to procure a ticket, and it was this cloak of secrecy over the two-thousand-seat tent that tantalized the local press. Ticket holders entered the CCC circus on September 9 through an international midway of booths decorated to represent different nations. There were Chinese tea servers, an Egyptian cigarette girl, and Turkish fruit vendors, as well as a lemonade stand and a peanut stand—to keep things totally authentic. The dog man, the frog man, the Zuni Indian snake dancer, and the Gypsy band performed for the audience. So did Margaret and Barbara, accompanied by Sir Paul, who rushed from the piano to change into his gymnast's outfit for his act on the rings. A month later, he and Margaret would be en route to Europe for their clandestine honeymoon, but on this night they were two stars in an elaborate, wildly successful show that surpassed everything the club had put on to date.

When the circus tent folded and the baseball season came to a close, things in Nyack tended to quiet down in the fall and winter. But early in 1923, two itinerant music teachers broke the monotony when they drove their auto trailer onto the main lawn and wandered into the clubhouse. After teaching stints at Juilliard's precursor, the Institute of Musical Arts, in Manhattan, and at California State University at Berkeley, Charles and Constance Seeger had been on the road with their three sons—Charles, John, and Pete—hoping to bring Bach and Beethoven to the countryside. This turned out to be an ill-fated venture, and so the family was looking for a place to rest and retrench with their vehicle full of fiddles and flutes.

"I was three years old, and I was left in the trailer," recalled Pete, who went on to become the legendary folk singer. "My parents had gone inside and I could not sleep. And I could see all the lights on in the buildings. So I walked over and into one and a Chinese cook gave me a banana and I went to look for my parents. In one of those rooms, everyone was sitting around in a circle and listening to Dr. Bernard speak. I ran across the room over to my father and into his arms. I remember everyone laughed. Then, my father wrapped me up in a blanket and put me to sleep."

Music was as much a part of the club's identity as yoga and baseball, and when the regulars returned for the warmer months, the Seegers happily found themselves in the company of Stokowski, Frijsh, and other talented performers, who routinely put on original four-hour theatricals for their fellow Tantriks. There was also a new generation of musical virtuosos interested in exploring the music of our own country—Ivy League musicians like Barty Bartholomew as well as renowned folk artists like John

Jacob Niles, who had just published his first collection of Appalachian songs.

Blanche DeVries, who'd become integral to the entertainment aspects of the club and its summer music school—the dances, the follies, festivals, and bazaars—persuaded Connie Seeger to give violin lessons and help Barty with his orchestrations. Shiny recalled bouncing young Pete on her lap and struggling along with Connie to teach wealthy amateur musicians to carry a tune.

The Seegers also fit neatly into the demographic of the growing Clarkstown Country Club membership: talented young people a bit perplexed by the times and bright enough to be interested in the larger matters of life. The terrible futility of the Great War had given rise to serious philosophical yearnings for Connie and Charles, as it had for many of their contemporaries. In Bernard they found not just a teacher, but a veritable savior. Charles Seeger was impressed with Bernard from the first, when he had seen him privately perform the Kali Mudra and the tongue-skewering exhibition. Charles took to mastering asana and pranayama, which he did quite easily, and could eventually hold his breath for fifteen minutes. But, he also noted warily, Bernard "had very strong control of the members. There was no questioning it." He later told his son Pete that Barty had given him a warning early on about dealing with Bernard. "The doctor is half saint and half devil," Barty said. "He's the boss. Don't try to change him or the club. If you don't like it, you can go somewhere else."

The Seegers didn't go anywhere else. Instead, they became devoted members of the CCC, and they would spend the next five years living in Nyack. Even after their marriage ended in divorce, they continued to frequent the club with their children. "I was always amused to see Dr. Bernard smoking regularly," Pete Seeger later remarked, "while he was advocating clean and healthy living for everyone else."

The strange playfulness that characterized 1920s life for many Americans began in earnest in 1923. "Yes, We Have No Bananas" blared from the radio in the remotest farm towns, and that spring Sir Arthur Conan Doyle introduced his spiritualist obsessions to a rapt audience at Carnegie Hall, claiming that his late friend and editor W. T. Stead had spoken to him from beyond the grave. F. Scott Fitzgerald famously called this era the Jazz Age, but he added these words: "It was an age of miracles, it was an age of art; it was an age of excess and an age of satire." The loosening of Victorian morals and manners was transmitted to the citizenry by an expanding national media which guaranteed that the flapper's lingo was readily decipherable in any rural backwater with access to a twopenny weekly. It also paved the way for a new appreciation of the occult, for which taboos suddenly seemed to have been lifted in a spirit of "why not?" Bankers trusted astrologers, U.S. senators consulted spirit mediums, and table-tipping séances were reported at the White House. Even the *New York Times* delivered the news of Arthur Conan Doyle's paranormal conversations with a straight face.

Magical thinking was everywhere—on Wall Street, in popular music, in the churches and temples of new religions. Who was to say what you could and couldn't believe? An ideological free-for-all was taking hold of the nation, and Bernard—who'd once been lampooned for his iconoclastic practices—gladly partook of the booming fusion of spirituality and play.

Nowhere could that fusion be better seen than at the club's first annual Spring Festival, an all-night bash to celebrate the birthday of none other than Buddha himself. On May 19, two hundred members of the club came together for an evening of music, dance, theatrics, food, and philosophy. "As an excuse for a party suitable to the joyous Springtime," the invitation beckoned, tongue firmly in cheek, "we discovered that one Gautama, alias the Lord Buddha, alias Prince Siddhartha (a Swedish gentleman, we are told, and not well known in the West), is supposed to have been born on or about the nineteenth of May. Thereupon, it was decided to celebrate *Buddhamas.* This accounts for the oriental character of the costumes and for the nature of the supper which will be served during the midnight intermission." If these playful associations gave the impression that the evening's festivities were meant to be ironic or frivolous, the invitation made certain that everyone knew the spirit of the fete was indeed central to the club's mission and identity, "a place where the Philosopher may dance and the Fool be provided with a thinking cap."

Dancing philosophers? Introspective fools? Sincere, earnest spirituality on display cheek by jowl with music and choreography? Here, then, was the totally weird (and obviously charming) admixture of playfulness, religion, and creativity that was beginning to define Bernard's club as a creation of its times. All truth is sacred, Bernard taught, and so there was no dissonance in mixing religious traditions, or even mixing the sacred with a little of the profane. Sir Paul Dukes, back from his honeymoon tour with Margaret, had composed an opening prayer that combined Buddhism, Hindu Vedanta, and Christianity. When the guests were settled down, he assumed the role of First Priest and began his recitation in great reverence before a living statue of the Lord Buddha, surrounded by a group of comely CCC dancers:

"Oh brethren, let us contemplate the eternal laws of Brahm; whose bounteous hand Dispenses with benevolence the gifts of Nature; whose mind inscrutably Directs the stars and planets."

Following the invocation, the stage was turned over to the members of DeVries's Inner Circle Theatre, who delivered on the program's warning to newcomers: "wild orgies of auditory and visual entertainment for the edification of its members and friends." Costumes were then provided for any guest who thought he or she had sufficient talent or was "willing to have his shortcomings subject to public scrutiny across the footlights." At midnight, a supper was served. Like the circus the previous fall, the Spring Festival was closed to the press and the general public, who were fed morsels of information just tantalizing enough to draw more and more interest in joining this organization that seemed to be squarely in the pulsing center of an age when séances were held in speakeasies and Harry Houdini's fans waited for spirit messages from his dearly departed mother.

That summer the club went into high gear and newcomers poured in week after week to see what it was all about. Bernard and DeVries made plans for an elaborate open-air dinner and costume ball in a tent on the Bradley estate lawns. The preparations and rehearsals were quite intense, and in July, Bernard insisted on a break, taking thirty-five club members on a boat ride up the Hudson to see a semipro baseball game in Haverstraw. The satellite efforts of Shiny and the other young teachers who'd spent the winter months teaching yoga in other American cities had begun to work their magic. The CCC filled up on most weekends with a Chicago contingent that included both Fred Upham, the treasurer of the Republican National Committee, and the renowned lawyer Clarence Darrow, defender of the underdog. There was another mini-invasion of European guests, including Countess de Korzybska of Poland and Lady Alastair Leveson-Gower, a widow of Scots gentry, both of whom signed their names in blood to join the rolls of Bernard's Tantrik Order.

To Cheerie and the other early adoptors, the idea of a small inner circle of devotees was now mere memory. Everyone was welcomed, it seemed, even the simply curious. Bernard, as usual, displayed peerless timing: his club had matched its offerings precisely to the intertwined desires of the age—to a rising generation's spiritual quests as well as their hunger for creative—and even outlandish—fun that was made possible by the growing prosperity of the decade.

Bernard would have been acutely aware of the American entrée that Anne Vanderbilt's other protégé, Emile Coué, had made that very spring. The Frenchman arrived to great fanfare and soon became a household name in the United States. He wrote a newspaper column and established Coué Institutes across the country that spread the word of his affirmative psychology. "Day by day I am getting better and better" became the mantra of his legions of followers, who were usually portrayed as quite solemn about their regimen. Meanwhile, in Nyack there was thriving a brand of self-help that looked to be just as successful and a lot more enjoyable.

While Bernard's circle of influence widened to greater and greater distances, he kept most of the local populace at a safe distance. He remained in the good graces of Rockland County's judges, politicians, and other leading lights by inviting them to the occasional CCC event, but the average Joe—or the average Joe who didn't work as a club employee—resented the exclusive nature of Bernard's Nyack empire. When Bernard ran his club treasurer, Morris Whitaker, against the baseball-hating Frank Crumbie for president of the Upper Nyack Board of Trustees earlier in the year, his influence peddling backfired, and the irascible Crumbie beat him (albeit by a single vote). The townies began to resort to pranks and nuisance making.

"My older brother was in school at the time," Pete Seeger recalled, "and somebody put manure in his desk, because we were associated with the club." As pranks and harassment became more frequent, Bernard was forced to employ night watchmen and guard dogs to keep vandals away from the expanding number of properties under his control. But one rainy September Saturday in Nyack, two local men managed to sneak into Sir Paul and Lady Dukes's garage at the Farm House. The famous couple was in Paris at the time, and the lone watchman was known to be off-duty between 7 p.m. and 10 p.m., a window of opportunity to push the Dukes's new Buick Roadster down the hill, jump-start it, and careen north in a joyride. Of course, they crashed the car, after which one of the thieves phoned a garage purporting to be Sir Paul himself, seeking roadside assistance. When the tow truck arrived at the scene, the mechanic was astonished to find the Buick sitting on the side of the road fully engulfed in flames, its doors still locked. One of the police officers surmised that a time fuse and dynamite had been used to destroy the car, and eventually, after much carrying-on by Bernard on his cherished members' behalf, a local boy was charged with the theft.

Ultimately, however, these petty incidents did nothing to stall the momentum the CCC had attained. The annual circus was put on hold that year, not because of the locals but to make way for efforts to install an indoor heated swimming pool, which would open the next winter. Bernard, reelected to the board of governors of the Nyack baseball club, ran the club again, with his midget second baseman as manager.

In the fall of 1923, they put on not one but *two* masked balls in celebration of Bernard's Halloween birthday. Members from Cleveland, Philadelphia, and Chicago who'd arrived a few days after the first party had insisted on a second one, and Bernard and DeVries not only obliged them but hand selected a costume for each member to wear.

The enhancements to the theatrical side of the club grew even more elaborate the next year. Professional costumers and scenarists from the theater district in New York were summoned to Nyack to lend a hand. Amateur enthusiasts from all over the country showed up as well, eager to be part of the fun. E. Warren Everett, the lead prosecutor in the infamous Teapot Dome scandal, took a break from the case and rented a house on the club grounds with his wife, Ruth. Fred Upham returned to host a series of summer parties, and more and more actors, painters, writers, and musicians filed in from as far away as San Francisco.

By this time the lead-up to the 1924 vaudeville supper and dance was at full steam, and the atmosphere up on the hill could only be described as high hoopla. Armed guards stood sentry around the big tent as it was rolled out on the Bradley lawn, and at 9 p.m. on August 30, the circus ringmaster boomed out a warning to his audience of lucky ticket holders. Everyone in attendance was hereby "initiated" into the Tantrik Order—he informed one and all that they wouldn't be allowed out of the confines of the tent before dawn, and that the orgy to come would test their endurance and break up many a happy home.

The 1924 show began with a burlesque play on *Hamlet*, followed by Memphis Mable Man and his singing hound. There was original music and clever choreography, including a piece called *The Jazz*, in which DeVries and her female choristers performed in oilcloth costumes strung with soup cans, their labels bearing recognizable household brands, while the men onstage were depicted as victims of the emasculating ravages of modern life and the mass consumerism that had taken hold of America.

As if to illustrate the CCC cure for these woes, Sir Paul then stepped into the amber glow of the spotlight, flipped onto his head, and brought his feet into the air in perfect alignment, demonstrating for the crowd *shirshasana*, the yoga headstand. Dropping to a shoulder stand, he then drank -a glass of grape juice—"unfermented," proclaimed the ringmaster—while inverted. Ruth Bartholomew climbed a rope into the highest reaches of the big tent while her brother Marshall directed the orchestra below.

Margaret performed a song-and-dance number that she had written herself, accompanied once more by her husband on the piano. Bernard, in overalls, ran around the tent the entire evening, making sure that the mechanics of the performance went off smoothly. An intermission dinner for all broke up only after the first sunlight hit the Nyack hills.

"Annual Orgies of Oom Witnessed by Hundreds in Big Top on Club's Grounds" read the headline of the *Nyack Evening Journal*. Even the local press, it seemed, was willing to go along with the ringmaster's joke.

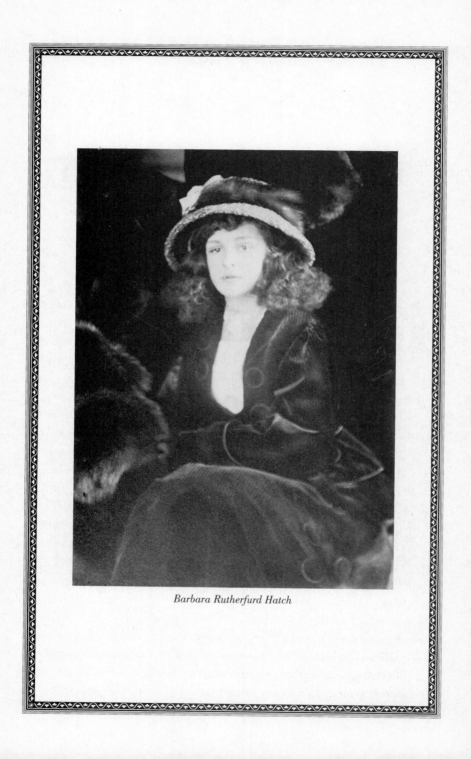

Barbara Rutherfurd Hatch

Chapter 16

THE VANDERBILT KNOT

ife at the club—the baseball, the jazz bands and circuses, the yoga lessons and the search for meaning—proceeded uninterrupted by the comings and goings of Anne Vanderbilt and her daughters. By the spring of 1924, Anne found herself satisfied enough by Barbara's progress in Nyack to purchase a large riverfront estate near the CCC. This home, she thought, would in time—and after much needed renovation—serve as a permanent residence for Barbara and her seven-year-old son, Rutherfurd, who'd been in Anne's care during the past three years. The $200,000 Moorings estate was officially signed over to Paul Dukes, who would oversee the improvements on its three Tudor homes and seven acres of land. In June he turned over the deed to Barbara Hatch, a recognition from her family that perhaps her course of treatment with DeVries was successfully nearing completion.

Anne's affection for DeVries had only grown during these years, and her regard came to encompass Mrs. Bernard's latest crop of female yoga students. Just as Anne had taken a motherly shine to the young Cheerie and Clara Thorpe at the Fifty-third Street center, she had now come to think of Ruth Bartholomew and Mildred Ryder as part of her family. These young women of character—steady, disciplined, kind—possessed the qualities she wanted so desperately to graft onto her own daughters.

But that spring, Barbara revealed that she had discovered an altogether different remedy to cure her attraction to Povla Frijsh—and it wasn't a result of her daily regimen with DeVries. Barbara Hatch was pregnant, and the lucky father was none other than one of Bernard's longest-standing and most trusted associates, Winfield Nicholls. Perhaps this was Nicholls's first and only betrayal of Bernard's trust—or perhaps it was a well-hatched plan on the part of the Great Oom himself: to steer his lovelorn charge into the orbit of his number one seducer. Bernard claimed to be able to "cure" homosexuality; maybe he simply engineered this match to keep Barbara's mind away from her opera singer.

Whatever the motives at work, the end result was that the Moorings estate became Barbara's wedding present. On August 11, 1924, while the Tantriks were preparing for their all-night extravaganza, Barbara and Winfield were married quietly, their union a secret from all but a few club members and her immediate family. But two weeks later, someone leaked the news to the press, and the combination of the Great Oom and the great Vanderbilt name once again guaranteed gossip at the national level: "Vanderbilts Join Cult by Marriage," read the headline in the Gettysburg, Pennsylvania, *Times*.

It's unknown whether the newspaper coverage forced Anne to reconsider her plans for Barbara and Nicholls at the Moorings estate or the renovations simply took longer than expected, but the couple never moved in. In fact, Winfield Nicholls never shared a home with his wife, the mother of his children. Instead, Barbara was relocated to a single-room apartment in the club's headquarters. When the Orgies of Oom went on in August, she watched quietly from the stands, and in September, in a letter to her mother, she spoke of her daily regimen as if she were not married and expecting a baby at all. In fact, it seems her life had simply continued apace as it had for the past three years:

SEPTEMBER 18TH, 1924

Darling Mother,

This being the first letter I have written [it] will probably come as a great surprise, but I am sure that owing to the nature of the news I have to tell you it will be a very pleasant one. For the first time in my life, I have made a definite and practical change in my mode of living. . . . Having already gotten such benefits from the change, I simply marvel that it was not made possible 2 years before this. The nature of the news is this: I am here living at the Bradley in a modest one room compartment but [with] a very extensive and varied plan of action for each day. Doctor Bernard made this move possible for me which [is] not as simple as it seems since DeVries is personally conducting my entire program [of] physical care and training and plan of action for some time to come. I consider it a great favor on DV's part as she has absolutely refused to undertake any other personal work for the past year and a half. . . . A short list of my activities will show you that I must be resigned to start from the bottom up, knowing it is after all, the shortest way to the top.

My day includes cooking lessons[,] typing[,] business (what do I mean by that? Being responsible for all my material assets, keeping books, accounts, etc.) Organization, mantra, dish washing & all such delicacies. . . . Errands, memorizing music; to be still more specific, I am on the mat at 7:30 every morning. The enclosed slip will show you in detail what happens. Of course, what will make this part of my real character is repetition. I know that this means hard work for me in the future. DeVries can show me the way, but I have to put in the time and effort, no one can do this for me. I seem to be talking a lot about myself, but I do want you to understand what I am trying to do. Have you had a pleasant and profitable summer? Are you feeling well? When are you coming back? Soon, I hope; my middle name will be EFFICIENCY by the time I see you again and my first name VITALITY. And now mummy dear, I must skip, this is my 4th venture on the type writer, not so bad is it? Lots and lots of love and many thoughts, devotedly,

Babs

Barbara's progress report was no doubt a public relations effort meant to soothe her mother, and in retrospect it betrays a certain jumpiness on the part of her custodians, who clearly had a hand in its composition. There is no mention of Nicholls, who seems to have vanished temporarily from Barbara's life. In fact, the main point of the letter is to communicate to Anne that all is well—that Barbara's education had entered a new and accelerated phase at the club. What is more likely is that Bernard and DeVries had judged the young woman still too unstable to function independently in the final months of her pregnancy. And there were real questions as to whether Barbara was emotionally ready to run a household and to become a mother for the second time.

⬛

But Nicholls was not entirely out of the picture—yet. On January 26, 1925, Barbara gave birth to fraternal twins, a girl they named Margaret and a boy they named Guy Winfield. But his role as a father would end there. It was arranged that Ruth Bartholomew and Mildred Ryder would take care of the babies in their first months. By May, allegations had begun to surface that the Nicholls's marriage had unraveled. The newlyweds were not even living together—had never lived together—it was whispered. And it was true. Barbara, who'd fallen into a postpartum psychiatric relapse, had fled to her mother's new home on Sutton Place in Manhattan, leaving her husband and babies behind in Nyack. Bernard fabricated a story for a trusting *Evening Journal* reporter, claiming that the couple was getting along fine, that Nicholls maintained an apartment in New York City, which he used when he stayed over in town taking a chemistry course. "Mrs. Nichols [sic] and the two babies, which were born in January, are staying at the home of her sister, Lady Dukes," Bernard said, adding that Barbara's place, the Moorings, had been leased to the club for the next five years and was presently undergoing renovations. "Sir Paul and Lady Dukes sailed for Europe last night and Mrs. Nicholls is conducting her sister's household during her absence," he went on.

In retrospect, it was obvious that Anne Vanderbilt felt compelled to swoop in and remake the plans for her daughter's new life. Bernard's outing of her family's personal affairs only made things worse. Though he had tried to put the best face on what was turning out to be a very bad situation indeed, Bernard's temerity in speaking to the press about a sensitive family matter would this time cost him Anne's favor for good.

In Fifth Avenue's mansions and Newport's bathing clubs, her peers tut-tutted furiously about these developments. Who was this man who spoke for her and for her daughters with such confidence? And why had she involved herself with this scandalous practice of yoga and those who believed in it? While Bernard held forth with the press, Anne was subjected to no small amount of ridicule over the public disclosure of her involvement with the Great Oom and his club. She was a woman who could endure extraordinary hardship with grace and aplomb, but the public airing of her private affairs was an affront she would not brook.

While Barbara languished at Sutton Place, her twins were promptly moved to a newly acquired property across the Hudson River in Westchester, where they were left in the care of professional nurses and kept hidden from their father. Her firstborn, Rutherfurd, remained in Anne's care, as did Barbara herself, and at year's end the Moorings estate was turned over to Pierre Bernard for an undisclosed sum.

By then, Anne and Barbara were long gone, having boarded an ocean liner for France, where the family's situation deteriorated further. In early 1926, Barbara landed herself in jail for physically striking her mother, and she would remain incarcerated—first in prison, then in sanitarium lockdown—for the rest of her life.

<hr/>

The family Bernard and DeVries had managed to woo back to Nyack had packed up and gone. In Anne's eyes Bernard had committed the single most grievous sin by dragging the Vanderbilt name into the newspapers with his crowing about Barbara and Nicholls. Moreover, he had allowed her daughter's pregnancy to happen and engineered a marriage—or at least consented to it—simply to garner publicity and perhaps to manipulate Barbara's fortune. At best, he was simply neglectful of her daughter's true needs.

Even Sir Paul and Lady Dukes had exited the CCC stage, the 1924 circus having so inspired them that they'd decided to launch real artistic careers of their own in Europe. The husband and wife were training intensively and rehearsing for their performance debuts, she as a ballet dancer, he as a composer and conductor, and in 1925 they turned over their Nyack home, the Farm House, to Bernard and DeVries as a parting gift, adding to his collection of estates.

But as the unlikelihood of Barbara's recovery became obvious, and the strain of tending to her became more profound with each new crisis, Margaret began to worry obsessively that her sister's mental disorder was hereditary and would soon infect her—a self-fulfilling prophecy if ever there was one, though an auspicious turn for Bernard.

In February 1927, after a month of fainting spells and weeping fits that not even a week on the French Riviera could cure, Margaret and Sir

Paul returned to New York. Anne Vanderbilt met them at the docks in a foul mood, suspecting that Margaret's true destination was Nyack and the real reason for her return was to see Bernard. Anne informed Sir Paul that if Margaret so much as contacted Bernard, she would disown her. Anne then brought in the best doctors in the city, who one by one assured her that Margaret was physically healthy, if stressed to the point of distraction. Margaret, in turn, took to her bedroom, and gave orders that no one but her doctors and nurses and husband would be allowed upstairs. One early morning, in a desperate state, she demanded that she "must see P.A. at once" and that it must be immediately, in her mother's house, and that her husband must arrange it.

Anne remained implacable. "Now understand that Bernard shall never put his foot inside this house, or if Margaret sees him I shall never give her any more money," she reiterated to Dukes. Even his offer to secure a suite of rooms at the Gladstone Hotel as a neutral meeting ground was met with her obstinate refusal.

But eventually, Margaret's obvious anguish forced Anne's capitulation, and Sir Paul was permitted to arrange for a visit. He called Bernard, who agreed to drive down to the city at once, arriving at eleven the next morning to sequester himself with Margaret. He worked on her one-on-one, guru-to-student, peered deeply into her eyes and soothed her, slowed her breathing and with his unquestionable authority convinced her that she was healthy and would soon recover. He answered to her satisfaction all of her medical questions regarding her mental condition, hereditary risks, the utility of her yoga and meditation regimen.

Predictably, Margaret showed immediate improvement, and as soon as her guru left, she promptly fell asleep. Mrs. Vanderbilt stayed away from her home until late in the afternoon, and on returning indicated to her son-in-law that she had indeed changed her opinion of Bernard once again. "She rather expressed herself as very satisfied [that] Margaret had seen him!" Dukes wrote in his journal. "She merely wanted an assurance that P.A. wd. not come again or use the incident for publicity."

Five days later, also predictably, Margaret relapsed. Despondent, she sat looking out her bedroom window at the East River through blue spectacles. Eleven days after Bernard's first visit, she asked for written messages from him, and she sent Sir Paul off on clandestine visits to Nyack to collect them. When Anne had to return to Europe to tend to Barbara's latest crisis, she repeatedly cautioned Dukes not to allow Margaret to fall once more into "that man's clutches." She warned him, too, to keep the news of Barbara's situation a total secret to all but the immediate family.

In Anne's view, Winfield Nicholls was decidedly not a part of the immediate family. When he pressed Dukes to give him any news at all about his wife and twins, Sir Paul wisely refused, but unwisely asked Margaret to ask Anne what answers he *might* give her brother-in-law, who after all deserved some small courtesy. At this request Margaret flew into a rage again and then collapsed into depression. More secret visits and letters from Bernard followed, and after each one, Margaret recovered for a few days, then relapsed precipitously.

By April, she was accusing Sir Paul of being after her money. "A hard, strange look came over her when I approached," he noted, and frankly, he should have seen the rest coming. Five years into her first marriage, Margaret had handled her unhappiness in the relationship by collapsing into a nervous exhaustion. Now, five years after the start of her second marriage, she was going cold on Sir Paul. The couple agreed to separate. Sir Paul wished to live in Europe, where he continued what would become a lifelong pursuit of hatha yoga, while Margaret settled in New York, where her affections quickly found a new target: Charles Michel Joachim Napoleon, a French royal known as Prince Murat. Happily, the separation was a friendly one; the following spring, in fulfillment of her show-business dreams, Margaret made her New York City stage debut with the Gavrilov Ballet Moderne, while her ex-husband conducted an original score for the company that night.

Matters weren't so harmonious between Barbara and Winfield Nicholls, however. The wistful sentiments he'd expressed in 1927—that "it is quite possible that the onrushing stream of soul and desire may carry the two [of us] apart, for the best good of each"—had in 1928 hardened into self-protection. Anne Vanderbilt had rebuffed Nicholls's final attempt to obtain any information about the condition of his wife and his children. He sued for an annulment in New York State Supreme Court, charging that Barbara was insane when they were married and that her true mental condition was concealed from him at the time, and when that attempt failed he decamped to Nevada to pursue divorce proceedings there. It took him two years to untangle his Vanderbilt knot, and he returned afterward to the safety of the CCC, where he would remain in residence until the late

1940s. Margaret, meanwhile, did marry her French royal and upgraded her social status from Lady Dukes to Princess Murat.

All ties to the CCC were now thoroughly severed, including Anne's participation in Bernard's Biophile Club Company, which carried on without her. In her royal marriage Margaret found contentment without the constant attentions of Bernard, while Barbara was in effect never heard from again; she would move from one institution to the next, dying tragically young in a sanitarium in Cannes, France, at the age of forty-four. During this time, her children were left in the care of Anne, who provided them with trust funds upon her own death in 1940. They had nothing to do with Bernard, DeVries, or the Clarkstown Country Club.

Though they'd finally broken free of Bernard, Margaret and her mother did not abandon yoga; together with Margaret's stepbrother, Harold Stirling Vanderbilt, they remained avid practitioners for the rest of their lives. Mother and daughter both would eventually resume friendships with DeVries and other club members, but it would take years—and another breach within the CCC—to bring this about.

The family had, by anyone's account, given more than sufficiently to the yoga cause in its establishment phase. Their financial generosity had single-handedly allowed a man considered a scoundrel by much of the world to set himself up as the biggest landowner in Nyack. Without them, it's doubtful that Bernard could have attained so much so fast, or even achieved any success at all.

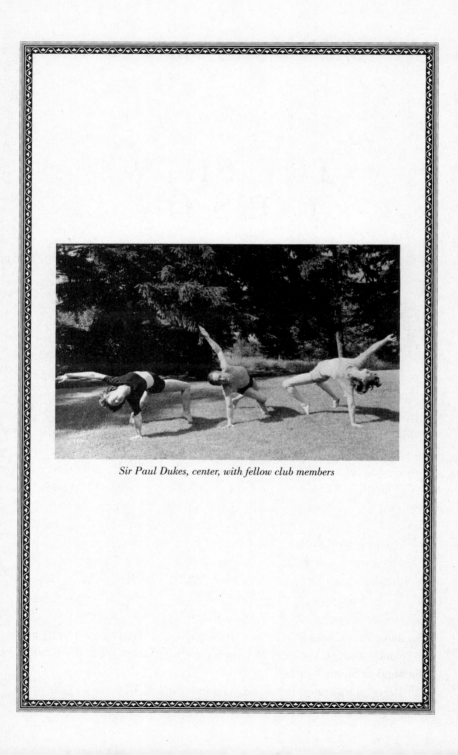

Sir Paul Dukes, center, with fellow club members

Chapter 17

THE SHOW
GOES ON

ccustomed to wild reversals of fortune from his early days, Bernard always seemed to have alternative plans cooking. Long before Barbara, Margaret, and Anne cut off all ties to the CCC, he had firmly established a self-sustaining educational empire that would thrive with or without the Vanderbilts' support. And he never ceased in his pursuit of even larger aspirations for himself, for yoga, and for the club. He needed to take the CCC's operations to an even higher level, the better to attract attention and new wealthy members. So each season, the parties and entertainments became larger and more outrageous, and the club demanded more and more of his attention.

Something had to give, and it turned out to be baseball—at least the semiprofessional variety. In March 1925, Bernard resigned as president and chief benefactor of the Nyack Athletic Association, the sponsor of the village's semipro baseball team for the past four years. He had lost money for several seasons, and with no profit in sight, he decided to step back and reclaim his weekends. He told the local sportswriters that he was curious to see if anyone else could do a better job for local baseball fans. Nobody stepped forward, and within weeks, the directors disbanded the association, thus ending the short reign of Bernardian semipro ball in Nyack—though his amateur games continued unabated at the Bradley diamond in South Nyack.

Bernard had other things on his mind. First of all there was the massive ongoing project of upgrading the huge Bradley property—there was additional landscaping to be done, as well as the preparation of the fields for the growing season—he had, after all, inherited a gentleman's farm. Wheat, melons, corn, and tomatoes were planted. A dairy herd could be seen grazing in the fields, along with chickens, ducks, pheasants, goats, and horses. Bernard himself tended to the fruit trees, vines, and other matters of husbandry that he had taken up as a passion since his move to Nyack in 1919.

That spring, too, he and DeVries revamped plans for the season's shows and other entertainments. In May, they put on their first annual Spring Frolic and Gambol. The clubhouse was hung with silk and satin tapestries and lit by professional stage lights. Hundreds of costumed partygoers wandered the lawns in robes, sandals, turbans, and sequins. There were senoritas, milkmaids, and Gypsy queens in gowns of silver and gold. The buzz surrounding this new costume ball had attracted a procession of Manhattan's new show-business royalty, including Major Edward Bowes, owner of the Capitol Theatre in New York and president of the Metro-Goldwyn Film Corporation. But the most honored guest at the ball was Pierre Bernard's own mother, Kittie, who'd come east with her husband, Robert Martin. The couple, now in their seventies, had moved to the CCC this year, making the club their permanent home for the rest of their lives. Bernard, the good son and family man, had once again stepped forward to take in kin who needed him. He was pleased to do so, as he approved mightily of Kittie's husband, who was, like Bernard, a high-ranking member of the Masonic lodge. The Spring Gambol would be their first gander at a CCC spectacle.

Prior to the festivities, in what was becoming a CCC ritual, Bernard conducted private consultations with each partygoer on his or her choice of costume. Often he dictated the selections himself, based on his intimate knowledge of each member's personality. He decided which of his women guests secretly wished to be seen in public as queens and which of them wanted to be slave girls. In his role as a theatrical psychotherapist, he provided each woman with the thrill of revealing some hidden, perhaps naughty, side of herself. The men came out of their consultation dressed in upscale versions of themselves as elegant diplomats and admirals or as fierce Apaches and gangsters. And Bernard alone knew the emotional resonance behind each choice.

At midnight, after two hours of dinner and dancing, Bernard called the party to order and started the show, which didn't break up until 4 a.m. Even Kittie and her husband stayed till the very end.

<hr />

That summer, Bernard's ambition went into overdrive. He installed a commercial-grade film projector in the Inner Circle Theatre, where first-run movies were screened on the weekends—by invitation only, of course—for members and guests. He purchased another sixty acres of land adjacent to the club. There was weekend baseball—club members and amateurs only—whenever time permitted. With the crops in the ground and the animals fed and happy, Bernard's operation had become something close to a self-sufficient village, and the labor this required tied in perfectly with his therapeutic vision: for his students and members, working in the fields was presented as a privilege, a form of healing, a way to tamp down outsize egos with manual labor. There were, however, plenty of professionals and tradesmen on hand to make sure things were done to his satisfaction.

To celebrate its abundant harvest, the club skipped the circus that fall in favor of a Thanksgiving celebration with an elaborate feast. "We harvested the last crops, baked pumpkin and mince pie[s]," recalled Cheerie. "We transformed an old barn into a pioneer scene with bundles of straw and lighted oil lanterns to add to the old time feeling. . . . Even P.A. entered into the party [spirit], dressed cowboy style, boots and all. While Stokowski played the fiddle, P.A. called the square and the round dances. All in all we had a wonderful life, healthful foods and a garden of Eden, our home. No wonder no one wanted to leave."

In the spirit of keeping everyone guessing as to what could possibly happen next, a month later Bernard and DeVries hosted a madcap Goth-flavored tenth wedding anniversary for Mr. and Mrs. Alfred G. Kay of Pittsburgh, who were longtime yogis and extremely wealthy sponsors of the club. Outside the big house on the Bradley estate, guards and dogs kept the curious at bay. Inside, costumes were assigned once more; some of the female guests dressed up as nuns, and the men wore Oriental robes over their evening clothes. The wedding procession began as a funeral cortege, with Mr. and Mrs. Kay preceded by nuns and monks carrying tall candles and wheeling two coffins draped in black. "We'll make this wedding the funeral of the dead past," Bernard announced. "And the dead past can bury its dead." When the banquet commenced, the coffins were flipped over and turned into dining tables, to the horror of some and the delight of Bernard.

A flurry of holiday banquets followed, culminating in a fourteen-act New Year's Eve vaudeville show that launched the Tantriks into 1926. Winter, it seems, was no longer keeping the seasonal guests away.

What could the CCC do to top its 1925 exploits? In the spring an entire orchard of 125 mature fruit trees was transplanted to the Farm House property, while construction crews were busy making preparations for the arrival of a forty-foot snake and a baby elephant. The acrobatics studio in the Brick House gymnasium was enlarged and improved, with improved tumbling mats and a new set of safety devices and harnesses designed to help beginners fly without fear. To head up the studio, Bernard hired circus veteran Eddie Evans—an old "twister," as he called him—who'd been a tumbling specialist for Barnum & Bailey and many other circuses.

Everyone was back in Nyack for the 1926 Spring Festival party on June 5. There were again fourteen acts on the bill that night, including original song-and-dance sketches called the *CCC Male Orgies* and a satire described tongue-in-cheek as *The Love Cult*, which poked fun at the club's new tabloid tormentor, the *New York Daily News*.

Promising newbies drawn to the naughtily named production included Tommy Jackson, an ambitious New York City actor with dreams of becoming a producer. He'd come to Nyack with his costar in the show *Broadway*, looking to flirt with pretty girls, blow off some steam, and see what everyone was talking about. What he found hooked him immediately. Jackson was bursting with the kind of energy that endeared him to one and all at the club, but especially to Bernard, who rarely let down his guard among members and students.

The actor never treated Bernard like a revered guru, Cheerie noted, "and even dared to kid him and got away with it." The new friends played baseball by day and cards on Sunday nights. They went to Madison Square Garden and the Hippodrome to see the fights—Bernard's longtime passion. Cheerie wisely observed that the pair "had one thing in common— both men were actors."

<hr />

Bernard was nothing if not a canny chameleon, capable of holding forth on ancient Hindu texts one night, throwing back peanut shells with Broadway showmen the next, then welcoming a Unitarian congregation to meet on Sundays at the Brick House in Upper Nyack. And with his right-hand man lost to the Vanderbilts, he proved himself equally adept at rearranging his leadership slots to accommodate the new generation of loyal adherents.

When Sir Paul turned over the Farm House to the CCC, he'd also relinquished his role as president of the club, a title Bernard passed along to Professor Lester M. Wilson of the Teachers College at Columbia University. He named another loyal number, Percival Whittlesey, assistant treasurer, reporting to longtime club secretary Edmund Dana. Then he turned his attentions outside the club grounds to what would become his first joint venture since his mortgage interest with Anne Vanderbilt in the Biophile Club Company. From Alfred G. Kay, whose anniversary had just been celebrated at the club, Bernard had secured $3.5 million in seed money to build and operate a chemical facility to make additives to poison industrial alcohol, to prevent it from being hijacked for bootleg alcoholic beverages. Once again, he'd found a way to capitalize on his philosophical tenets, this time through the caprices of Prohibition. Kay Research, as they called their venture, had already procured $5 million in federal contracts. Ground was broken for the factory in West Nyack in October, and it began operating in March 1927. Three years later the company moved a few miles north to Haverstraw and was incorporated as Kay-Fries Chemicals, Inc. It continued as a thriving business well into the Great Depression—and past the end of Prohibition—providing Bernard with yet another income stream.

<hr />

Bernard's distaste for booze obviously didn't carry over into his views of sex, but neither was he the free-love maniac he parodied in his shows. He was, in truth, a cheerleader for inspired coupling, and few things delighted him more than to preside over unions that had been initiated under his watch at the Clarkstown Country Club. "Until one has loved, the years are wasted," he told his flock one Saturday night.

That year, Bernard toasted the marriage of Leopold Stokowski to the heiress Evangeline Johnson. He hosted the wedding of Ruth Bartholomew and Oliver Judson, a good-looking Yalie who'd first come to the club in 1922 to get a handle on his drinking, and he blessed the engagement of her much-sought-after friend, Mildred Ryder, to a serious young man named

James Love Gillingham, whom she would marry the next year in a full-scale party and ceremony at the club.

But Bernard was equally wary of outsiders' claims on his most cherished members, and he didn't hesitate to step in to deter them from what he thought were bad choices. About that time, Cheerie became enamored of a handsome townie named Frank Perrino, whose family ran the taxi service in Nyack. He wanted to marry her, but she was wavering. "Again not trusting my own judgment, I asked P.A. to see me," she wrote. "With caution not to mention Frank, I told him I felt it time I should think of marriage. I didn't plan to live as a nun. I needed a normal married life. Surely yoga believed in a good marriage and I asked him as my guru, what advice could he give me in regard to marriage."

She'd found Bernard smoking a big cigar in his office, where he usually received visitors, and as she spoke, he looked at her quizzically. "I sensed his mistrust and didn't want to be caught in a trap, so I mentioned my brother was getting married and that made me think about my own future."

Visibly relieved, Bernard responded with good-natured, avuncular advice. "Cheerie, anyone can get married," he told her, "but with your training here and advancement in yoga and your talent you would soon find it a humdrum experience. You will need a husband to challenge you, someone to live up to and respect, someone having all the qualities you lack. Otherwise boredom would end in divorce and I don't want that for you. You are not ready yet. I'll find the right person for you."

Though she declined Bernard's offer to arrange her marriage, Cheerie heeded his words and put Frank on ice—a wise decision, for she was really in love with Tommy Jackson, who was also secretly smitten with her. Late one Saturday night, during her shift serving hot chocolate and doughnuts at the Cat's Whiskers, Bernard and Tommy Jackson came in and pulled up chairs at the big round table, talking about the importance of love in a man's life. Jackson, carried away with emotion, declared loudly enough for the entire room to hear: "Cheerie, I'm going to marry you." The young woman turned crimson and rushed away to the kitchen, not knowing whether this handsome, powerful, and influential man of the theater was serious or simply fooling around.

He was quite serious indeed.

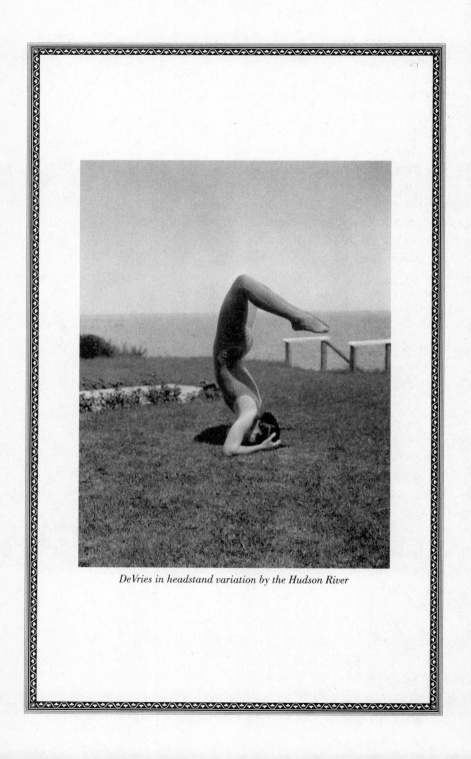

DeVries in headstand variation by the Hudson River

Chapter 18

BLUE SKIES, BIG PLANS

t the age of fifty, Bernard was as vigorous and fit as he had ever been—and brash enough to imagine new beginnings, not just for his young followers but for his relentlessly enterprising vision. He'd dipped into the manufacturing business with his joint venture with Kay Research and grown his menagerie to include pheasants, monkeys, goats, horses, a baby elephant, and a forty-foot South American snake. After Colonel Charles Lindbergh flew nonstop to Paris in thirty-three and a half hours and returned home an undisputed hero to "oceans of upturned friendly faces," Bernard, too, began to look skyward. It was the spring of 1927, and the entire nation had good reason to look up. The economy was beginning its furious ascent, drawing millions of first-timers into the market; waitresses and bus drivers were buying stocks on margin—sometimes with no money down—expecting risk-free dividends and unending gains. Ever the spiritual pragmatist, Bernard thought, Airplanes need places to land, don't they? And so he embarked on the biggest expansion yet of his club's activities: his own airport and flying club.

In those days, even without Anne Vanderbilt's help, money was not a problem. The wealthy members of the next generation, like the Wertheim sisters, played their part willingly, paying a financial bonus for his personal attention. For mere financial mortals and most other students, Bernard never charged more than $100 a year in dues to join the club (plus $2.50 a night to visit). To grow and build and flourish—to extend knowledge of "the work," as he would have put it himself—it was necessary for yoga to

have an influx of new American Medicis as well as new attractions for this
full-speed-ahead, thrill-seeking age.

Tommy Jackson was rarely seen up at Nyack in 1927, with *Broadway* in the
middle of a long run that had made him the toast of Manhattan. He'd begun
taking his girlfriend Cheerie Smith deeper into his world, escorting her to
the Rose Room, where Tommy bantered with the likes of Robert Benchley
and Robert Nathan, to Cheerie's astonishment, along with Scott Fitzgerald, Sinclair Lewis, Irving Cobb, Dorothy Parker, and Edna Ferber.

That year, her friend Clara Thorpe, the most talented dancer of all
the Nyack yoginis, decided to go into show business in a serious way herself. While Cheerie was dating Tommy Jackson, Clara had met a fellow
dancer named Richard Stuart at the club in Nyack. The two formed a
professional partnership as ballroom dancers and were married the next
year. As Lea & Stuart, they combined asanas with artsy, modern pas de
deux, reuniting yoga with popular dance on the stage, as Ruth St. Denis
had some twenty years before.

Then in March 1928, on a Saturday night in Nyack, it was Cheerie's
turn at the altar—*finally*, in her opinion. Bernard and DeVries stood as
joyful witnesses to the marriage of Llellwyn "Cheerie" Smith and Thomas
Jackson. Cheerie had been living with Bernard for more than eight years,
and told all who asked that everything she valued in life she had learned
from him. She asked his blessing this one last time, and he gave it, holding the ceremonies at his and DeVries's home, the Farm House. With the
departure of Clara and Cheerie, the first generation of America's trained
yoginis had flown from the Bernard-DeVries nest.

Bernard, now fully immersed in the face-lift he'd designed for the CCC,
had enough energy left over to get in on the new craze for flying. "Two
factors in our civilization have been greatly overemphasized," wrote
E. B. White of the year 1928. "One is aviation, the other is sex." Boosters
of amateur aeronautics assured the public that flying was easy. The gung-
ho slogan of the American Society for the Promotion of Aviation was "An
airport in every town." The society set about selling do-it-yourself aviation
to the general public through the formation of boosterish flying clubs all

across the nation—from Harvard to Hollywood—promoting amateur air shows and stunt pilots, along with dreams of long distances and shorter times. Everyone, it seemed, wanted to at least go up for a ride; every day the papers ran pictures of the floppy-helmeted, goggled, and bescarfed young heroes of the skies.

Nobody seemed to understand this better than Bernard, whose life had been devoted to the close study of desire and other flights of the soul. As a fan of science and technology as well as a Tantric yogi eager for new experience, he, too, sought the experience of flight. But Bernard had by this time conjured a more fully formed picture of the skies of the future. Even the dimmest Babbitts of the land could foresee that there would soon be huge sums of money to be made in airmail, air freight, and airlines for passenger transport. He saw like-minded men and women coming together under his leadership, starting a school to train pilots and then other teachers and then, perhaps, building an airport that would put little Nyack on the national map. Since Bernard was known as something of an organizational genius in the lower Hudson River Valley, nary a soul objected when the Rockland Aero Club, after two initial meetings in 1928, moved its headquarters to the guru's Clarkstown Country Club. And nobody objected—in fact, quite the contrary—when Bernard was persuaded by popular vote to accept the presidency of the club.

First grow the club, Bernard commanded as their president; then incorporate, get as many members as possible licensed and up into the skies, start a school, and then you can brag about your town as one of the nation's new air traffic hubs. The Friday night meetings filled up, the gung-ho audience roared with applause at the films and lectures; the immediate goal to recruit a hundred members to the Rockland Aero Club was easily surpassed by the end of March. Just as he had created the Tantrik Order three decades earlier and organized semipro baseball at the start of the 1920s (not to mention the shows and circuses), he now re-created himself as the aviation czar. He appointed the Aero Club's committees, wrote the charter for incorporation, hired his friends as lawyers, publicists, and trainers, and opened up lines of communication to the federal government—all of which was merely a prelude to finding a suitable training field, a mission that one local flier had tried to accomplish for more than three years, and failed. Now the job was put in Bernard's hands, and frankly, everyone expected nothing short of total success.

His first act was to volunteer the services of two club members: the musician John Jacob Niles, who, in addition to being a popular figure at the CCC music school, was a veteran World War I airman with the American Expeditionary Forces in Europe, and the English author Major Francis Yeats-Brown of the Seventeenth Bengal Lancers, who as the CCC's soldier intellectual—the Sandhurst version of Sir Paul Dukes— was Bernard's ideal Tantrik hero. Yeats-Brown was a thinking man of action who had studied yoga in its birthplace, India, and had publicly endorsed "Bernard's insight into the true meaning of the ancient Sanskrit texts." And the major had flown missions with the Allies in Mesopotamia, thus making him the perfect partner for Niles to lecture, teach, and explain firsthand the wonders and exigencies of motorized flight. It's likely that Bernard did not dwell upon the fact that both had suffered harrowing, near fatal airplane crashes in their short flying careers.

Bernard also pulled from the large pool of Great War veterans in the area—various Brits and Aussies among them—as well as European nobility like the Italian flier Count Ernesto Casamello. Every Friday night that spring, Bernard hosted his flying buddies and ran the meeting. His plan was to avoid associating with the bumblers in other amateur clubs; instead they would partner with the U.S. government, who would surely be the biggest player in air traffic. Bernard announced that his flight school would certify pilots of all kinds, "transport pilot, limited commercial pilot, industrial pilot or private pilot." The members heard lectures about all types of aircraft—blimps, dirigibles, and gliders—and how to fly them. They cheered the films of Byrd's and Amundsen's polar flights and Lindy's triumphant puddle hop. In April, Bernard was reelected to the presidency of a permanent organization.

Even the Saturday night yoga lectures were fodder for Bernard's aeronautical ambitions. The club was fairly empty in winter and early spring—many of the well-to-do members were in Palm Springs or Palm Beach—but the hard core were present for Bernard's new take on the old Tantric values of *experience* and *imagination*. To be a true Tantric yogi, he explained, is to approach life as an art, something to be learned—like aviation. Go flying if you like, he said; race cars, grow flowers, dance, sing, walk the tightrope, but do something. Tantriks are interested in every aspect of life, Bernard explained—"all departments are encompassed within the underlying principles of growth, health, and betterment."

On May 7 Bernard squinted into the afternoon sky at the sound of a small biplane approaching his home. As it came closer and circled his property, he realized that here was indeed the sign: The deal was done! He and his boys had pulled off the impossible. They had acquired the sixty-acre plot they were seeking, just eight miles from Nyack and three miles from the Hudson River. Not only did they get the beautiful flat land at Schomberg Farms for the first airport in the county; they had leased it for six years—with no rent due the first year.

Preparations began immediately to prepare the field for takeoffs and landings: volunteers filled and leveled the ground and put up lights and markers. A local farmer, whose own spread was close by, was bought off with a membership in the club and the right to sell snacks and gasoline.

The new Rockland Airport opened Memorial Day weekend to great, noisy fanfare. Twenty-five hundred attendees watched more than fifty aerial stunts; the bravest spectators went up for their first airplane rides. Fliers buzzed the crowd and performed barrel rolls, half rolls, loops, and tailspins, even the dangerous "falling leaf" stunt, designed to give shivers to the uninitiated. Three powerful new Waco planes flew in from Curtiss Field on Long Island to do the opening-day honors, and the celebration went off without a hitch until late in the rainy afternoon, when the main attraction, a young parachutist, slipped while exiting the cockpit of his airplane and fell to the earth, his chute unopened.

Bernard helped take the body back to Nyack, and he called his fliers together to lead them in a unanimous vote to purchase a wreath to send to the dead man's mother. He reassured the Aero Club members that field conditions were perfect, despite the rainy weather, and that the organization bore no responsibility for the accident. The parachutist's death, however tragic, was considered a mere bump in the road of local aeronautical progress. The memory of the young man's death was drowned out by day's end in a drumbeat of stories about progress at the airfield.

Eight of the club's pilots, who had pooled their assets to purchase a $6,000 three-passenger transport plane, asked that they be allowed to form a school. At the time, a pilot's license required only ten hours of solo flying, and the motion passed easily. Niles and Yeats-Brown had plenty to do—and both had day jobs, to boot—so Bernard installed as vice president a British aviator from Upper Nyack with the wonderful name of W. I. N. Strong. Space was provided for Strong to set up an office at

Bernard's Moorings estate, the property formerly owned by Barbara Rutherfurd, though the large meetings would still be held at the Eagle's Nest. Plans were then made to start an informal passenger service, with Bernard's guests and yoga followers first on the list.

"Have you been up yet?" That was the question on everyone's lips in Nyack by the fall of 1928. Every Saturday, some fifty-five people paid their $5 and took in a bird's-eye view of their county, swooping along the length of Rockland Lake and over Hook Mountain, the glacier-carved hills and valleys rising up like storm-tossed oceans. The spectacular new point of view had made the town flying crazy.

The club began bringing to its meetings the most renowned Great War heroes. René Fonck, the French "ace of aces" who had dispatched more than forty German warplanes—including a record six in one day with only fifty-five bullets!—came to rub shoulders with Bernard and the locals. "Dr. Pierre Bernard, president of the club, is greatly interested in getting all the national and international aces possible to lecture before the club," said the *Evening Journal*, "for the personal acquaintance with the boys."

Life at the CCC continued, with yoga in the morning and acrobatics classes every afternoon, personally coached by Bernard. DeVries was occupied with completing interior design work on the new Washington, D.C., home of Frances Payne Bolton, whose husband, Chester, had just been elected to the U.S. Congress. Most nights in Nyack, however, there were clubhouse card games into the wee hours, usually hearts. On Friday nights, Bernard introduced his European aces and showed war films to the Aero Club. On Saturdays, the lectures returned to the subject of yoga and its relationship to the good life, which, in keeping with the predominant salutary fads of 1928, was to be approached through "the power tube"—Bernard-speak for the colon: "Auto-intoxication, in the world at large, exists to a point that is unimaginable," he said. "When you have cleaned up the blood stream and established healthy habits, there is little more necessary to be done. The colon is not a warehouse—but only an exit. Keep it empty. Fifteen minutes of daily abdominal exercise will do more for your gut than a sixty mile walk. . . . Don't mope around in pathological states—take a Hi E."

These were the glory days of internal cleansing, the hallmark of John Harvey Kellogg's Battle Creek, Michigan, sanitarium, where five enemas a day were recommended for beginners. But for Bernard, the idea of internal purification was more than just commonsense plumbing: it was closer to a yoga sacrament. "An enema, thoroughly given, requires a good hour's work, and both the operator and the patient will be perspiring," he said. "If you are Monistic and have studied matter and its constitution, you will see how romantic it is. Matter in its last analysis is so fine that it can be termed pure force. The Vedic concept is that we come out of food, live through food, and when we die, return to food. In this light, the whole world is food. . . . The saying of 'Grace' may be for the purpose of producing in us a certain state of mind and heart towards the food we eat. We have a duty towards food after it goes into the mouth—there Yoga can teach us what it is! . . . What you put into your tube, becomes you."

By late October, as president of the Rockland Aeros, Bernard had completed a deal with the U.S. Department of Commerce to use his airport as a way station and emergency landing field on the New York to Albany to Montreal and Buffalo mail route. The federal government would maintain the field, pave it, light it, and spend $25,000 for improvements, all of it a giant boon for the county. And the best part? "Under the terms negotiated by Dr. Bernard, club members will continue to have the use of the field for their private flying and meanwhile obtain these enormous advantages for nothing," reported a local newspaper.

While thousands of communities across the nation were still dreaming of an airport, the guru of Nyack had pulled it off, the local paper noted. "It will put Rockland County on the new aerial map of the United States in which the progress of this country is being written today with amazing speed."

Bernard, who turned fifty-two on October 31, 1928, had attained the respect of the entire Nyack community, which now regarded him as the organizational magician who had brought baseball and air travel to Nyack. His stature as a solid citizen was so well established that year that nobody gave it a second thought when a famous Unitarian minister named Charles Francis Potter came to the club in April to speak to the congregation that had been meeting in Tantrik territory for about a year.

Potter and Bernard would go on to become close friends, but for the moment the clergyman's reputation was useful for Oom's latest academic venture. In October 1928, Bernard marshaled his wealth and his connections—including Potter—to begin his most ambitious effort yet to legitimize yoga. At the monthlong First India Conference, held in New York City, he introduced the International School for Vedic and Allied Research, ISVAR, whose mission was to promote better understanding of Vedic culture, especially hatha yoga, which was still misunderstood in the West. ISVAR would seek to establish professorships at major universities, publish scholarly works, create student exchange programs (something Bernard had been doing on his own for years), and set up educational programs in Europe and India. Bernard agreed to fund these efforts and pay the salary of an Indian scholar named Pandit Jagadish Chandra Chatterji, who would lead the group's efforts in the United States and overseas. ISVAR attracted to its board heavyweight scholars from major American universities and began its work in an office in the Times Tower in midtown Manhattan.

The staff was populated with Bernard's friends, including Professor Sunder Joshi of Dartmouth and Viola Wertheim, who signed on to be Chatterji's assistant, commuting from Nyack to Manhattan when she was needed in the office.

ISVAR's animating idea, and Bernard's as well, was to promote respect for India's ancient culture and for yoga as a practical science—a technology for living a better life—the modern way to health and happiness.

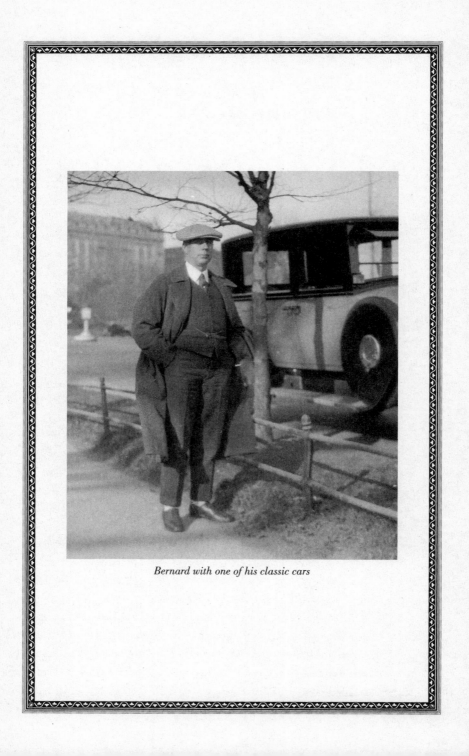

Bernard with one of his classic cars

Chapter 19

A LEAP OF FAITH

y 1929 American culture was besotted with the proposition that what was new had to be good. The Museum of Modern Art opened its doors in New York City that year, and that quintessentially modern trope, the "sexual revolution," first appeared in popular print in Thurber and White's book *Is Sex Necessary?* which poked gentle fun at the shift in morals that had already taken place.

Of course, it paid to be modern in 1929. That year saw the height of what came to be generally known as "new era investing," a modern economic fable that fueled Wall Street's Great Bull Run with the promise of never-ending growth in stock values. Radio went from a public service to a profitable entertainment, and the print media reinvented itself once more with a raft of new magazines for movie fans.

The new era at the CCC, heralded by the brochure for the summer 1929 season, was a bounteous menu of physical exercise, learning, and entertainment. "We advise you to enlarge your health program," Dr. and Mrs. Bernard wrote. "Take advantage of the scope of our libraries and cooperate with us in our attempt to provide deluxe service in all departments." They rechristened yoga studies the "physical re-education program," and their extracurricular options expanded well beyond the baseball diamond and the airport. There was the enclosed swimming pool, four professional tennis courts, and this year a private forty-eight-foot yacht named the *Queen of Spades*. The place was truly becoming what Bernard had always dreamed of: a completely idiosyncratic institution of learning, an academy for life. There was the Seymour Music Summer School for children and adults; the Inner Circle Theatre, whose members taught dancing of all kinds from tap to ballet to acrobatic; and Eddie Evans's circus skills studio, where lessons in acrobatics, tumbling, and tightrope walking were given. Another veteran circus performer, Josie DeMott Robinson, taught equestrian stunt riding, including bareback acrobatics on moving horses. There was Bernard's lending library, now grown to seven thousand volumes. The club maintained its own herd and dairy, ice-making machinery, orchards, and farm, providing fresh butter and cream and fruits and vegetables for meals and selling the rest down in the village.

The members particularly enjoyed the weekend Open Forum lectures, which gave them a chance to see and hear esteemed speakers interact with Bernard. On one such night in January 1929, the topic was phrenology and the speaker was Miss Jessie Fowler, the last of the Phrenological Fowlers. The acclaimed Miss Fowler, seventy years old, commenced her reading extemporaneously as she traced the bumps, contours, and peculiarities of Bernard's skull.

> More than average energy—Pep—Development of executive ability—Much will, likes his own way. Full development of self-esteem. Likes to plan own efforts, and goes from one subject to another in a very effective way.

Fowler was "reading a head," in the parlance of phrenology. With her sterling lineage—her father and uncle were renowned in the field— decades of experience, and a large collection of animal and human skulls, she radiated authority. In London, she'd read the skulls of Mark Twain and Sir Arthur Conan Doyle.

A reading didn't predict the subject's fate but merely directed him where to concentrate efforts in self-improvement—an approach that placed her philosophically right at home at the Clarkstown Country Club. She continued with Bernard.

> Very conscientious—has the consciousness of right and wrong, duty and obligation. Desires to do the right thing—does not want to do business [with anyone] who makes a promise and breaks it.

Tremendous degree of honesty. . . . Able to understand the needs of other people—will make sacrifices himself to gratify the needs and desires of others. . . . Head very high. More than average veneration. Perceptives very well represented. Thinks, plans, arranges, solves problems with anterior part of brain. Should invent things. Such as some device to keep autos from going so fast.

Fowler's reading must have set off a few chortles in the audience. First of all, it couldn't have been more accurate, as those who knew Bernard could attest. He admitted that she got him just right—him, Bernard, the unerring reader of the character of others. And the next month's big excitement—a police chief's drunken trespass on the CCC flower beds—would no doubt have made Bernard recall her words and wish he had invented a device to slow down a speeding car.

On February 15 Bernard awoke to an explosion of shattering glass. A runaway coupe, occupied by three drunkards carrying a cargo of bootleg liquor, had driven past the gates of the club and plowed through flower beds and landscaped gardens until finally it crashed into the glass-covered swimming pool. Bernard ran from his bed and over to the club grounds in his pajamas, in time to watch the runaway car revving up for another pass.

He telephoned the South Nyack police, and within minutes a squad car came roaring up the driveway, sirens blaring, the officers with guns drawn. Shots rang out—one, two, three, more—but the little coupe refused to halt. Bernard watched in mute horror as the policemen in their pursuit doubled the damage to his gardens. Finally the vandals' coupe slammed into a wire fence, recoiled into the air, and landed upside down.

Laid out on the ground amid Bernard's shredded shrubs, flat on his back in full uniform amid gallon jugs of apple whiskey, was Harold Nutter, the unpopular chief of police of a neighboring town called Grand View—*hated* was more like it, because Nutter and his force had a reputation for handing out speeding tickets with egregious frequency for their tiny jurisdiction. With him were two inebriated deputies, who were, they tried to explain to the arresting officer, delivering a load of hooch to Bernard. Chief Nutter, too drunk to walk, had nearly as much trouble speaking. "Came to deliver applejack t'oom," Chief Nutter said to the arresting officer. "T'Oom. Tuh Oom it may concern."

Confronted with a list of charges that included driving without a license and trespassing, Nutter burst into tears and was led away to a holding cell. In the judge's chambers, a hearing determined that the chief was lucky to be alive: during the chase up South Mountain, six bullets had actually penetrated Nutter's car, one punching through the windshield and another penetrating the gas tank. Bernard appeared in court to tell the judge he had not ordered the applejack—his club was dry and everyone knew it—and there was not a person in the hearing room who doubted his word. It was a coup for the new local news czar, Robert J. Setchanove, a sworn enemy of Bernard, whose story starring the Omnipotent Oom, the corrupt Chief Nutter, and a load of black-market applejack played to the blue-collar locals who still harbored a distaste for the guru on the hill. But Bernard himself laughed off the incident and refused to press for damages.

In March, celebrating a decade of growth and prosperity and a healthy sense of self-effacing parody, the club staged the CCC Orgies of 1929. This particular production was subtitled *A Chauve-Souris*, after a popular European touring company that put on a revue of twenty speedy scenes in two acts. But for this, the most elaborate production yet of the Inner Circle Theatre Company, the Nyack troupe would present its evening of international merriment in "forty rounds," a nightlong boxing match of singing and dancing, with Bernard as referee and Alfred G. Kay and Lester Wilson as judges. Most of the old gang made it back to Nyack to perform in the event—Diana and Viola Wertheim, Percival Whittlesey, Constance Seeger, Clara and Richard Stuart, Marie Louise Schreiner, the Powell sisters, Millie Ryder and her new husband, James Gillingham, along with a distinguished new member, Henry Goldmark, close chum of Teddy Roosevelt and designer of the locks for the Panama Canal, who acted in a skit called *The Three Musketeers*.

DeVries took charge of the choreography, costumes, and stage settings; Di and Vi wrote the lyrics for the original songs, which poked fun at phrenology and the popular press; and the evening concluded with a Russian-inspired feast at midnight. Right before intermission Bernard brought in Baby, the young elephant he'd been training for the past three years.

Two of Bernard's favorite people, leading performers that night, had circled each other romantically for years. Diana Hunt Wertheim and Percival Wilcox Whittlesey made a striking physical match. "She was very tall," according to her daughter Joan Wofford. "Five feet ten or eleven. I could always find her in a crowd. He was six feet. He was very attractive, with light blue eyes and sandy hair, a good deal older than she, 12 years older, and very bright." They both held Phi Beta Kappa keys; each was curious, rebellious, and headstrong; and Whittlesey had just been promoted from assistant treasurer to executive VP of the CCC.

On Memorial Day, they took the plunge. More than two hundred guests, including dozens of club members, traveled by private rail car to Elburon, New Jersey, for the wedding, which was covered in the *New York Times* society pages. The writer Hamish McLaurin took time out from a book he was writing on Bernard and yoga to stand in as Percival's best man. Viola was Diana's bridesmaid.

Over the past two years, Bernard had formed strong ties with the First Unitarian Church of Nyack, the liberal-minded Sunday tenants of his meeting room at the Brick House. Bernard, who had little use for most organized religion, began including news of their meetings in his club newsletter, celebrating the "eminent visiting ministers" who addressed the congregation and expressing the high regard he held for them. The Unitarians, he wrote, "have incorporated as much of Eastern teachings as the West can stand. They seem to want as much Yoga as they can get." It was something of a love match: Unitarians believed that the combination of Eastern wisdom and Western practicality, Bernard's specialty and life's work, would yield great benefits to those of all religions. "Yoga doesn't present itself to any one group of people from a blood standpoint," Bernard wrote. "But it appeals only to a certain grade of body, heart and mind. It pierces the orthodoxy of all religious systems, and may be called the philosophy of mental medicine."

Echoing a belief of Carl Jung, who had, incidentally, begun to experiment with Tantric yoga in Switzerland, Bernard maintained that if yoga was presented in a Christian context, it would be a success. And so he cultivated his budding relationship with Charles Francis Potter, a virtuoso of Christian language, whom he had conscripted the year before to help out with ISVAR. A liberal even among Unitarians, Potter had achieved a national reputation in 1923 for his role in a series of widely covered public debates dubbed "The Battle over the Bible." His opponent was the fundamentalist Baptist preacher Dr. John Roach Straton. Darwin's theory of evolution had fueled the confrontation, but the debates mainly addressed the larger question of whether the Bible was literally true and historically accurate.

It was billed as science versus religion in four rounds, the debates broadcast on the fledgling WTKK radio network while thousands attended in person. This early Bible battle set the stage for the national interest in the Scopes Monkey Trial in 1925, and Potter had been there for that, too, sitting at the counselors' table, providing expert guidance to Clarence Darrow as the court decided the fate of John Scopes, who dared to teach the theory of evolution in a public school in Tennessee. So the Reverend Mr. Potter had something of a reputation to think about when he arrived in Nyack to preach at the CCC, which for all Bernard's recent successes hadn't entirely shaken itself of the risqué reputation that had colored its early years.

Potter had certainly heard the rumors, perhaps from Darrow himself, who'd visited the club in the early 1920s. "Strange tales were told me of the weird rites and unholy orgies of a secret inner circle," Potter wrote. "It was said to be a love-cult where adepts, under the hypnotic eye of the Ever-loving Guru of Tantrik Yoga, pranced and danced naked in mystic gyration."

Potter had just finished writing a book called *The Story of Religion*, for which he had immersed himself in the historical facts about the lives of the major figures of the world's faiths. Now he was intent on sizing up this Oom character himself, to take his measure man-to-man. Potter didn't realize that in his early visits to the club, *he* was being sized up by its resident manager. "He always liked to puzzle people a bit when he first met them," Potter wrote. "It was, as I learned later, a part of his system of measuring their IQ and reaction time."

Evidently Potter fared well enough in this first test, for Bernard welcomed the preacher into the fold and gave him the run of his club, his library, and his thinking. Potter in turn came away from these early meetings with increasing respect for a fellow student of the world's religions.

Many late-night discussions followed, and Potter came to the conclusion that Bernard was truly a genius in the rough: "He was both prophet and showman who could lecture on any religion with singular penetration and discernment, and, with equal facility, could stage a big circus, manage a winning ball team, superintend the construction of a large building, or put on an exhibition of magic which rivaled Houdini. He knew the human body, anatomically and every other way, to such an extent as to amaze veteran surgeons and physicians."

In September 1929, Potter took a leap of faith, bewildered his friends, and moved his family into one of the club's residences in Upper Nyack. The preacher had so thoroughly gained Bernard's trust that he was commissioned to write a history of the CCC and allowed to interview some of the recovery cases at the club, which had continued to function as a retreat for the addicted and emotionally disabled. Potter assessed that Bernard was "particularly successful with nervous cases, such as neurasthenia, melancholia, suicidal mania and the like, and he will be looked back on a few years hence as a pioneer in the methods of treating sexual pathology. Part of the talk about love cults doubtless originated from his work in that field." But the great majority of members, Potter found, were healthy, curious individuals in serious pursuit of their yoga studies, and Bernard's advice, he noted, went a long way toward easing their anxiety as they pushed away from the moorings of their old-time religions. "In yoga training you must pass through the 'crying period,'" Bernard said one night. "You can't duck the tears—sometimes this period lasts months or even a year. Then the tears stop. Later you no longer look through a fog, but can see clearly. When the heart helps you see, the mist clears, you understand, and have an infallible, unshakeable Faith. The formal must pass away before you can reach the essential."

<hr />

While Potter was buffing up Bernard's spiritual credibility, Blanche DeVries and her entourage were preparing for a CCC circus of unprecedented scope. All two thousand $10 tickets to the September 7 social event of the year were sold out in advance. Musical groups were booked from India as well as from the southern United States for two performances, one in the late afternoon and one in the evening, after which well-connected Rocklanders and New Yorkers would revel until breakfast was served under the big top at dawn. Bernard was planning to let audiences see a few of the new tricks he'd taught Baby, now dubbed the club's official mascot.

Two days before the opening of the circus, however, weather reports for Saturday cast an ominous shadow on the coming days' activities, and worse, a gossip reporter from the *Daily News* uncovered details of the program's main events and began to embroider them into a tabloid fantasy: "As darkness falls on Oom's domains, DeVries, who is the wife of Oom—whose earthly name is Dr. Pierre Bernard—will offer the pièce-de-résistance. Garbed in a wispy shroud designed to make any ghost feel cool, DeVries will arise in a casket twisting her torso and moan 'That man has got the whole world in his hands.' . . ."

Next, the reporter wrote, a troupe of "colored ballet dancers imported from Dixie will pound their heads on the floor before DeVries and croon a dirge. As DeVries settles back into the coffin, Oom himself will go into his dance," signifying to his adoring cult that he, Bernard, is "that man" who holds the world in his hands.

At least the weather report turned out to be accurate. The skies stayed clear in the early part of Saturday, and the first show went off without a hitch, lasting until midnight. But then the rains began, followed by severe thunderstorms, and the rest of the evening was canceled. Robert Setchanove's *Rockland County Evening Journal*, still the declared enemy of Oom and his club, reported the canceled show on Monday with malicious glee, noting that the torrential rains, in a sign of disapproval from the heavens, had not only stopped the show but nearly torn down Bernard's big top.

The second-show washout turned out to be a portent for debacles of much greater consequences. On September 3, the stock market had reached its all-time high, but from that day forward Wall Street had begun to wobble. On October 24, over 12 million shares were sold, prices fell swiftly, and thousands of investors appeared to be wiped out. A late-day rally turned the market around, but something palpable had changed. Fear, the uninvited guest, had insisted on being factored into the sunny calculations of "new era investing." The bubble was about to burst.

There was little immediate reaction to Black Tuesday, October 29, in small towns like Nyack. Life went on, since fewer than 1 million Americans, less than 1 percent of the U.S. population at the time, actually possessed the stocks that fell victim to the Wall Street crash. The cascade of economic damage began stealthily, with dwindling share prices wiping

out the capital needed to run corporations. Within months, rising unemployment had cast its pall on the Hudson Valley; the word *relief* began
appearing with some regularity in the pages of the *Evening Journal*.

In Nyack, however, Bernard displayed nothing but faith in the
future. He added to his automobile collection one of the largest and
most extravagant cars ever fabricated: a new baby-blue Minerva with
mahogany-trimmed interior and African-ivory window and door handles.
As cavernous as a limousine-and-a-half, the Minerva featured a foldaway
dining table and a full set of Wedgwood china for auto-camping in deluxe
style. Bernard's land and his property, estimated to be two hundred acres
at this time, were all his, owned outright. The number of wealthy folk who
were coming to his club was still growing. To his favored few he spoke
of his grand plans for further expansion. He envisioned a great sports
center that would draw people from all over the state—to watch boxing,
baseball, wrestling, to attend state fairs and outdoor theater. And he was
already planning with architect Howard Greenley the construction of a
new, modern, and up-to-date clubhouse, the centerpiece of the Clarkstown
Country Club properties.

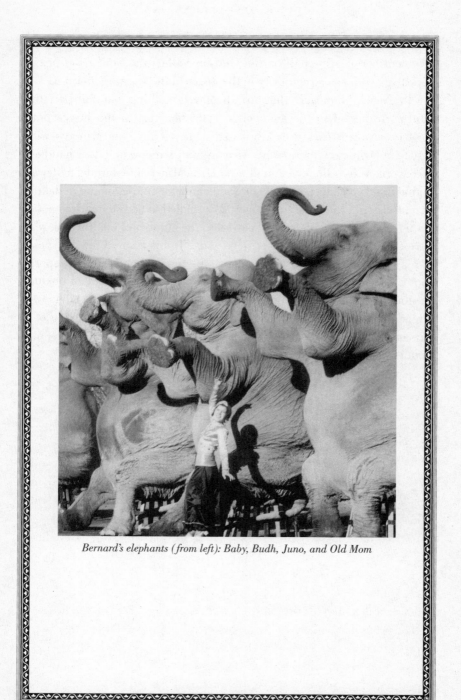
Bernard's elephants (from left): Baby, Budh, Juno, and Old Mom

Chapter 20

GOOD TIMES, BAD TIMES

It feels funny to take money from elephants. But what can
you do in hard times like these?

—Pierre Bernard

verybody lies a little, especially when Uncle Sam comes
snooping around. On April 28, 1930, a U.S. census taker
passed through South Nyack, totting up the particulars of
this Hudson River village of some seven hundred homes and
two thousand citizens. This year, along with the usual data collected on
household size, occupations, and property values, the federal government
wanted to know how many Americans were in possession of the technological marvel of its day—a radio receiving set. Bernard didn't mind answering that one truthfully—and affirmatively—or including his mother,
Kittie, and her husband among the members of his household. He listed
his occupation as teacher, and with a straight face claimed he was paying
rent of $250 a month for his mansion and thirty-nine acres on the hill.

These humble personal statistics aside, Bernard's ambitions that year
were as grand as ever, the Great Depression be damned. New discoveries
about the history of early Vedic civilizations in archaeology and philology circles increased interest in the work being done at his yoga think
tank, ISVAR. He encouraged his man Chatterji to establish branches in

Benares and in London, fund archaeological digs, publish journals, and start a speakers' bureau. In this ongoing attempt to find legitimate contact points between the ancient civilizations of Asia and the modern West, Bernard sought to enlarge the school's reach to a global level.

Chatterji himself had his own ideas, however. He had blown through $31,000 (the equivalent of $350,000 today) in Bernard's seed money with casual accounting and not much to show for it. He insisted on running ISVAR as a dictatorship and refused to answer to anyone—not the board, not even Bernard, his chief means of support. When Chatterji remained obstinate, Bernard finally cut off funding and dissociated himself from the group. Chatterji, outraged, began demanding even larger sums of money, in addition to the promise of inheriting Bernard's entire Nyack real estate holdings. The hotheaded Indian scholar threatened lawsuits, more bad publicity, and reprisals if he didn't get his way. When Bernard stonewalled him, Chatterji tried to blackmail Potter, warning that he would seek to damage the clergyman's reputation unless he took sides against Bernard. ISVAR soon collapsed, but in the end it wasn't just the internecine squabbling that killed it, but the economic morass of the times. Viola Wertheim, who'd served as Chatterji's assistant for two years, returned to the Nyack fold, continuing to work with DeVries in her decorating business and pondering what to do about her own career.

By the autumn of 1930, the Depression had settled into Rockland County. One by one, small businesses along Broadway and Main Street in Nyack fell on hard times, shuttered, and closed. What few opportunities arose for working-class people, like the Orangeburg Hospital construction project, drew applicants from as far away as California and Canada. There was an occasional suicide attributed to "financial matters," and sad, random acts of desperation—fake Salvation Army collectors going door-to-door in Nyack, a husband and wife leaving six starving children behind to look for work in New York City. The need for "relief" was by now a drumbeat in curbside conversations and in the news.

In October, Governor Franklin Delano Roosevelt came to Nyack and presided over a capacity crowd at a rally to whip up support for his re-election. It was hardly necessary; Rockland County, like the nation, had lost faith in Herbert Hoover and his party, and the November elections reflected this. The Democrats swept to power across the state of New York, with FDR leading the charge and winning every township in the county.

Bernard was aware that tough times had hit, but his response was to charge into an uncertain future with the most aggressive building project of his career. By January 1931, the plans were finalized, permissions granted, and the work commenced. The new Eagle's Nest was going to be an extravagant $3 million affair, partly of Bernard's own design, a short distance from the stately old Bradley House, which would later be razed.

Bernard and the members stayed at the Bradley while the construction got going. Club activities were held to a minimum—it was the dead of winter, after all—but the Nyack community was basking in the windfall of the sudden appearance of more than a hundred new jobs for local laborers at good wages of $4 a day. Like many Americans, Bernard felt that the bottom of the stock market would soon be reached, and the economy would recover in due time. He would be ready for this new dawn with a freshly revamped institution. A new nationally known headquarters for yoga? He was a gambler by nature, but this seemed like a sure thing.

On March 12, his mother, Kittie Martin, died at her son's estate. She was seventy-five years old. Kittie left a modest legacy—a savings account and an *Encyclopaedia Britannica*—to be divided among the four sons she bore with her second husband, John Bernard. These men—Glen, Ervin, Ray, and Clyde Bernard—had settled in the West and lived modest, anonymous lives that had nothing to do with Pierre. Two of them owed money to Kittie at her death. In excluding Pierre from her meager life savings and set of books, she knew there would be no chance of hard feelings. She'd seen with her own eyes the luxurious life enjoyed by the son she had named Perry, the son whose generosity extended not only to her but to her husband, Robert, both of whom had lived with him for the last years of her life. On the other hand, Kittie's death failed to bring her sons together in any meaningful way. Even Glen, who shared Pierre's love of yoga and had joined the Tantriks in the West for a time, had parted company with his brother more than twenty years before and never let go of his old grudges against Pierre.

At Kittie's funeral, Charles Potter comforted Bernard and stood with him next to the elaborate, cost-be-damned copper coffin Bernard had chosen for his mother. Potter listened to Bernard's tales of Kittie and life on the old Iowa farm and again noted to himself what a warm, open, and misjudged man this was.

In April, during the quiet months before the summer season

began, Potter sought out an open-minded reporter from the *New York World-Telegram*—it was probably Joe Mitchell, writing anonymously—and on May 7, 1931, for the first time ever in a New York City newspaper, Bernard was granted a sane and literate defense of his life and his devotion to yoga. "Oom Is a Sound Theologian, Not a Charlatan, Says Dr. Potter, Promising to Explode Accounts of Nyack Cults and Orgies."

After studying Bernard and his yoga club for more than a year, Potter attested that he found no evidence of fishy stuff—Bernard's people were puritanical even in their devotion to health. He went so far as to say that the guru of Nyack had "all the earmarks of genius" and compared him to the major religious figures in his 1929 best seller, *The Story of Religion*, which included Jesus, Mohammed, and Gautama Buddha. He pointed out that Professor Lester Wilson of Columbia University had been the Clarkstown Country Club's president for the past five years, and that Bernard's influence was growing far and wide. "There are groups of yoga students acknowledging [Bernard's] mastership in Florida, California and elsewhere in the country," the story concluded. With his wholesale approval, the well-respected Potter bestowed on Bernard a legitimacy that would fend off his detractors for years.

That same month Bernard let it drop that he had secured for himself a seat on the board of directors of two reputable banking institutions in Rockland County: the Ramapo Trust Company of Spring Valley and the State Bank of Pearl River. Yogi, aviation expert, animal trainer, baseball manager, architect, and now banker—there wasn't a single aspect of Rockland County's civilian life that Bernard didn't dominate. At the same time, the construction of the new forty-three-room clubhouse was under way and more than one hundred local men were still busy at work. And not to be lost in all the hoopla was the midyear arrival of a second baby elephant, named Budh—short for Buddha—who joined Baby in the club's elephant barn at the Bradley estate. Budh, born in Nepal, was said to be a gift of one of Bernard's oldest Indian friends, Dr. P. C. Banerjee.

Bernard continued to acquire and sell small parcels of land whenever opportunity permitted, even as he gave up his interest in the airport property because of thorny legal issues that had made his investment of time and money futile. And then, without his leadership and support, the Aero Club simply dissolved, just as the Nyack Athletic Association had six years before—nobody, it seems, could match his energy or fill his managerial shoes. In June, Bernard purchased a beautiful twenty-two-acre plot on the side of South Mountain, across South Highland Avenue from the main grounds. He sold part of the land to Diana's mother, Emma Wertheim, and she began to build a palatial Tudor-Norman home that she named Sky Island—primarily to be near her daughters. The two young women were spending nearly all of their time in Nyack these days, and her eldest, Diana, was thinking about starting a family.

Viola, meanwhile, had spent much of the last six years immersed in the club and was getting restless. After her stint at ISVAR, she'd decided that she wanted her own career, something serious and perhaps even academic. And though she had been assisting DeVries in running her interior decorating business, this was not the life for her—though she'd put her skills to use helping her mother and DeVries decorate Sky Island.

Viola also joined in the festivities celebrating the natural conclusion of another club romance. That summer, thirty-five-year-old Marie Louise "Shiny" Schreiner married fellow CCC member Morris "Whit" Whitaker in Greenwich, Connecticut. Whit was fifty-eight and recently divorced. It was another union cultivated and encouraged by Bernard himself, who went so far as to suggest how many children Shiny should have—one. The new Mrs. Whitaker took her guru's advice and made sure Sara was her only child.

On July 11, Baby and Budh embarked on their debut as performers with a tour of New York State. Traveling in a specially outfitted moving van, the two young elephants performed at Playland amusement park in Rye and at fairs in Oneonta, Cortland, and Ithaca, picking up good notices along the way. They were scheduled for a brief rest at home before heading south to a Shriners Convention in Philadelphia, and then on to Atlantic City, New Jersey, and Luna Park in Coney Island, collecting $400 a week for their services. Bernard told a local newsman with a wink, "It feels funny to take money from elephants. But what can you do in hard times like these?"

By the early autumn, Bernard had opened his home to two more elephants: another youngster, named Juno, and Old Mom, the largest performing pachyderm in the country, as the circus men liked to put it. Old Mom was of Indian origin, thought to be somewhere in the neighborhood of eighty years old, and weighed 8,200 pounds. She had first arrived in the United States back in 1893 to perform at the Chicago World's Fair and had traveled with the Sells-Floto and Ringling Bros. circuses. Along the way Old Mom had acquired a reputation for surliness; in her youth she had killed a trainer by accident, and some circus people were wary of her. Bernard, who was seemingly unafraid of any animal, set about integrating her into his herd, and she quickly became the natural leader among the young bulls. When she ambled down South Mountain from the club to the main streets of Nyack, the huge old elephant made many a villager do a double take. When Bernard put her to work two months later, it wasn't for profit but for charity, performing at halftime at the Rotary-Lions benefit football game for the unemployed.

October 31, 1931, was a day of triple celebrations: Halloween, Bernard's fifty-fifth birthday, and the official opening of the new clubhouse, a structure of stone, stucco, and timbered rectangles arranged in a cruciform pattern that mimicked the shape of ancient Vedic altars. Club members descended noisily on Nyack from across the nation for the opening, an all-night dinner party for 217 revelers, who danced to the McGill-Ricci orchestra from New York City. During coffee and dessert, the curtains covering the entire east wall of the new dining room were flung open, and seen coming up the steps of the bluestone terrace was Bernard's herd of four elephants, Old Mom in the lead, carrying on her head the tiniest little girl dressed as a circus performer.

The guests gasped as expected, applauded, and after dinner moved over to the studio building, where dressing rooms were provided for the guests to change into costumes for a masked ball. The Swedish muralist Olle Nordmark, a new club member, had been busy for days decorating the assembly room with ghosts, witches, and strange, batlike creatures.

It was another evening of entertainment that would have been considered a little too outrageous for most American country clubs. Performers included a Swedish opera star and a Creole singer from New York's Cotton Club. The lead act—giving a one-woman, one-act mini-play— was Willette Kershaw, famous at the time for staging banned plays in Paris. "Kentucky mountain and plantation songs" were performed by Barty Bartholomew, and a first-run film, Will Rogers's *Young As You Feel*, was shown. After the entertainment a midnight supper began, and the festivities kept going till 6 a.m.

In December, Joseph Mitchell, the young staff writer for the *New York World-Telegram*, paid another visit to Bernard. Mitchell was then only two years out of college, and Bernard turned avuncular around him, calling the reporter "my boy" as he directed him around the properties. Mitchell in turn composed a favorable portrait of Bernard and his club, this time stepping out from anonymity to take the byline.

"He has become conservative, reticent, and he no longer wears a turban and robe," Mitchell wrote of Bernard, "but dresses in expensive English tweeds and carries a briar cane." Mitchell noted that Bernard's enterprise employed 120 local people and dropped more than $250,000 in local stores and businesses. More than a dozen Manhattan families had built homes to live near their guru—who was now a bank president, the treasurer of the Rockland County Chamber of Commerce, a director of a trust company in Spring Valley, and a junior partner in a chemical plant.

Mitchell, even at his young age, possessed an uncanny ear for the defining quote and an empathy with outsiders that would garner him a peculiar kind of journalistic fame later in life. He took the CCC tour, scribbled down the details, but kept listening, waiting, wanting to be the first reporter to crack the code of Oom's true identity and real motivation. The best he could get was Bernard's tossed-off assessment of himself as a "curious combination of the businessman and the religious scholar." On Mitchell's way out of town, he collared a ticket agent at the South Nyack railroad station for one last try. What do folks around these parts think of the Omnipotent Oom? the reporter asked.

"Nobody knows if he's got religion," the man replied, "but everybody knows he's got money."

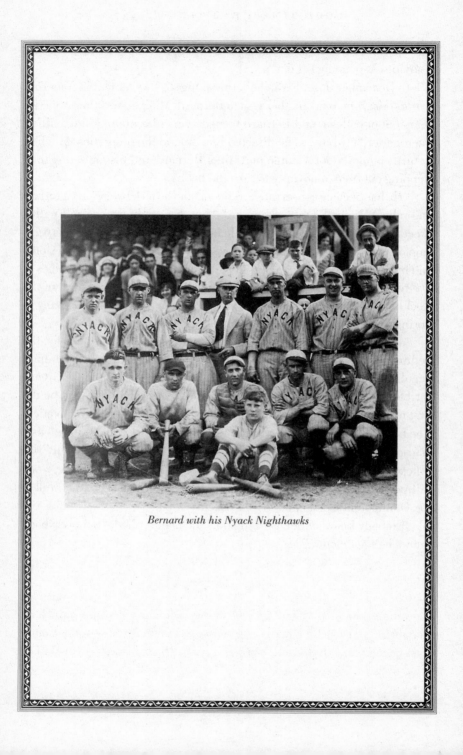

Bernard with his Nyack Nighthawks

Chapter 21

CITIZEN OOM

efore ringing in 1932, and the promise of a new year, Bernard headed down to the same railroad station to say good-bye to Old Mom, Baby, Budh, and Juno. His four elephants were preparing to board their own sixty-foot, steam-heated railroad car, followed by nine crates of props, four elaborate silk-and-velvet-cushioned howdahs, a road trainer, and four assistants. This assemblage, known to booking agents as Bernard's Educated Elephants, had been contracted to perform for the next fifty weeks in circuses, benefits, and fairs across the eastern United States. First stop: New York City, where they would headline a sixteen-act show for the benefit of Great War soldiers and sailors. Before she departed, Old Mom delighted the local children by leaning her huge head against the railroad cars and moving them down the tracks.

Bernard liked to say that "everyone worked at the club," and the elephants were no exception. In between gigs, they hauled boulders and entertained the children of the guests as well as curious young Nyackers. Old Mom, especially, was adopted by all of Rockland County. In their downtime, the elephants frolicked in the swimming pool Bernard built for them, and together they—the animals and Bernard—worked out a fast-paced and entertaining routine of stunts. Soon enough the news had spread that this was no amateur act. The Ringling Bros. Circus dispatched a couple of scouts up to Nyack to take a look. Their report was so promising that John Ringling himself came up to check it out. Then, in April,

Fox Movietone, the newsreel company, shot three thousand feet of film of the elephants going through the choreography that Bernard had lovingly taught them. The film was shown in theaters across the nation in June.

All four elephants played a set of musical chimes with their feet; Baby rode an oversize tricycle; Juno learned how to box with a single big glove tied on the end of his trunk. He would lay out his trainer with a comical uppercut; then Old Mom would amble over and save the man, picking him up gently in her mouth and carrying him to safety. But the jaw-dropper of the show was little Budh's "tightrope walk," in which the two-thousand-pound elephant sauntered back and forth on a twenty-foot-long plank of seasoned hickory that was four inches wide and suspended ten feet in the air. For his finale, Budh paused dead center on the "rope" and did a gymnast's turnaround, balanced at times on only one foot.

John Ringling was so impressed that he asked Bernard to lend him the four elephants for the length of his circus's stay at Madison Square Garden in May of 1932. This request was major news in the circus world, since it shattered a long-held precedent that Ringling's used only its own herd of fifty trained elephants. DeVries designed the costumes for the animals and trainers, and circus people praised Bernard's crew as "the best elephant act ever developed." In no time Bernard was elected to the membership of the Circus Saints and Sinners Club, a benevolent association of old big-top vets that staged charity events to raise money for injured and indigent performers.

Bernard's elephants were not just groundskeepers, entertainers, and status symbols, however; they were also pedagogical assistants and therapists who worked hand-in-trunk with the guru. Like the Himalayan-turned yogis of antiquity, Bernard continued an ancient tradition of teaching humans the wisdom of animals. He and his followers already knew that the postures and breathing exercises of hatha yoga were based on close observation of the natural behaviors of animals. The asanas were even given names like downward dog or serpent pose; there were pigeon, rabbit, cobra, locust, crow, eagle, frog, and scorpion poses, too. "The old Vedic observers noted certain physical attributes, characteristics and powers in different species of animals, which they wished to possess," Bernard said. The ancient rishis "experimented not on the guinea pig but with themselves. . . . As we learn to fly and swim from the birds and fish, so they studied all sorts of lower animals, learning from them powers of agility, strength, repose, peace of mind, etc.—control through ordered discipline."

Charles Potter recalled that Bernard would typically greet a newly arrived guest-patient with a hearty command to come out and see the elephants. The guest was usually skeptical of such an invitation, knowing only that he had booked a room at a rest farm. Out on the lawns, Bernard would call out to the elephants, and a sea of gray—eight or so tons of friendly pachyderm—rumbled over, an impressive enough sight. Then Bernard would put them through their paces specifically for the entertainment of the new guest. After the fun and games, he would dismiss the three young bulls—Baby, Budh, and Juno—leaving Old Mom, the leader of the herd, on center stage for the lesson.

Bernard would then turn to the newcomer. "Here, take this stopwatch and count the respirations per minute of that big old lady elephant over there." He would show the man how to locate the rise and fall of Mom's diaphragm.

"Eleven per minute, did you say? Well, perhaps Mom is a little excited today. Now count your own. Twenty-eight, eh? Well, Big Mom will live to be a hundred and twenty five, probably."

"And how long have I got, Doctor?"

"You? Oh, well, I'm no fortune teller, but I'd say six months, maybe eight if you're careful. You don't even know how to breathe."

After that encounter, Bernard walked away, no further health advice proffered. But any visitor who spent more than a few days at the CCC could not help noticing other people—men and women in their fifties and sixties and older—turning cartwheels on the gymnastics mats, playing baseball, planting vegetables, or pitching hay in the fields. And then the newcomer would notice there were actually classes teaching yoga breathing and postures, as well as tumbling and dance and music. Thus would a sick, nervous man or woman receive the message about the relationship of deep, slow breathing to good health and longevity—the kind of respiratory control called pranayama by the Hindus, but hardly ever called that by Bernard. Suddenly the newcomer wanted to learn how to breathe.

The theory at the Clarkstown Country Club, according to Potter's observation, was that the patient must first find the desire for good health, then learn what he or she must do to get it, since revitalizing a sluggish body requires effort and sacrifice. Then the newcomer would attend the lectures on discipline and patience, eat meals and mix with the other members of the club. There were no exceptions to this rule: alcoholics, drug addicts, people who were profoundly mentally ill worked, studied, and entertained one another with the rest of the guests—Betty Ford Center–style, but with the extra kick of vaudeville, parties, wildlife, and circuses.

◈～◈～◈～◈～◈

Tending to the ailing local economy, that spring the Nyack chapter of the American Legion declared "War on Depression." The legion had already drummed up work for 225,000 American men, and the goal was a million jobs in all. Still, the new employment opportunities seemed to materialize at a trickle of one or two at a time, while entire businesses continued to fold. In January, Woo Hang Sang, the proprietor of the local Chinese restaurant, filed for bankruptcy. On Main Street, the Surprise Store, a variety retail outlet (linen knickers for boys, 25 cents; dresses in extra-large sizes, 39 cents) lost its lease that spring, too. Personal bankruptcy notices were becoming a recurring feature in the local papers. Bernard's Educated Elephants had rung in a rocky year, but at least they had jobs.

In good times and bad, Americans wanted to be entertained. If anything was more popular than circuses it had to be baseball. And the latest hook for the national pastime was the advent of night games, which sometimes commenced as late as 9 p.m. to better show off the lights and gather a crowd. Though it was expensive to power up three or four big banks of incandescent bulbs, night ball was the child of Depression-era invention. On Long Island, one bright freelance electrician began transporting whole lighting systems (poles and a generator) around on a flatbed truck to illuminate baseball games and other public events. This was visionary thinking in the history of sport; it would be a few more years before even the first major-league stadium offered lighted night games.

That summer, Bernard, too, decided to take a gamble with night ball. He began talking with a local man named Skee Watson, one of the most talented semiprofessional outfielders ever to play the game in the Hudson Valley. Watson, whom old-timers knew by the name of "Jigger" Graham, accepted Bernard's offer to use the CCC field. Bernard in turn would set up poles for lights and pay for electricity and new grandstands. The seating had to be good enough to charge admission, of course.

The first night baseball game was set for July 11, and the drumbeat began in the sports pages: Bernard pays New York Telephone to put up six poles for the floodlights . . . Bernard builds a new grandstand adding 750 seats . . . Bernard's men test the lights and prepare the field . . . and finally, the season opener, complete with elephants. The West New York Red Sox arrived to defend their Hudson County Championship title against the Nyack team, which was now fully under the stewardship of Jigger Graham. The mayor of Nyack, William E. Mott, was spotted practicing with village trustee Bunny Haire down on New Street—hoping not to look like a clown when he threw out the first ball. And so it started. Though the hometown boys lost the first game, the evening was a smash.

What better symbol could there be of Doc Bernard's status as local hero? The summer sky glowed above his club, the illumination visible for twenty miles: down in the flatland villages of the Nyacks, across the Hudson in Tarrytown, as far up the river as Sing Sing prison. A young baseball fan trudging up South Highland Avenue in 1932 would have widened his eyes at the setting: a professional grade baseball diamond set in a dark, bosky amphitheater of towering oaks, pines, and cedars, the smooth orange of the infield dirt, the white chalk lines and green grass of the outfield glowing surreally under 100,000 watts of illumination.

From the start, the crowds came, and the players loved the field's leafy backdrop, which helped them keep track of the ball in the glare of the lights. The great barnstorming clubs returned to Nyack to play at night. Bernard met the Detroit Clowns with his herd of elephants, and he donned wig and paste-on beard to play with the House of David.

As the season went on, Bernard invested still more money in the field. Additional bleachers and grandstands were built—crowds were turned away from the early games—and the little club field was soon enough seating two thousand paying spectators. There was enthusiasm to spare and only one way for this project to go, Bernard felt: bigger, bigger and better. He went looking for more land.

The Rockland County Chamber of Commerce proclaimed rightly that Bernard had once again put the community on the map. Bernard in turn granted the use of the lighted field at no cost to any charitable organization that asked (even as he continued to lend the project increasing sums of money). He booked a few boxing bouts and a major wrestling card for Rotary Club charities. He would even throw in the elephants—no charge. And though the Nyack baseball team wasn't exactly world beating in its first season, the games sold out.

One night that summer the action on the field paused for a moment, and fans looked up, squinting to see past the lights into the dark sky. It had to be an airplane, from the sound of it, traveling fast and coming in low. If folks didn't know it then, by the next day everyone knew it was Major Jimmy Doolittle, the holder of every airspeed record a pilot could claim. Major Doolittle, on a mad, fourteen-state sprint, swooped in low over the glow of the CCC field, and the crowd, the reporters, and Bernard himself couldn't help interpreting this as a benediction from a hero of the skies.

Back at the club, things were changing with the times, too. A working health farm and yoga ashram by day, the CCC by night was turning into something resembling a PBS marathon, with a wide range of programming spanning the arts, sciences, and current affairs. Explorers, doctors, yogis, experts of all stripes came to speak and mingle with the members. The actress Beverly Sitgreaves performed a series of readings that brought to mind her mentor, Sarah Bernhardt. The Hungarian count Victor de Kubinyi, an artist whose work was on display at the Museum of Modern Art, arrived to explain his new "psychograph" paintings. There were presentations from the likes of Arthur Terry, the U.S. marshal for the Indian territories in the Pacific Northwest and an expert on the Eskimo peoples. Brahmin musicians Lota and Sarat Lahiri played Tchaikovsky compositions on Indian instruments as a warm-up to an evening of full-out Indian ragas.

In August, as the Democrats nominated New York governor Franklin Delano Roosevelt for president, Bernard and leading financiers of his community—fellow bank presidents, politicians, and religious leaders—pooled their resources to create a privately run financial salvage operation they named the Rockland Reconstruction Corporation. This was a private economic stimulus program, capitalized at $500,000 and designed to bail out the county's troubled small businesses.

But Citizen Bernard, distracted as he may have been by night baseball and Rockland County economics, was still at heart a Tantric yogi. And if anyone needed reminding of that fact, they needed only turn to a new book called *Eastern Philosophy for Western Minds*, published that same summer by one of the CCC's most stalwart members, the writer Hamish McLaurin.

Dedicated "to P.A.B. with admiration and gratitude," the book was a Sanskrit-free introduction to Bernard's version of India's wisdom, the only book of its kind ever written for the American public. It boasted a preface by fellow CCC member Francis Yeats-Brown, whose memoir, *The Lives of a Bengal Lancer,* was an international best seller.

Indeed, of all the Vedanta Centers and dharma practices then flourishing under mega-successful swamis like Paramahansa Yogananda, only Pierre Bernard and his disciples were engaged in the systematic teaching of hatha yoga. Hatha yoga was viewed by Yogananda and other swamis as a low-class, mumbo-jumbo waste of time that had long fallen out of favor even in India, and it was McLaurin's mission to spread Bernard's view that hatha yoga was actually the *key* to a good American life. In fact, after generations of neglect in India, hatha yoga was now in the midst of a revival in its homeland, claimed as a point of national pride by India's Home Rule movement as it sought independence from British occupation.

Still, even the most renowned hatha yoga practitioners who'd arisen in this new generation of Indian yogis were kept away from the United States by a series of harsh anti-immigration laws put in place after World War I. So despite the growing fame of figures like T. K. V. Desikachar, B. K. S. Iyengar, Pattabhi Jois, and Indra Devi—who would prove influential in the West later in the twentieth century—the *only* working hatha yoga ashram in the United States was still Bernard's Clarkstown Country Club. And McLaurin was its resident scribe.

Eastern Philosophy for Western Minds was published to favorable notices throughout the country, from the *Los Angeles Times* to the *Hartford Courant,* and though it wasn't a national best seller, it gave a persuasive public face to a practice that Bernard had until then kept protected from the uninitiated. McLaurin employed the wise tactic of keeping the book free of Vedic texts and diagrams, instead focusing on pragmatic, closer-to-earth descriptions of philosophy, monism, karma, morality, and the varieties of yoga practice. Only late in the book did McLaurin address the physical practice of yoga—thirty-two postures of note and twenty-four sequences—and even there he emphasized the scientific rationale for the exercises as a means of self-healing.

For the first time in his career, Pierre Bernard had seen his philosophy validated in print by a reputable writer. Now his version of Americanized hatha yoga was available to anyone willing to purchase McLaurin's easy-to-read adaptation. When added to Charles Potter's vigorous defense of his ethics and morality, this blast of good publicity gave the guru of Nyack enough confidence to begin speaking of yoga outside the confines of the CCC walls—if he could find room in his schedule.

Flush with his summer successes, Bernard found himself even busier that autumn. He remained president of the State Bank of Pearl River but stepped down from the board of the Ramapo Trust Company to give more attention to the Rockland Reconstruction Corporation. He retained his positions on so many other corporate, real estate, and arbitration boards that months passed without a free weekday night. Meanwhile, he entertained offers to bring Monday night football (along with Friday night games) to Nyack in October. He began planning the construction of a new sports stadium, one that would dwarf his little CCC ballpark. Even after the completion of the new clubhouse, the Clarkstown Country Club employed on average sixty-two men every day in addition to the eight full-time office employees. "Without the club, Nyack would have seen a far worse phase of the depression than it has," one local leader said, which everyone knew was putting it mildly.

DeVries should get credit for that, too—and she was just as busy as her husband. A gifted administrator and hostess, DeVries kept the club running like a top, even as she pursued her interior decorating sideline, which over the past decade had designed homes in Washington, Cleveland, New York City, and Westchester County. (She later boasted that she had over 150 rooms in her decorating portfolio.) The asana, mantra, and breathing classes kept to their schedules, as did the theatricals and other performances. Viola Wertheim had joined DeVries as her assistant in some of these ventures, as had Diana and a half dozen other dedicated young women, whom DeVries trained to pursue excellence in whatever career they engaged in. In fact, it was through DeVries's chief admirer, Frances Payne Bolton, that Viola was able to embark on her illustrious career as a psychoanalyst, continuing the arc of the work she had been introduced to by Bernard and DeVries.

A victim of not just the anti-Semitism and gender discrimination of the time but a woeful academic record, Viola had been rejected by Yale, New York University, and Cornell Medical School before Frances Bolton intervened. Heading to Cornell directly from an African vacation, Mrs. Bolton laid out some obvious facts. The dean, well aware that one of Frances's relatives was William Payne Whitney, was reminded that Whitney had just donated $40 million to the college. The dean suddenly understood Mrs. Bolton's concern and remarked, "Isn't it just terrible, Mrs. Bolton, that the candidate that you and I both care about so much should be the subject of a clerical error?" And with that, Viola went off to medical school and later became a distinguished psychoanalyst and professor at Columbia University, where she founded the School of Community Psychiatry.

<hr />

Bernard's weekly lectures on yoga, meanwhile, had begun to taper off—by 1933, it seems, they'd come to a complete halt. If he was free on weekend nights and not lecturing on yoga to community groups outside the club, he served as the CCC's emcee, introducing distinguished guests like the nineteenth-century ivory hunter and movie star Alfred Aloysius "Trader" Horn, along with experts in Russian affairs, botany, African tribal culture, bridge building, and medicine. Later in the evening he would conduct public conversations with them, bringing the subject around to yoga in the most casual fashion. Outside the club, however, his once unconventional views were suddenly very much in demand. A few days after Thanksgiving, he spoke to the Rockland Chamber of Commerce about his Vedic vision for the financial future of the county, stressing the interrelatedness of all people and the unity of purpose in the physical world. He heralded a future of true community—cooperation based on a new translation of a time-honored American ethic. "I don't know who started it," he wrote, this notion "that every American citizen was born equal and free to do as he damn pleases. Well there never was a more mischievous theory set on foot. Some call it rugged individuality—it's rugged all right and obstructive. Others call it liberty when it is nothing more than a common ordinary license to do as one pleases irregardless [sic] as to the injury that this reckless person does to his neighbor. This spirit is more likely to prevail in the wide open spaces like Rockland than in the metropolitan centers where of necessity they must live and work closer together." Rocklanders, he warned, should hang together or hang separately, as Ben Franklin had once put it.

These were increasingly difficult times for his neighbors in the wide-open spaces in the weeks after Roosevelt's election. A palpable feeling of panic was descending on everyone—householders and businessmen alike—driving a few to grab what they could by hook or by crook. Bernard insisted that such an individual "must be shown that even his personal material welfare will be enhanced by working with others to make Rockland a land that desirable people will want to settle in."

Then in January of 1933, Bernard returned to the scene of the crime, in this case, the fourteen-year-old assault on his life's work. In the parish room of Grace Episcopal Church, the very house of worship whose pastor had tried to drive him out of town in 1919, a serious-minded standing-room-only crowd welcomed him. Bernard spoke of his lifelong love for this "philosophy reduced to practice," as he called yoga. He described to his white Anglo-Saxon Protestant listeners the comforting nineteenth-century belief—still held by many academics at that time—that yoga was the creation of the Aryans, a light-skinned nomadic Indo-European tribe who spoke and wrote in Sanskrit, the language of the Vedas and mother tongue of European languages. He also addressed the reigning prejudice against yoga, as laid out in the American press, as something unnatural. "Its teachings in no way violate the well known laws of anatomy, physiology . . . as now known in the modern medical world." There were quite a few local doctors in the audience that night, and one of them rose to call for a vote of thanks for the esteemed Dr. Bernard. The question-and-answer session, set for a half hour, continued for ninety minutes.

<hr />

The clerics and the doctors had listened to Bernard's wisdom, and now the bankers were paying attention too. By the time FDR took office in the spring of 1933, the nation's banking system was in chaos. Some five thousand individual banks had failed, and millions of Americans had simply lost faith in the system. Roosevelt set forth in his inauguration speech the idea of a "national bank holiday"—four days during which federal

inspectors would examine and relicense healthy banks. During this turmoil, Bernard's State Bank of Pearl River stayed solvent and profitable—it
was the first Rockland bank to reopen the day after the national bank
holiday. And the hundred or so people who depended upon him for their
livelihood missed not a single paycheck.

Characteristically, Bernard continued to find opportunities in the
sinking local economy. That winter he'd sold one of his Upper Nyack properties and bought the Brush estate, an uninhabited eleven-acre hilltop just
to the west of his main holdings, which would be the site of his latest field
of dreams. In March, an army of men and machines could be seen whit-
tling away at the peak. On most days they could be heard, too. The hiss
and slam of compressed-air drills and the roar of diesel-powered steam
shovels and earthmovers ceased only when the operators jumped from
their machines and beat a retreat to a safe distance. Then the explosives
crew hit the plungers, and the short silence was shattered by the sound of
dynamite cracking loose a few more cubic yards of rock from this ancient
ledge. It was slower going than anyone expected, but, as the saying went,
"Hey, that's why they call it Rockland County." Despite the cold and the
smoke and the noise and the flying shards, the men on the hill considered
themselves lucky to find decent-paying jobs.

The laborers knew little about the project, only that they were bringing
to life the latest of Doc Bernard's schemes, and the strange yoga teacher
from Nyack paid his bills. Not content with his modest little jewel of a ball
field on the club's grounds, Bernard wanted to upgrade to a world-class
sports stadium with acres of parking, grandstands for eight thousand fans,
bigger and brighter lights, restaurants, and concessions—an attraction
that would bring them in from all over.

Clearing the trees and brush proved to be merely the opening act.
For the next several months, it was Oom vs. the mountain. Tons of jagged
traprock had to be drilled and dynamited and then turned into retaining
walls. Ever the showman, Bernard trotted out his elephants, including Old
Mom, to haul boulders, as the now-welcome newspaper reporters shook
their heads and took their photos. Then, slowly, to the amazement of some,
but just as Bernard had predicted, a new skyline sports stadium began to
emerge like a vision from the flattened and manicured hilltop. Bernard
convinced the engineering shop of Rockland Power and Light to build

him four new sixty-foot-tall light towers, fabricated from the same cross-hatched steel that carried the electric power for the entire county.

Bernard was justly proud of this accomplishment, said Charles Potter, but "I have noticed that the thing about it that he most frequently emphasizes is the fact that it took eighteen-hundred cases of dynamite to blow the top off a rocky hill and reduce it to a huge baseball diamond and football gridiron. He likes dynamite—because he has a lot of it in his blood."

On the clear, starlit evening of June 22, 1933, Bernard presented his new Clarkstown Country Club Sports Centre to the people of his community. Its scale was shocking to some, dwarfing his old field even before it was finished. It would be years before it would turn a profit in this economy, but on that warm, clear, and glorious summer night, any naysayers were shouted down by the whoops of the crowd of 3,500 who cheered Bernard's elephants as they transported onto the field the new home team of the CCC Sports Centre. . . . *Ladies and Gentlemen, the Nyack Nighthawks!*

Then a lone figure walked out to the pitcher's mound. It was boxer Jack Sharkey, a Boston sailor who eleven months before had defeated Max Schmeling to become heavyweight champion of the world. Dressed in a white linen suit and wearing a flowing orange necktie, the champ wound up stiffly and flung the ball wide of the plate. The crowd cheered him on to try again, and this time he let it fly into the catcher's mitt. "I don't know how I am about throwing a baseball," Sharkey said into the public address system, "but I sure can use these." He held up his big fists and the fans roared their approval. In the audience this June night were political insiders of both parties: sheriffs, postmasters, attorneys-general, as well as assemblymen, the state Democratic chairman, and a state supreme court justice. Peanut vendors worked the crowd, and "near beer"—the low-alcohol brew permitted under Prohibition—was sold for $2 a glass. (Bernard's no-booze policy at the club, it seems, had slackened for the public.) All the CCC mainstays helped out; manning the ticket booth were Percival Whittlesey and the Misses Powell. The evening was a resounding success, except for the hapless Nighthawks, who were "rocked in the trundle bed of defeat," as a local sportswriter wag wrote, going down 6–5 to the Brooklyn Winchesters.

That summer Bernard produced soccer, boxing, and wrestling matches and staged professional theater at the sports center. "He has thrown rather a large pile of chips into the pot for Rockland County and taken a magnificent gamble," a fellow businessman wrote. Even *Fortune* magazine took notice, describing Bernard as "a shrewd and level-headed businessman."

On August 8, General Hugh S. Johnson, President Roosevelt's newly announced head of the National Recovery Administration, made his desire known that he wanted Bernard and the Rockland County Chamber of Commerce to take charge of the federal relief activities in the county. The chamber accepted unanimously and began organizing and planning a mass rally. Johnson, who the month before had appeared on the cover of *Time*, was one of the New Deal's most public figures, and in his letter he asked the Rockland businessmen to fully focus their efforts to "speed the return of prosperity through the expansion of consumer purchasing power." Bernard was charged with securing and preparing the Sports Centre for a five-thousand-person event.

So Pierre Bernard turned fifty-seven in a celebratory mood on October 31. After thirteen months of additional work and $140,000 spent on labor alone, the Sports Centre was finished. Newly added were a four-acre extension to handle even bigger crowds and more parking, along with new roadways and a raised staging area for smaller events. The grateful men of the work crew pocketed their last paychecks and took one long look at this vast thing they had created.

But the biggest birthday present was a place of honor, shared with Old Mom, at the head of Rockland County's parade in support of Roosevelt's National Recovery Act. All over the United States, there were NRA marches that autumn to celebrate solidarity with the president's plan for fair wages and just prices. In New York City, 250,000 people marched in September, wearing armbands decorated with the NRA's blue eagle. In Monroe, Georgia, that same month, more than four thousand marched. In Tarrytown, New York, the parade stretched for four miles, and three thousand marched. Rockland decided to forgo the planned rally at the Sports Centre and march through the streets, too. New York's governor declared October 31 a county holiday so kids and families could turn out for the festivities.

Old Mom was dressed in her finest howdah and silks, wearing big, painted eyelashes on her face. Eighteen-inch-tall letters spelling out N-R-A were printed in blue on her sides, and large silver stars were affixed to her hindquarters. But Bernard's good mood was soured when Old

Mom, being led to the street, refused to walk down the hill to the village. Sensing her fear even from a distance, the other three elephants began to bellow. Bernard and the trainers quieted them down, but Old Mom, clearly in physical distress, would not be forced to walk. She was led back to her berth in the elephant house, and the NRA parade went on without her.

Five days later, she collapsed in her stall, sustaining internal injuries and lying helpless in her berth. Bernard rushed from a board meeting to be at her side and quickly realized the seriousness of her situation. Baby, Budh, and Juno were moved to a garage a distance away, and the elephant house was transformed into an oversize intensive care ward. Local vets arrived to advise, electric heaters were brought in, and two block-and-tackle devices were arranged to turn the 8,200-pound elephant in order to prevent her from catching pneumonia.

" 'Mom' lies on a dozen mattresses placed upon a solid foot of hay . . . with thirty-odd bags of hot sand about her body," the *Journal-News* reported a week after she refused to march. "Treatment of the sick creature has included intestinal irrigation with twenty-five gallons of water in which potassium permanganate was dissolved. Through a hosing inserted into her stomach by means of a wooden gag to keep her jaws apart, she was fed last night ten gallons of pureed vegetables. She has night and day nurses on constant duty; her two keepers alternate in the sick quarters . . . and Dr. Bernard is always on call."

The story, elephantine enemas and all, seemed to engage readers with its pathos. In the next few days, reports on Mom's condition appeared in papers across the nation, from Charleston, South Carolina, to Billings, Montana. Mom was responding to treatment, and her old friend Courtney Ryley Cooper, a former circus clown who had written about her in several books and more than a hundred articles and short stories, rushed to Nyack, trailed by a phalanx of city and entertainment reporters, who dispatched daily reports: Mom was dehydrating and getting sicker. . . . She must be turned upright to be fed. . . . Bernard ingeniously rigged up a new rope contraption to help her sit up. . . . Twenty men, nurses, and keepers worked day and night to save her. . . . Bernard, at his creative best, converted two hydraulic truck jacks to keep her hindquarters raised so she might take sustenance.

"There's life in the old girl yet," Bernard announced on November 8.

She ate a bucket of bran, and one and all sighed with relief. The chef of the CCC mixed up a pail of her favorite soup.

Then suddenly Old Mom took a turn for the worse. The next day Bernard sat by her for eight hours, but Joe Hansen, the trainer who was busy with the other elephants, had a terrible premonition. He was tending to Baby in the garage when the young bull let loose a bone-chilling howl. Joe dropped the water pail and raced over to the elephant house. He found Bernard and an assistant named Olle on his knees beside Mom, who was still and silent. On Saturday, a week after her collapse and eleven days after her NRA no-show, Mom had died. Olle was stroking the giant gray head and half sobbing: "Never mind old girl—you let the world go by."

Mom's death brought out reportorial poetry in the *Journal-News*, where Winifred Van Duzer wrote, "With a final gallant flirt of her trunk and a flicker of fast-glazing eyes toward Dr. Pierre A. Bernard, her master and friend, the great creature late yesterday afternoon set out on the long trail to those celestial jungles where all good elephants go in the end." An autopsy, supervised by Bernard, revealed that Mom's brain weighed thirteen pounds, her heart twenty-seven, and she appeared to be much older than her purported ninety-two years.

<hr />

Despite Mom's absence, Rockland's NRA parade had been a resounding success, with twelve thousand marchers and three thousand cars, Bernard driving an automobile that was decorated to look like an elephant in Old Mom's honor. When Roosevelt repealed Prohibition the next month ("I think this would be a good time for a beer," he said as he signed the legislation), Bernard used the change in national policy to shepherd in a new era at the CCC as well. Not only would wine be served at dinner—for the first time in club history—but "whatever aspect the famous club has had as a sanitarium, medical center, asylum or convalescent home, ends with the year 1933."

He was growing older, he said; he felt that his time was at a premium. His real interest was not in the heretofore secret work of curing well-heeled mental patients, but in adult education of the type that he had been providing with his Open Forum lectures every Saturday night. Time had changed the man and the club once again.

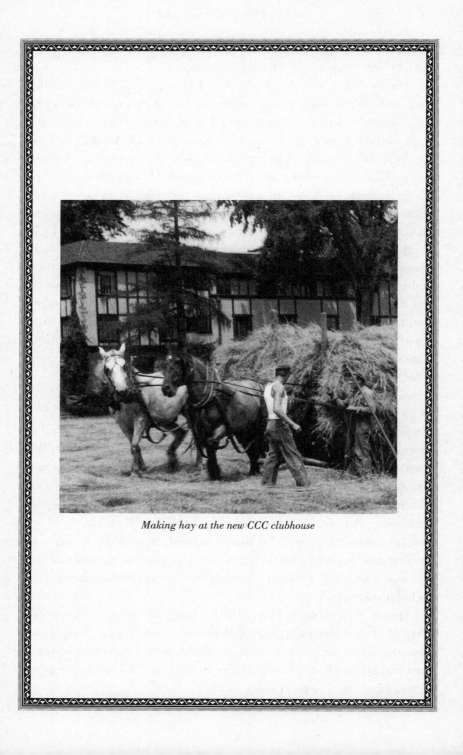

Making hay at the new CCC clubhouse

Chapter 22

THE MESSAGE GETS OUT

reed from his caregiver role at the CCC, Bernard became something of a roving ambassador for hatha yoga. He parlayed his business success into an all-access pass to the precincts of power and influence. In January 1934 he was welcomed as the guest speaker at a Yale Club luncheon in New York, where he proclaimed that yoga was simply part of an advanced and modern approach to living. Health care should be preventive, he explained, not illness-oriented, and people should be concerned about internal as well as external cleanliness. He denounced fads in diets and preached moderation in all things, especially exercise. Eat anything you want, he told the men in his audience—even pie and cake!—as long as the amounts are appropriate for each individual and you get off your couch every day.

Other Bernard disciples besides Hamish McLaurin were getting the message out, too. Major Francis Yeats-Brown, having settled himself in Hollywood to advise on the movie version of *The Lives of a Bengal Lancer*, so impressed Gary Cooper, the film's star, that Coop began experimenting with yoga then and there. Cooper in turn convinced the film's director, Henry Hathaway, to try it, and soon there were others on the set trying out yoga and meditation. According to the *Los Angeles Times*, Yeats-Brown made "a lot of converts" during his stay in L.A.

Evidently, so too did Anne Vanderbilt and "Princess Murat"— Margaret Rutherfurd—who, despite having cut off contact with the CCC, continued to share what they learned from Bernard with any and all willing to listen—including their friend Elsie de Wolfe, the famed decorator who had become an influential Hollywood insider. Not only did she decorate the home of Mr. and Mrs. Gary Cooper and other Hollywood lights; she boasted about her morning routines of asana and meditation, practices "introduced to me by Anne Vanderbilt and her daughter, Princess Murat, who were ardent disciples of Yogi-ism and can stand on their heads with the facility of any professional acrobat, as I also am able to do."

Suddenly it seemed permissible to reveal that Mae West, Greta Garbo, and Maureen O'Sullivan were also practitioners of yoga, as were dozens of other stars and starlets whose names are now forgotten. Could it be that yoga actually made people healthier? Happier? The press was suddenly keen to give the question serious thought as the public relations efforts of the Nyack team began getting some traction. Bernard was out on the hustings as often as possible, introducing the subject to the uninitiated at churches and synagogues; at meetings of the Lions Club, the Unity Club; to Rotarians and Yalies.

Progressively and definitively during these years, the health and beauty benefits of yoga were being separated from the idea of the evil occult swami. Positive press accounts began to outnumber the negative in the 1930s by larger margins as the decade—and the Depression—wore on. In 1934, readers all over the nation read a wire service story with the unprecedented headline "Scientists Study Yoga Breathing," which reported that the practice of pranayama actually oxygenates blood to higher levels, lowers blood pressure, and elevates mood.

But a major pivot in the cultural history of yoga in America can be traced to a do-it-yourself article titled "Yoga for You," by Major Yeats-Brown, which appeared in the April 1935 issue of *Cosmopolitan* magazine. Yeats-Brown wrote it as an adaptation from *his* literary contribution to the cause: *Yoga Explained*. Unlike McLaurin's brainier take on the subject, the best-selling author wrote a guide to actual yoga practices that could be undertaken *immediately* and without the benefit of a teacher (though he cautioned that a teacher must be found as quickly as possible). *Cosmopolitan*'s sexy female models illustrated the serpent pose, the lotus seat, the shoulder stand—and the whole package hit the right note at the right time, summoning the do-it-yourself spirit of American women in search of health and beauty in tough times. The *Cosmo* story was further condensed and syndicated, redistributed to hundreds of newspapers under the head-line "Yoga Is Helpful to Mental, Physical Powers." The irony could not have been lost on Bernard: William Randolph Hearst, *Cosmopolitan*'s new owner and Bernard's antagonist for more than three decades, was suddenly on Oom's bandwagon, spreading the good news.

***

Back in Nyack, however, the CCC was morphing again, adding to its iden-tity a new function as celebrity rest retreat, catering to some of the old lions of American culture. If yoga seemed to be taking a temporary backseat, perhaps it was because the place that incubated Bernard's vision no longer needed to work so hard to cultivate it. The message had gotten out.

The playwright Augustus Thomas and his family, who'd been fre-quent guests for some time, decided to spend the winter of 1934 in Nyack. Seventy-seven years old and in poor health, Thomas was universally known as the "dean of American playwrights," having written some sixty-five popular theatrical entertainments, including *The Copperhead*, which in 1918 had made Lionel Barrymore a star. And the fact that Gus Thomas felt comfortable enough at the club to live out his days under the care of Bernard and DeVries drew others to the CCC for the same reasons.

Thomas was joined in Nyack by his friend of sixty-five years, sculp-tor Frederick Wellington Ruckstull, who had created over twenty major public monuments, including the bronze *Solon* in the Library of Congress in Washington, D.C. Together these old artists could often be found sitting in wicker chairs on the clubhouse patio, shooting the breeze with Major Yeats-Brown when he was back in town from Hollywood. Thomas died on August 13, 1934, but his widow stayed on in Nyack for years, and their presence brought many other theatrical lights to the club.

The CCC occasionally hosted actress Helen Hayes, the "first lady of American theater" and playwright and Pulitzer Prize winner Maxwell Anderson. And, together with Diana Whittlesey and other club members, DeVries and Bernard worked hard to make sure that high-quality theater found a welcome home in the Hudson Valley.

In fact, sleepy little Nyack had become a veritable refuge for show-business A-listers in theater and film. As renowned Oscar-winning script-writers Charlie MacArthur and Ben Hecht drew other talent to their rented space at the old Nyack Girls' Academy, Rockland County took on a Hamptons-like allure. "Noël Coward is out there most of his weekends when he's around New York," wrote syndicated Broadway columnist James Aswell. Movie magnate Adolph Zukor presided over a 1,500-acre spread nearby, and Katharine Cornell (another first lady of the theater) lived there, too. Aswell gushed about the "unique quality of Nyack as a sort of Broadway, Park Avenue, Greenwich Village and Summer-Winter resort rolled into one."

The place, he wrote, "crackled with celebrity."

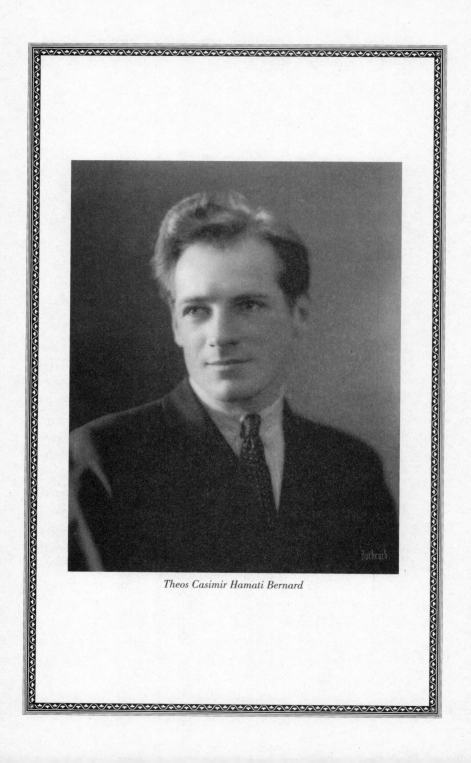

Theos Casimir Hamati Bernard

Chapter 23

CHANGE IN
THE AIR

he first generation of American yoga teachers was long gone. Cheerie Jackson and her husband, Tommy, were living happily in Hollywood, raising a family while Tommy took supporting-actor roles and Cheerie taught dance. Ruth Bartholomew, married to club member Oliver Judson, had three children, raised chickens in Nyack, and had opened a yoga and physical culture studio of her own down in New York City. Millie Ryder Gillingham had gone west to Carmel, California, with her husband, James, and their young son, Peter. Florin Jones, one of Bernard's San Francisco converts, had drifted away from the club, leaving only Winfield Nicholls from the early days.

While Bernard and DeVries maintained ties to departed club members, Bernard had kept up little contact with his blood kin, though he occasionally exchanged letters with his Hoffman cousins in Iowa, a family of well-to-do lawyers. But after his half brother Glen's departure from the Tantriks in 1906 and Ora Ray's elopement in 1913, there is no evidence of any interaction among the Bernards or the Bakers. Even Kittie's funeral, it seemed, couldn't bring them together.

In fact, as Bernard was about to learn, Glen had not only kept his distance but kept his old grievances very much alive. Throughout years of working as a chemist to bankroll his trips to India and his long periods of solitary yoga practice, Glen had never changed his dark opinion of his older half brother and his glamorous life. Now, after thirty years of estrangement, a ghost from Pierre Bernard's past was catching up with him, and the smiling messenger would be none other than Glen's only child, Theos Casimir Hamati Bernard.

Theos Bernard had not spent his childhood with his father, who'd abandoned his young family when his son was a toddler. He grew up instead with his mother and a doting stepfather and stepbrothers in Tombstone, Arizona. It wasn't until his first year in college, while Theos was reading law at the University of Arizona, that Glen made contact with his ex-wife and son; coincidentally, at about the same time, Theos encountered the philosophy and spiritual thought that had drawn his parents together thirty years earlier.

Theos had come down with nearly fatal inflammatory rheumatism, and during his recovery in his mother's care, he immersed himself in her old spiritual books, combing the texts for wisdom—an activity that compelled him to change his plans from legal to metaphysical pursuits. As it had for many seekers before him, Theos's illness had served as his spiritual initiation, and he was suddenly hungry for knowledge about the meaning of life and death and the other big questions. When he gained enough strength, he returned to his favorite haunts in the high-desert Dragoon Mountains, and it was there, taking in the clear, high air, that the young man received word that a stranger, a spiritual teacher known to his family, wished to see him. "He was a rather elderly man, of heavy stature and sensitive features, radiating spiritual strength," Theos later wrote. The visitor was from India, passing through Arizona, and promised the teenager a single evening's audience.

It turned out to be an all-night session. The older man, whose identity Theos never revealed, counseled the revved-up young seeker to be patient—to forget about results and learn to enjoy the years of training he was about to begin. "All action without the guidance of intelligence is futile," the teacher said; forget the arrival—enjoy the journey. We live in the Kali Yuga, Theos was told, a dark age for mankind according to Hindu history. The way to truth during this time of droughts, famines, floods, hurricanes, earthquakes, and war—when the dharma has been destroyed—is to study the Tantras. The way to gain liberation is "through the practice of yoga."

As the sun rose in the sky, the guru began his farewell with these words: "Live free from malice, envy, hypocrisy, hatred, falsehood," and you will be safe in the Kali Yuga. "Be frank and honest and devoted to the good of others." Finally, as he took his leave, the man reminded Theos "to prepare [himself] . . . to be economically independent; for poverty was the worst of all evils. Poverty of the body, it was taught, led inevitably to poverty of the spirit." Study first, avoid women, then return to the world; marry and have a family; only when your wife and family are well provided for should you seek enlightenment full-time. "Patience and perseverance are the key to salvation" were his new master's final words.

Who was the Indian sage and family friend who dispensed this advice? Theos later referred to the stranger as the "family guru." He also identifies him as a Tantrik master who had been his parents' teacher. Sylvais Hamati would seem to fit the man's age and physical description, and the message—to study the Tantras and practice yoga—was identical to the one he left with Pierre. Did the Indian guru reappear in Arizona to ignite in Theos the desire to delve deep into hatha yoga—as he had for his father and his uncle?

Whoever dispensed the advice, Theos took it to heart. Once he'd acquired his LLB from the University of Arizona in 1931, he circled back to study for a bachelor's degree in philosophy, which he planned to use as a launching pad for a doctorate.

When Theos came east in the spring of 1934, he was twenty-five years old, fit and tan from another summer in the Arizona mountains. He was in something of a hurry, as usual, with dueling agendas for his short visit: He wanted to gain admission to Harvard College or Columbia University. He also wanted to lay his blue eyes on his illustrious uncle Pierre and check out his infamous ashram-on-the-Hudson. Pierre happily extended an invitation to the young man to come to the club for the weekend of the big Spring Festival of 1934.

DeVries and the club members had colored hundreds of Easter eggs, cut flowers from the gardens for baskets for every table and room, and nursed dozens of tiny yellow chicks and white rabbits for the weekend's live entertainment. Inside and out the place was freshly painted and spruced up.

But it was Pierre's wavy-haired nephew who struck the most marked impression that weekend—especially on the women. "He was young, he was beautiful," said Viola Wertheim, back in Nyack on a break from Cornell Medical School. "He was handsome and he was tremendously interested in all of this yoga business," she added. His combination of spiritual and physical gifts created a powerful magnetic field for Viola: "We were drawn to each other," she said—though what turned out to be a decisive moment in Viola's life could only later be seen as the first crack in the foundations of Bernard's fortune.

On Easter Sunday, there was a cross-country walk, a late afternoon tea, and a banquet in the evening, followed by a lecture on religion in art. Theos and Viola barely noticed the festivities. In her second year of medical school, Viola had found her career—her true calling. And now finally, she had found love—which every student of Sigmund Freud knows is the one-two combination for happiness.

<hr />

After the Easter weekend, Viola returned to New York City to classes, and Theos to Arizona to finish his exams and collect his second degree. Four days after his graduation, he hitched a ride back to New York, where he and Vi quickly made plans to marry in August. Seeking to assure her brother Maurice—the financier who after Jacob's death had acted as the Wertheim paterfamilias—that Theos was not marrying her for her substantial fortune, she felt it necessary to slightly embellish the groom's credentials, claiming in a letter that Theos had been accepted at Harvard and owned "considerable zinc holdings in Arizona, which though less lucrative right now than in the past (obviously) are still adequate to make him financially independent."

Theos had not been accepted at Harvard—he'd only just entered Columbia as a master's student in philosophy—and was never close to being financially independent, no matter how much mining stock he held. What was indisputably true was that Viola Wertheim's fiancé was headstrong and independent and that their connection was real and immediate.

But news of a hasty wedding was not welcomed by Dr. Bernard. He disapproved of their plans entirely and told the couple so in no uncertain terms. He advised them to stay with him in Nyack, to forget about useless advanced degrees and other such matters, which are the epitome of maya—worldly illusion—though he may have also desired to keep Viola's generosity close at hand. The couple listened not at all and conspired behind his back.

Viola was no longer impressed by the grand improvisation that had characterized Bernard's fifty-eight years; nor was she charmed by his multiple masteries as yoga teacher, bank president, real estate mogul, sportsman, elephant trainer, entrepreneur, visionary, rescuer of souls, and savior of ailing corporations. "He was a promoter, an entrepreneur, he was a public relations guy," she said. "But the most embarrassing kind of public relations."

If she hadn't completely turned against the man who had for ten years been her greatest influence—to whom she had once bequeathed her entire inheritance—Theos volunteered to finish the job. In a rambling early morning letter that suggests father and son were not only acquainted but in cahoots in a scheme they'd conceived well in advance, Theos wrote to Glen:

JULY 20 1934

Dear Dad

It is a little after 4 a.m. but I must give you the latest developments. Vi and I have just finished a long conference with P.A. who has been on his high horse. We did not give into [sic] anything—but did get him quieted down. Glad to report she is with me—says if she breaks up with P.A. she will try not to bring me into it. At present— and has been of this opinion for sometime—she feels that P.A. is doing everything to keep her around for *her money* (you know the answer however)[—] she is still feeding him. . . . The way it is—I am always going to have to do a certain amount of "playing the game"— however—it is probably worth it—I am getting ahead—& she is with me 100%—He had better never get too funny. If he plays right—& we support him—he (*might*) will the place to me—God knows who he could leave it too [sic]—and it is a beautiful place. . . .—a luxurious country estate with our other one next door. I wonder if P.A. would be that decent—to ever think of me—my wife has virtually made him. . . . We have been working on the will lately—she is cutting the sum in half that she originally left to P.A. & giving the other half to DeVries—her first step away from P.A. . . . it makes me *sick* to see this girl made such a sucker—she has had so damn much money that she does not know what it means to figure with dollars—It has always been with thousands. She actually *wants to be*

broke—& earn her own—She thinks it would be easy—She once offered to give all she had to P.A. & he refused it—she says she knows
why now—she was under 21. . . . We went cruising today over into L.
Island Sound—about 100 mile trip and a grand one. So I play and
work at the same time.

Love,

Theos.

⬤⬤⬤⬤⬤

Giddy with late-night possibilities—paramount among them the idea of
rescuing Viola's millions from his uncle—Theos was jumping the gun in
every conceivable way. In addition to inheriting his uncle's two-hundred-
acre property, he imagines annexing it to Emma Wertheim's Sky Island, the
estate he blithely describes to his father as "our other one." He and Viola
are not even married yet, and Viola's mother is still alive. Theos must know,
however, that Emma has just returned from the Kellogg health farm in
Battle Creek, Michigan, fighting the breast cancer that will take her life.

With the wedding day fast approaching, decoy plans were dropped
into phone calls to fool the Nyack operators still eavesdropping for the
New York papers. The event went off without a hitch on August 1, at the
Wertheim family home in New York City, with Diana as maid of honor.
While the newlyweds embarked on a quick, monthlong tour of the western
United States for their honeymoon, the New York tabloids had a feast:
"Bernards Flee to Oom," read the headline in the *Daily Mirror*. "Viola
Wertheim, Disciple of Oom, Weds a Bernard," read the *Daily News*.

Diana and her mother, on the other hand, remained staunch advocates
of Bernard, DeVries, and the CCC, as did Diana's husband, Percival Whittlesey. Di had taken a job as Charles Potter's associate editor at his new
magazine of ideas, *Tomorrow*, and signed on as a founding member of the
Gypsy Trail Club in Westchester, a rural retreat for the well-to-do, where
she skied, hiked, climbed, and kept her horses—even in such dire economic times as these. In fact, Diana never lost her faith in Bernard, who
with DeVries had encouraged her to expand her writing talents on behalf
of the CCC cause, inspiring her to write, with Potter's help, a book about

it. *Life at the Clarkstown Country Club,* which Diana had self-published in 1935, was even that year more an exercise in nostalgia than a testament to the CCC's growing appeal in the midst of the Great Depression. By 1937, with Theos's fame on the brink of eclipsing Bernard's hard-won renown, it was a veritable relic, full of images from the glory years of the circuses, theatricals, masked balls, and past members like Sir Paul Dukes and Princess Margaret Rutherfurd Murat.

Despite Theos's obvious designs on his uncle's empire, the young man had made off with no more than one half of the Wertheim sisters—and whatever financial perks Viola's presence at the club had brought Bernard. But it seems that Theos had taken his uncle's good luck away with him, too. The storm of economic misfortune that had been bearing down on most Americans now descended upon Bernard's operations. His stature in the community, the hope and enthusiasm embodied in the Sports Centre that had opened a year earlier, his growing renown as the expert on a pastime that was suddenly no longer taboo—these achievements didn't assuage the fact that the rich were cutting back sharply on leisure-time pursuits. Bernard's Educated Elephants may have been bringing in $1,000 a week while on tour, but at home in Nyack, there were no longer dewy young applicants lining up outside the CCC gates, pledging to sign over their financial legacies if only they could be stripped of their egos and taught how to breathe. At the same time, Bernard had also lost the support of a number of existing wealthy patrons, preeminent among them the Alfred G. Kays, who had moved their primary residence to Palm Beach, though Alfred maintained his position as president of Kay-Fries Chemicals. The McLaurins were in the process of relocating to the West Coast permanently. Others, like Frances Bolton, had left Nyack disillusioned with Bernard and DeVries for reasons unknown. Meanwhile, property taxes, of great importance to Bernard as an owner of two hundred acres of prime real estate, also doubled in the early years of the Depression. And the coup de grâce? The top income tax rate had been raised from 25 to 63 percent in 1932 and would be raised again to 79 percent in 1936.

So by June of 1935, not two years after he'd opened the CCC Sports Centre to great fanfare and sold-out games, Bernard was forced for the first time to downsize his holdings. He leased the Rossiter House, with its eighteen rooms and acres of fields, meadows, and playgrounds, to a man named John Karkos, who wanted to start a new boys' school. Everyone else at the club did what they could as well to bring in money for their own survival.

Marie Louise "Shiny" Whitaker, a new mother of the child Bernard had advised her to have, began a home business making jams and jellies for sale. Her Yale-educated architect husband ran street maintenance crews for the Works Progress Administration and picked up whatever other work he could. The couple created an apartment on the street level of their Nyack home, which they rented to help cover the mortgage, but every month pushed them further behind. "In the apartment, the Kelvinator's motor burned out, and the company replaced it," their daughter, Sara, recalled, "but when it burned out again, they didn't. Without a fridge, the tenant wouldn't stay and we lost that income. My father had been selling Band-Aids door to door, anything he could find."

He wasn't alone. By 1935, unemployment had reached 17 percent nationally; in New York City, thousands of men and boys waited overnight in lines for the remote possibility of temporary work the next day.

Everyone needed to blow off some steam, so Ben Hecht and Charlie MacArthur, the entertainment barons who were Bernard's Nyack neighbors, hatched a plan over a boozy late-summer night at the 21 Club: a charity baseball game to be held at Bernard's Sports Centre—proceeds to the Nyack Rotary Club . . . or maybe it was the Lions or the Community Fund or the YMCA. Nobody really knew after a few more drinks, and it mattered little once the publicists got to laying on the ballyhoo and the celebrities started signing up. By October 25 the gossip columns were pumping up the event as the "baseball game of the century."

In early November on a particularly blustery day, a motorcade of buses, limousines, and cars headed north from Manhattan, led by a police escort. The passengers were a raucous bunch of celebrities, playboys, movie stars, Broadway actors, journalists, and boulevardiers, accompanied by a gaggle of chorus girls from the Stork Club, the Paradise, and other haunts of the hip and moneyed. The face-off pitted the Nyack Eagles, managed by homeboys Hecht and MacArthur (Helen Hayes's husband) against the 21 Club Hangovers. The Fox Movietone newsreel team set up out by third base to capture the whole thing. Herbert Bayard Swope, the famed war correspondent and editor of the *New York World*, volunteered to adjudicate over the rulings of the *ten* umpires.

Bernard made sure there was a glorious welcome awaiting. Two brass bands boomed and strutted around the circumference of the Sports Centre. His elephants, brought home to Nyack for the occasion, circled the field twice, one of them carrying the tiny Billy Rose, the well-known composer who had that year opened the Billy Rose Music Hall at Fifty-second and Broadway. Coffee, hot dogs, and cigarettes were sold in the stands—proceeds going to the charities—and lots of beer disappeared. The actress Helen Hayes led the cheering section for her husband's team, along with the Whittleseys, the McLaurins, and other CCC members who'd come out for the festivities.

For unknown reasons, the Nyack Eagles were dressed in sailor suits, except for a few who wore complete admiral getups. The lineup included gossip columnist (and later TV host) Ed Sullivan, comic Arthur "Bugs" Baer, and heavyweight boxer Jack Dempsey. They were joined by Walter Huston, Bert Lahr, Ernst Lubitsch, Charlie MacArthur, and the noted painter Henry Varnum Poor. Harold Ross and James Thurber, editor and cartoonist from the *New Yorker*, came to play, drink, and clown around, as did columnists Walter Winchell and Damon Runyon, Adolph Zukor, and some thirty others. With this kind of depth, Eagles manager MacArthur made frequent substitutions, including at one point sending the elephants in to bat.

The 21 Club Hangovers, dressed in red socks and jerseys, knickers, and football helmets, included Humphrey Bogart and Algonquin Round Tabler Heywood Broun, writer Erskine Gwynne, professional celebrity and restaurateur Prince Mike Romanoff, actor Ernest Truex, tennis stars Francis T. Hunter and Big Bill Tilden, Hollywood dabbler Cornelius Vanderbilt Whitney (son-in-law of CCC member Beulah Norton), and dozens of others.

Roughly, it was the artists versus the writers, but the reporters dubbed it a "basebrawl," which was a fair enough approximation of the contest that transpired that day. "A consensus of estimates places the score either at 47–19 in favor of the Eagles or 38–14 in favor of the Hangovers," wrote syndicated columnist Paul Harrison. "There were, in all, five home runs, two touchdowns, one grand slam . . . and three goals in the final chukker." There were kegs of beer at every base. Georgie Jessel pitched *and* umpired, and Rose, among others of short stature, insisted on batting from second base. "Billy Rose of music hall fame and Harold (Hill-billy) Ross, editor of the *New Yorker*, were the heavy hitters for the Eagles. . . . Ross played second base and a Paradise blonde for all he was worth. He fielded his position well, missing everything but his front tooth."

There they were on Bernard's home field. The name-dropping accounts of that day included Bernard as the generous soul who lent his brio, his field, and his elephants to the festivities and whose name carried equal weight in the columns, even among such a gallery of star-dusted swells. A few of the writers referred to him as Oom the Omnipotent, but the nickname was bestowed with fondness—a little jab for a beloved eccentric. Despite his recent belt-tightening at the club—and the loss of one of his prized heiresses—the old guru was still able to rise to an occasion.

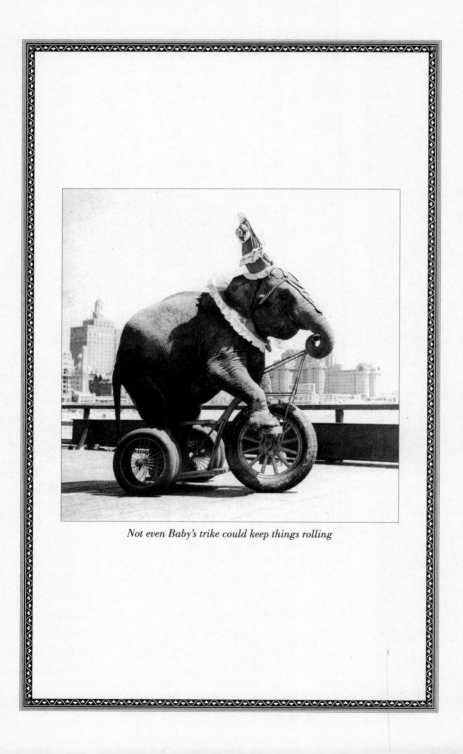

Not even Baby's trike could keep things rolling

Chapter 24

RUNNING OUT
OF TRICKS

ven a four-alarm fire couldn't discourage Bernard for long. At 1:45 in the morning on a chilly March night in 1936, he was awakened by the news that his Rossiter House, now the home of a boys' academy, was fully engulfed in flames and burning to the ground. Nineteen schoolboys held hands and trod the snowy lawns in single file, led to safety by volunteer firefighters, who fought the blaze until well after daylight. Bernard dressed and arrived at the scene, where he promptly gathered up the children in a makeshift caravan and brought them up the hill to the club. He gave them all beds and blankets in his lecture room. The boys were undoubtedly disappointed when he told them that classes would go on at the club until their school was rebuilt.

That spring, he announced that the CCC Sports Centre would be the new home field of the Black Yankees semipro baseball club. His previous attractions, the Nyack Nighthawks and the Winchesters, had failed to draw large enough crowds, and neither did the boxing and wrestling cards he'd put on. The early results for the Black Yanks were not at all promising, either. In fact, the opening night visitors were a no-show, and Bernard scrambled to fill seats by whatever means he could. In June, when the Heller-Acme circus and carnival came through for a week, he grabbed the chance to book them, pulling out all the stops once again: five-cent admission, free parking, fireworks every night. Everything for young and old was promised.

This included the elephants, of course. Juno rode the oversize tricycle to wild applause, and Baby performed his Drunk Walk, weaving back and forth while waving a bottle held in his trunk—evidently people were still cheering the end of Prohibition. The crowds came all week, despite the rain that cut two evenings short. But still, when the receipts were totaled against the bills, it wasn't enough to turn a profit.

So Bernard turned to the sport of donkey ball. The rules were simple: All players on the field, except for pitcher and catcher, were required to sit atop donkeys at all times. Batters would hit normally at the plate, then mount a donkey and ride. The defense fielded the ball mounted on their own donkeys. If a player was forced to dismount to pick up the ball, he had to keep hold of the animal's tether. The donkeys, needless to say, were usually less than enthusiastic about the team spirit required for this sport. They stalled, bucked, reared, swung their powerful necks, and threw more than a few players to the ground—to the delight of old and young, including seventeen-year-old Pete Seeger, still an occasional visitor to the club.

On July 8, midway through a donkey ball game, Bernard took the microphone and quieted the crowd for an important announcement. Tonight's game would be the last time baseball of any kind would be seen on this field, he began. From here on, work would begin immediately to transform the park into an even grander palace for what he mysteriously described as "another kind of diversion."

The truth came out the next day. The stadium was being leased to a syndicate that had previously operated dog-racing tracks in Florida and New Jersey. In Nyack, a new oval track would be laid atop the baseball diamond, and the seating would be reconstructed to make a large grandstand that stretched along the finish line. Three shifts of seventy-five men began working around the clock to have the whole show ready in a month, which was halfway through the dog-racing season in the Northeast.

Even if it broke Bernard's heart to give up on baseball, he could not avoid the hard facts. While he was laboring unsuccessfully to keep his venue profitable by juggling novelty baseball and circuses, not more than five miles away, crowds of up to ten thousand spectators were lining up each night to watch a pack of greyhounds chase a mechanical rabbit around an eight-mile oval. Dog racing, which had started in the United

States in the 1920s, may have been unregulated and quasi-legal, considered by many to be a low, mean pastime that tolerated fixers and wiseguys, but it never failed to pack them in.

Church groups and animal rights activists complained that dog racing was cruel to the animals, and that its real attraction was the gambling that went on at these tracks. Dogs were starved to keep them lean and fast, critics said, and killed routinely when they slowed down; there were persistent whispers that races were fixed by hard-hearted cheats who would slip a thumbtack inside a dog's harness to keep it from running full out.

Defenders, charging elitism, called it poor man's horse racing. Track patrons showed up to bet on the dogs with a form of wagering called "options betting," in which they joined the local kennel club with their admission ticket, making them friends for the night—gambling among friends was legal. Their wagers were considered "options to purchase" the winning dog, though the dog never actually changed hands.

Bernard, genetically programmed to plunge forward in the face of uncertainty, this time fell victim to bad timing and inauspicious politics. Even worse, he had thrown in his lot with unscrupulous company. The Nyack Kennel Club, a new public corporation that sought to operate the track, had already sold $22,000 in shares to the public based on an offering prospectus that claimed the sport of greyhound racing was legal. Not so fast, said one local judge. An immediate halt to sales of stock was ordered until the legal standing of the sport was clarified.

Damn the codicils and full speed ahead, Bernard's investors said. Dog racing was attracting huge crowds at fairgrounds across New York State. Despite occasional raids, the tracks had been operating for years and were wildly popular with working-class people. Moreover, the New York State legislature had passed a bill that legalized the sport and needed only the governor's signature to make it law.

On September 1, Bernard's dog track opened its gates to thousands of excited fans. The new sand oval glistened under the lights, and the crowd bunched up at the windows to place their bets. It was a great start, but after the eighth and final race, Bernard watched from the sidelines in horror as thirty deputy sheriffs and state troopers stepped up to the windows and politely closed the place down. Two track workers were arrested for organized bookmaking, and later that evening the general contractor for the track was arrested for passing a bad check for $1,600 to a local trucker.

The lawyers went to battle stations. Track operators filed injunctions, preventing the police from raiding again until state law was clarified. It was a political free-for-all until September 12, when the district attorney himself visited Bernard's track along with the county sheriff and state and local police. The lawmen sent all eight thousand spectators packing and shut the place down again. As the crowds slunk away into the night, boxes of betting slips were shipped to the state appeals courts; everyone held his breath, waiting for word from the governor. Each passing day was a slow death for Bernard and his partners at the Nyack Kennel Club, who were drained of income, unable to sell stock to raise capital, and facing a massive and growing debt.

By this point Bernard was in deep. His CCC friends and students wondered what in the world he was doing with this wretched dog-racing business. A succession of liens were filed against him personally and against his Clarkstown Country Club, his real estate company, the Biophile Club, along with his partners in the track. What was more damaging to his reputation was that the liens were filed by local contractors and workingmen who had been hired to build the new grandstand. The hero of Rockland County suddenly had a tarnished balance sheet. Bernard felt besieged in his adopted hometown, and even escaped for a few days to his real one— Leon, Iowa—to seek the counsel of his cousin G. F. Hoffman, who ran the family law firm in Leon, and George Baker, the county attorney who happened to be the nephew of Bernard's grandfather.

The visit, it seems, was fruitless, for he returned still stressed and angry. He flew off the handle at a reporter from the *Sunday Mirror*, refusing to answer the man's repeated questions about the failure of the dog track. Bernard shouted at him, "What the hell do you expect me to do— tear out my heart and throw it in your pocket?"

In October, Bernard defiantly celebrated his sixtieth birthday with one of the most elaborate parties the club had thrown in years. "In all there were about 175 present, including many leaders in art and education and in the professions, notably in the field of medicine," read the *Journal-News* report. Festivities began with high tea at five o'clock in the afternoon and progressed through a series of polished entertainments until everyone sat for dinner at midnight. A quartet from Harlem sang spirituals, concert pianist Pescha Kagan performed two Chopin numbers, and a soloist baritone with the Boston Symphony Orchestra sang "Carry Me Back to Ol' Virginny" to such acclaim that he was forced to repeat it. The Young Ensemble Players, Juilliard students under the tutelage of Constance Seeger, performed. Connie, although she had been separated from Charles since 1927, never stopped going to the club, even in its waning years.

Then came DeVries and her dancers—in a series of vaudeville numbers described as Spanish, Tyrolean, Russian, Gay Nineties, Halloween, and jazz. Guests and performers strolled through the night in elaborate costumes; Diana went onstage in whiteface for her Pierrot number. "You Must Never Forget How to Play," read the giant banner hanging across the proscenium of the theater.

Once the curtain fell, Bernard was forced once again to face more mundane, if no less pressing, concerns. He sold off nine cows to cut down expenses, and tried to dream up other ways to pay for the fifteen lawyers he had working on the fallout from the dog track, on which he had accrued $129,000 worth of liens.

In November, Millie Gillingham received a series of increasingly desperate letters written to her by her old friend Shiny, who asked if she and her daughter, Sara, could stay with them if things got worse in Nyack. "The club is almost extinct," Shiny told her, and "it seems as though everything I have ever counted on has gone out from under me."

> I guess you know what a struggle these last five years have been and we have been trying to get along and hang on to our place, like so many others. However, now, although Whit has work and we are in no immediate want, the Home Loan foreclosure on our property is a definite certainty, and any hope of realizing anything out of real estate here is quite out of the question, as taxes have piled up so. . . . [After] interest payments—there is nothing left for us. So some twenty thousand dollars will just have to be sacrificed and so goodbye to our resources. Whit's job of street foreman in South Nyack brings in only about enough for one person, let alone three . . . as he only gets paid when he works and where he has bad luck with

the weather, well he just doesn't get anything. Of course his age is
against his being able to get anything better here. . . .

Well, in short, things are so hopeless and the struggle has been
so long that I can't take it with any kind of spirit . . . the club is very
much on the downgrade & shows every evidence of an early demise,
which also renders my position more untenable. Can you picture life
in Nyack without it?

It seemed they would soon have to. In the club's year-end newsletter
to members, "The Pill," Bernard and DeVries announced, "Our Xmas
intention is to enjoy a very quiet celebration this year by our own fireside.
As postage has gone up we are not sending out cards!"

While DeVries and Bernard spent the year pruning expenses, Theos
and his new bride were energetically pursuing ambitious plans. That past
summer he and Viola set off for Asia, to celebrate her graduation from
Cornell University Medical College and his master's degree from Columbia University. The voyage would be their real honeymoon, an extended
spiritual retreat to India, China, and Japan.

"Be careful on your trip," Pierre Bernard had written gamely to his
nephew. "I know it will be marvelously interesting. If there is anything you
wish to talk about, get me on the phone before you leave and I can reply
to any requests by letter for addresses, etc." Bernard provided his nephew
with contacts and arrangements to see two old friends, Dr. Joshi and P. C.
Banerjee, and ended by giving Theos travel advice. "I'd pay a good visit
to Mysore University and all that constitutes it, as well as the town," he
wrote. "I would visit Puri, Kashmir Hill, Shrinigar and the entire Nadia
district in Bengal especially the *tols* or native schools in Bhatta Pali, just
to see the deterioration in Indian native school teachings."

Theos no doubt snickered at reading this. His uncle had never set
foot in India, and furthermore appeared blind in this letter to Theos's and
Viola's total lack of faith in him, not to mention their vague designs on his
empire. And despite Theos's disdain for Bernard, he shared his uncle's
focus in his single-minded spiritual quest. When Viola returned in November to begin her medical residency in New Jersey, he stayed behind
in India to undertake research for a doctoral thesis at Columbia on hatha
yoga. He was on fire to assimilate all he saw and heard, determined to sit

at the feet of every Indian yogi who would see him and pry from them the esoteric secrets of Tantric yoga. His extended travels were financed by his wife, who suspected—correctly—that she was also paying the freight for Glen Bernard, who had joined his son on the sly.

After training and initiation by a Tantric maharishi in Calcutta, Theos relocated north to Kalimpong, in the foothills of the Himalayas, to study Tibetan languages in preparation for a planned trip to that kingdom. There in the forbidden city of Lhasa, he was told, could be found the surviving bedrock texts of Tantra—not to mention the esoteric knowledge that was yoga's foundation—guarded jealously for centuries by the Buddhist lamas.

On March 6, 1937, Theos wrote to Viola from northern India, bursting with pride about a new friend, Charles Lindbergh. This new companion was "vitally interested in all that I am doing and is anxious for my return so that we can start some experiments on the breath for high altitude flying." Ten days later Theos assured her that he would join her in resigning from the CCC when the time was right, but warned her that he was a lot like his hardheaded uncle, who like all the Bernards, "lives on his emotions like a woman." Then on March 28, 1937, after idle chitchat about his inability to hold his breath more than a fraction (six minutes) of the time a Tibetan yogi could still his breathing (two hours), he revealed that he had arrived in Gyantze, Tibet, on Sang-Wa-Dubo, the anniversary of the Buddha's ascension into heaven, and managed to gain permission to enter the forbidden city of Lhasa. To his great amazement, he was welcomed—not just as an inquisitive scholar but as the reincarnation of a sixth-century lama.

Because of Theos's Tantric résumé, his hatha yoga training, his language skills, and his earnest desire to spread the news of Tibetan Buddhism, the high lamas decided that he would be the first outsider granted access into the sacred mysteries of their religious life. The Tibetans interpreted his unending questioning about Buddhism, Tantrism, and yoga as evidence of a past life attempting to break through to his present incarnation.

In the next five months in Tibet, he would participate in rituals and ceremonies never before seen by outsiders, tour forbidden temples, and document all of it with ten thousand still photographs and twenty thousand feet of color motion picture film. He would bring back beautiful images of a thousand flickering butter candles lit in his honor; "air burials," where corpses were eaten by vultures; and the whirling dervish–like Black Hat

Dances. In the end he was granted the ultimate honor: "I would become a full-fledged Buddhist monk, a Lama."

Now that Theos's hatha yoga credibility had far surpassed his uncle's, he and Viola chose this moment to quit the CCC and formally break off relations with Bernard. They knew this move would be interpreted as treason, that repercussions would follow, and they were right. "I got a line on the reaction to your resignation," Viola wrote to her husband. "P.A. got mad as hell & in a dumb mood of impulse tacked your formal letter of resignation (no sign of the personal one) on the bulletin board of the club house." Bernard stomped around the halls of the clubhouse, and only DeVries could convince him to take the letter down and consider the effect of such a public outburst on what little membership remained.

Viola went to Nyack and confronted Bernard herself. "I told him it didn't matter to us if he wanted to spread that sort of news," she wrote, "only we both were under the impression he preferred our keeping relatively quiet[,] so as not to confuse the minds of other members—including Mother and Di."

Perhaps it was the other wealthy members he'd already lost—the well-heeled Boltons and Kays—who came to mind as Viola spoke to Bernard. "He sputtered about your thinking you didn't need anybody ever just because you got into Tibet," she wrote to Theos. "It takes too long & is unnecessary to get across all the various shadings of this matter—in any case he has said nothing further & as so few saw it I'm letting it ride. . . . You've done the necessary step & that's that. And I'm glad it's done."

Frosty as relations were with Bernard, the couple maintained a cordial relationship with DeVries, who confided to Viola that after nearly twenty years of marriage, she had been having her own troubles with her husband. Bernard argued with his wife bitterly over what he considered her excessive spending. He pushed her to figure out a way to bring in some income—presumably the interior decorating commissions had stopped with the Depression—and she began to look into starting her own yoga studio in New York. But even as she herself seemed to be preparing an exit, she extended an olive branch to Theos on Bernard's behalf: "P.A. is doing lots of things," she wrote in a letter. "Perhaps both of us can be instrumental in his fulfilling his desires, if not satisfying them."

In DeVries's letter was a hint that her husband had not been entirely faithful to her. Satisfying his desires, he later bragged, took many lovers—a statement that suggests his stated views on relationships over the years did not fully embrace the idea of monogamy. Or perhaps he considered himself an exception. In any event, his own relationship was sounding rather worse for the wear.

A March letter from one of the club's accountants can't have helped the matter: "The present movement being one of 'immediate economy,' I am recording below suggestions, which, if followed in their entirety, will result in a very substantial reduction of monthly expenses." There ensues a painfully detailed list of ways to cut staff salaries, heating, electric and telephone bills, gas and mileage on his fleet of cars, and other labor costs. The biggest savings would accrue by closing down entire buildings, mainly the lecture hall and the billiard room, thus resulting in "the concentration of club life and activity in one central place, that being the main club house."

Though its financial footing had slipped, to the outside world Bernard's club was still considered a center of social life in the lower Hudson Valley. The ladies of the Nyack Morning Music Club met there regularly, as did the Women's Republican Club. The English department of Hunter College in New York City and the faculty of the new Rockland Community College held functions there, too. Though there were no longer any wild costume balls till dawn, there were three lectures a week planned for the CCC's fall and winter schedule. The place had become genteel, welcoming to the public at large—for a small fee, of course, and a per-plate charge. The secrecy and menace of the 1920s—"Live dangerously, carefully," Bernard had told his followers then—had long ago vanished. When a *New Yorker* "Talk of the Town" writer came to the club in September looking for any remaining evidence of sex and sin, he found nothing but propriety. Even the grounds, he wrote, may "at one time have been exotic, at least in decoration, but they are now conventional and pleasing in appearance."

In early December 1937, the *Queen Mary* steamed into New York harbor carrying among its passengers twenty-eight-year-old Theos Bernard, a freshly minted celebrity even before he disembarked. In London he'd been ambushed by reporters from the *Daily Mail* and the *Statesman,* who knew much about his stay in Tibet. The story of his extraordinary access had bounced from India to London and then to New York. He was interviewed on the ship-to-shore radio, and the *New York Times* previewed his arrival with a front-page story: "Buddhist Worship in Tibet Pictured: Young Explorer Is Returning Tomorrow with Results of Five-Month Study." When he walked down the gangway, Theos found himself greeted by other reporters, who would, in the next few days and weeks, extol his exploits.

The myth of the White Lama was born, perfectly timed to supplant Bernard's legendary fame as the once dangerous Oom the Omnipotent.

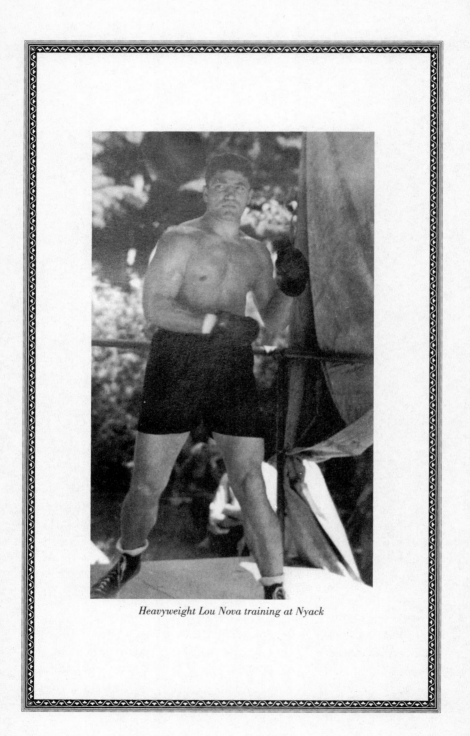

Heavyweight Lou Nova training at Nyack

Chapter 25

THE COSMIC PUNCH

ne day early in 1938, Bernard's fortunes lifted temporarily when a woman named Mrs. Power telephoned the club, insisting that she speak directly to the man in charge. There was urgency in the voice of this cultured and gentle woman, so the switchboard operator put her through to Bernard. He knew exactly who she was. Jeannette Power and her late husband, Walter, were the owners of a performing elephant act; well, not just any elephant act, but four of the world's most famous, beloved, and talented showbiz elephants: Lena, Jennie, Julia, and Roxie, who were respectively eighty-one, seventy-four, fifty-five, and fifty-two years of age. In its prime the quartet was known as Power's Dancing Elephants; now, with vaudeville virtually extinct, Mrs. Power realized all at once that she did not have enough bookings to support her animals. She had nowhere to turn; she needed a place to board them and had heard that Pierre Bernard was, as the *New Yorker* put it, "an almost rabid elephant fancier."

"Bring them right up, madam," Bernard told her on the phone. "I'd be proud to have them as my guests." Bernard subdivided his existing elephant quarters and made room for the four females and for Mrs. Power's son, Tom, who slept in the barn's loft with the elephants on many nights. Taking in orphaned animals appeared to divert Bernard's mind from his larger troubles. The number of human guests at the Nyack club continued to fall off; some of Bernard's original supporters who had made homes nearby were losing them to unpaid taxes and mortgages. The Whitakers were forced out of the house Whit had built for them, just as Shiny had foretold in her letter to Millie. The family headed north to upstate New York to find work and refuge with Ruth Bartholomew and Oliver Judson, who had moved to the Adirondack Mountains. In 1937, Emma Wertheim succumbed to breast cancer at home at Sky Island, tended to devotedly in her last days by Viola. Diana had been having marital troubles and had left her husband, Percival Whittlesey, in their Nyack honeymoon cottage. She took the children to the Wertheim family home in Deal, New Jersey, where she began the process of negotiating a messy divorce.

Through it all, the animals kept arriving, and Bernard could not bring himself to say "no occupancy." To keep company with the elephants, he had in recent years added ten ring-tailed monkeys, two mandrills, a llama, a lioness, peacocks and pea hens, an alarmingly large—160 pounds— bull chimpanzee named Mr. Jimmer, and a Canadian golden eagle. It was an impressive enough collection of exotic fauna, but when a professional big-cat trainer named Captain Roman Proske joined the club with his lions and tigers, Bernard found himself housing a proper zoo. "I remember there was an animal trainer there," Pete Seeger recalled. "Once he put his head in the tiger's mouth—and I was only ten feet away!"

The new elephants were put to work at circuses and fairs as often as they could be booked. At their new home, however, all the beasts played their parts in Bernard's latest scheme: a public attraction called the CCC Children's Zoo and Animal Park. A fresh coat of paint was applied to the whole place, and in a fit of whimsy, a giant dinosaur was fabricated in con- crete and placed in the middle of the elephants' swimming pool. Nervous neighbors could hear Proske's lions and tigers roaring and growling in the night. "The big opening of the Animal Park was, despite the clouded skies, fairly well attended by the traveling public," DeVries noted in her diary in August 1938.

<hr />

That weekend the woman who would become one of Bernard's more im- portant proponents in the human potential movement returned to the club, bringing along her husband and two sons. As a biochemist Ida Rolf had put in more than a decade of scientific work at the Rockefeller Institute, concentrating on chemotherapy and organic chemistry. In Europe she'd trained in homeopathic medicine, and when she returned to the States in the 1930s, she began in earnest her life's work: a new kind of body-mind therapy utilizing osteopathy, chiropractic, and yoga, along with more esoteric stuff on states of consciousness. She called her synthesis "structural integration," but the world, through her famous patients like Garbo and Georgia O'Keeffe, would come to know it as Rolfing.

During her time at the CCC in the 1920s, she'd become convinced that Bernard's brand of Tantric bodywork, accomplished through the use of yoga asanas, was actually a radical new form of osteopathic medicine. As a child, Rolf had suffered a near-fatal kick by a horse; she developed a raging fever followed by pneumonia that flooded her lungs. But when a rural Montana osteopath manipulated her spine, the fever broke and her breathing returned to normal—a spontaneous healing. Rolf had been introduced, the hard way, to a central principle of osteopathic medicine: that the alignment of the spine can affect overall physical health for good or ill.

This discovery eventually led her to Bernard, whom she referred to affectionately as her "Tantric yog in Nyack." She was drawn to the central tenet of Bernard's system of yoga—balance—and it was her 1920s experience with Bernard's brand of hatha yoga that made up what her biographer called "the cornerstone of her thinking" and led to the development of her famous "Rolfing" technique. To her own followers she quoted Bernard—"Worship the body!"—and preached his message that better bodies lead to better lives.

The next spring, to his great delight, Bernard had been asked to find room in his club's menagerie for a young heavyweight boxer from Alameda, California, named Lou Nova. After years of attending matches at Madison Square Garden, the Hippodrome, and the Coliseum—and hosting his own share of matches at his Sports Centre stadium—he would finally be given the opportunity to apply his hatha yoga to a willing subject who excelled in a sport he loved.

Nova arrived in Nyack with his manager, Ray Carlen, three sparring partners, and ten handlers, and for a time it seemed that the CCC was once again the object of the nation's attention. Nova's oversize entourage, followed by "a constant stream of reporters, photographers and sightseers, make the Clarkstown Country Club a lively place indeed," noted the *New Yorker*.

"He's about as fine a specimen as you could find to demonstrate yoga," Bernard said, directing all eyes toward the six-foot-two-inch, 210-pound, twenty-six-year-old Nova, who was billed in the fight game as the California Giant, but in reality was the college-educated son of a concert violinist. Nova, a former national amateur heavyweight champ, had gone undefeated in his first twenty-two professional fights and had earned the right to step into the ring against former world heavyweight champion Max Baer. The bout was to be held in six weeks' time at Yankee Stadium.

The winner would get in line for the dubious honor of challenging Joe Louis, the heavyweight titleholder now in the prime of his career. Baer, who was dethroned two years before by James Braddock, the Cinderella Man, needed a clean victory to earn his way back to a title shot. Nova needed to eliminate Baer from his path to Louis.

Bernard told Carlen that he had never trained a professional fighter, but if there was anything he could do to help, he would be happy to pitch in. So Carlen got an invitation, along with the fight's promoter, Mike Jacobs, to come up to Nyack for a tour. What the two men kept to themselves at this point was that they had no interest in the utility of yoga training, but saw Bernard and his fancy club as an easy way to generate publicity for the fight. Even so, after more than an hour touring the grounds, Jacobs appeared to have been stunned into silence. He said not a word as the trio passed the elephants' swimming pool, the lions and tigers in their cages, the forty-seven-room clubhouse, the theater, the library, the cows in the field, the bell tower, the gardens, the great lawn where the outdoor ring would be set up. In the end, the promoter was reduced to stammering, "What a joint! What a joint!"

Ray Carlen was impressed with Bernard's joint, too. "You ought to see the bedrooms," he exclaimed to reporters. "There isn't a hotel in New York that can touch them."

Bernard's lavishly appointed ashram for wealthy seekers provided the necessary publicity angle for the sporting press—and the proprietor himself got in on the act: "Sweat-shirted men carrying pails and smelling salts will move about with no embarrassment among the dreamy eyed students of yoga, and Dr. Bernard . . . will preside over all with beneficent eye."

The young boxer was provided with silk sheets, silver water pitchers, lamb chops with mint jelly, a seven-thousand-volume spiritual library, and a huge telescope, along with all the animals and the pretty yoga teachers walking around. He would dine on fine china, in fine company that included an up-and-coming soprano named Hazel Hayes, the famous bridge builder Gus Lindenthal, and the widow of Gus Thomas.

For Nova and Bernard, however, the yoga training was serious business. The two spent two hours together each day in intensive yoga instructions, and after three weeks of this, Nova's publicity machine invited the boxing press back up to check on the boxer's progress. "He is stronger, heavier and is hitting harder than ever," wrote Henry McLemore, the United Press man on the scene. "It is not difficult to imagine the revolution in boxing a victory for Nova would bring about. In the past training camps have been rugged places at best, where culture was limited to the artistic application of the hotfoot."

The *hotfoot*. You could almost see them chortling around their cigars in barbershops across the nation. Nyack was now crawling with sports reporters. Even the deans of the boxing press, Grantland Rice and John Lardner, came up to take a look. Bernard set out long tables filled with food and plenty of scotch and soda, and invited the writers to unleash their finest prose on his behalf. "'Oom the Omnipotent' Works Yoga Wonders on Lou Nova," read a typical response.

Bernard was again in his element. If things worked out with Nova, he said, he just might do it again—there was another heavyweight he liked, the ex-bartender "Two Ton" Tony Galento. "I believe athletics is a great character builder," Bernard said. "Nothing like the clean sport of prize fighting."

So the cameras clacked and the newsreels whirred, and the promoters watched from the sidelines with great satisfaction. Nova boxed with Bernard's elephants, posed with Mr. Jimmer and the llama, and entertained Yankee superstar Joe DiMaggio when he came up for a visit. On another day he was motored off in Oom's antique Daimler to West Point to bask in the adoration of thousands of U.S. Army cadets. And every day, student and teacher hit the mat.

Bernard showed Nova how to stand on his head, a practice the young boxer adopted for the rest of his career. Bernard taught him to sit motionless in meditation, legs crossed in *padmasana*, breathing so slowly and deeply that his lung capacity would increase fourfold, Bernard promised. Nova, entranced by everything he was learning, did what he was told and blended his yoga practice with his sparring and roadwork.

In the press, the high-low culture bit, along with the mystic overlay, had done its PR job: the Nova-Baer fight now had its narrative. The young warrior and his avuncular guru versus the popular vet who trained at Grossinger's and wore a Star of David on his trunks. (Baer, whose grandfather was Jewish, had worn the six-pointed star since his 1933 knockout of German heavyweight Max Schmeling—Adolf Hitler's great Aryan hope.) One inventive wordsmith noted that Bernard had armed his young charge with the Cosmic Punch. Lou Nova was Bernard's *vira*—"hero" in Sanskrit—a young athlete bright enough to understand the philosophy attached to the physical work. If Nova were to take on Joe Louis, Bernard vowed to be there with him, working on his body and his psyche, too. "I'll give him the whole works," Bernard said. "And he'll get it, too. He has a noodle that would fit a man of forty."

Nova's management purported to be happy with the results, though Carlen and his trainers secretly worried, as they would later admit, that they had lost control of the boxer to Bernard. Oom continued to play to the press, showering colorful quotes on his prize student. "Not for nothing have I baptized Nova by the name *Paramahamsa*, which in the ancient tongue of India means 'he who has achieved perfect balance of mind, body and spirit,'" Bernard boasted. "Hell, the kid is a shoo-in."

Thus the stage was set and the countdown begun. Even the venue was major-league—Yankee Stadium on a late-spring evening—and for the first time in history a heavyweight fight was to be televised over the National Broadcasting Company in New York—only a month after FDR opened the 1939 World's Fair with the first presidential TV speech.

On June 1, 1939, Lou Nova and Max Baer stepped into the ring in the House of Ruth for the much-anticipated fifteen-rounder. It was youth and yoga vs. experience and tradition. The seasoned, dangerous thirty-one-year-old Baer could hit so hard that he had already killed a man in the ring, but early in this fight, two things were made clear: Nova could take Baer's hardest punches and Baer had not sufficiently prepared for a long siege. Hoping for an early knockout, Baer threw everything he had at Nova in the first four rounds but failed to hurt him.

Then began a slow and bloody turnabout. Not only did Nova's Cosmic Punch prove to be as damaging a weapon as advertised, slicing Baer's face once, twice, then at will, but the younger man simply outlasted his opponent, as predicted by Bernard. Though the fight did not draw the expected crowd—it was competing with the World's Fair—it was distinguished by its brutality: "one of the most furious heavyweight battles seen in a local ring in years," said the *New York Times*. "Baer took the worst beating of his life last night. He was a horrible sight leaving the ring and an even worse sight in the dressing room."

Baer's face had been battered into a hideous new shape—beyond recognition; the veteran's left eye had completely closed and his lower lip had opened so extravagantly that in the early seconds of the eleventh round, the fighter's windpipe filled with a river of his clotting blood. Baer gasped for enough breath to go on, but the referee called the fight: a TKO for Nova.

It was a great, whooping victory for the power of yoga and Bernard. From then on, and for the rest of his life, Lou Nova was linked to yoga and branded a disciple of Oom. He practiced meditation and headstands before each contest and put himself into such deep pre-bout trances that his handlers had to scream in his ear to get his attention. In round after round, Nova demonstrated that he had learned how to endure pain and physical punishment with something akin to a yogi's detachment. He needed it in his next fight when he was nearly beaten into a coma by Tony Galento in a barely refereed match that *Sports Illustrated* later called "one of the goriest fights in ring history." Two years later Nova redeployed the Cosmic Punch to take down Baer for a second time, and thus earn his ticket to challenge Joe Louis for the heavyweight championship. The challenge was taken up on a cold night in the Bronx. Nova darted around the ring with great energy until the sixth round, when he paused to gather himself. Louis then hit him in the head with a single blow that stretched the challenger out on the canvas, immobile. It was reported that the right-hand blow that ended the fight sounded like a clap of thunder in the furthest reaches of Yankee Stadium. Nova said the last thing he remembered was that he forgot to duck.

But for all his success with Nova, Bernard's own ambitions to teach other boxers didn't take off after the 1939 season. For reasons that were never made clear, he failed to lure Tony Galento or any other fighter back to Nyack to set up a training camp. Nova's manager, Ray Carlen, jealous of Bernard, began turning against the CCC immediately after the first fight against Baer, telling all who would listen that the yoga-club living was a bit too soft for his taste, and the whole thing was done simply for

publicity. Later in 1939, he took his fighter to a woodsy, isolated camp
in Maine where there was no yogi in attendance, no culture to speak of,
nothing to distract Nova but the occasional hotfoot. In 1941, when Carlen
was suspended for his poor preparation of Nova for the Louis fight, he went
so far as to blame his fighter's defeat on the effects of the yoga training,
vowing that the name of Oom the Omnipotent "will never be linked with
Nova again." Carlen did not succeed in banning the association—Nova
himself brought up the benefits of yoga time and again—but Bernard was
never given the opportunity to train another boxer.

But no matter. By the summer of 1939 Bernard's focus had moved on to another heavyweight protégé. Not one to dwell on past victories, that summer
he'd welcomed his old pal Leopold Stokowski, who moved in as the Nova
camp moved out. Stokowski, the leader of the Philadelphia Orchestra,
possessed a superstar level of celebrity by this time. Recently divorced
from his second wife, Evangeline, the Johnson & Johnson heiress, he had
been spending much of his time in Hollywood. He had already appeared
in two movies—*The Big Broadcast of 1937* with Benny Goodman and *One
Hundred Men and a Girl* with singer Deanna Durbin—both times playing himself, Stokowski the flamboyant conductor. The international press
corps had recently shadowed him through Italy as he courted the world's
most beautiful woman, Greta Garbo. Now the Maestro was planning his
biggest coup, appearing (of course) as himself, in *Fantasia*, a collaboration with Walt Disney and Disney's cartoon empire.

For the first time in his life, Stokowski was considerably overweight
and wished to slim down in private at the club. But he was also nostalgic
for the memorable days he'd spent there in the mid-1920s, flirting, cooking,
lecturing on music and theater, and soaking up all he could about yoga.
And he wanted to use the time there to find his muse as a composer, something that had eluded him his entire career. Bernard set the conductor up
in one of the private houses on the grounds and began working with him,
providing him with poetry and prose to free up his imagination. DeVries,
who was spending more time apart from her husband at her yoga studio
on Fifty-seventh Street, feigned jealousy at not getting her fair share of
Stokowski's attention when she heard his plans. Before he even arrived in

Nyack, she wrote him a playfully threatening letter, casting herself in the role of Kali, the angry mother of Tantra.

> Dear Stokowski,
>
> The Goddess Kali is a rather difficult person to manage. Should the mood of that irate person be willing, perhaps before your departure we might hope for a talk at the address below, where, by the way, I am specializing in the teaching of physical yoga. Perhaps you will send a note in any case.

Stokowski got the joke and wrote back full of warmth and good tidings: "I feel we shall always be friends and hope you feel the same on your side. . . . I shall be happy to see you again and no matter how seldom we see each other I hope we shall always be friends."

Stokowski, true to his word, maintained a friendship with DeVries and Bernard both, though what he found at Nyack that summer was no doubt a diminished version of his memories. There were fewer young women and more widows at the Cat's Whiskers, and the place was badly missing DeVries's soothing touch. Time and the Depression had stripped away much of the glitter of the CCC, and this turned out to be Stokowski's last visit.

DeVries, meanwhile, was quite busy in New York, getting ready to move her yoga studio to a fancier location on Central Park South. It was becoming clear that she and Bernard were headed for a permanent separation, and that it was Bernard's inability to stay faithful that had brought them to this state. Most recently he had turned his attention to Jeanne Powell, the more devoted of the Powell sisters, both of whom had lived at the club since 1921. Jeanne's worship of Bernard, addressing him as "beloved" and vowing to be with him "always" in letters, had always annoyed DeVries. So when her husband started giving Jeanne a place of honor at the club, DeVries was so outraged that if she had occasion to telephone the clubhouse, she would not deign to speak to Jeanne Powell.

DeVries's scorn elicited Viola's sympathy, and she later wrote of Bernard: "I thought he treated her rather badly in a personal way, including humiliating her by having one of the other women in the group, suddenly treating her as though she was the chief lady." Though it would take a few more years for the breach to widen intractably, DeVries's love for her husband was by this time fatally ruptured.

<hr />

While Bernard was preoccupied in 1938 and 1939, training a fighter and slimming down a conductor, his nephew Theos had become the most celebrated American yogi of his generation. Upon his return to the United States in December 1937, the White Lama embarked on a frantic lecture tour, speaking about his Tibetan adventure and showing his slides and films. In Viola's view, though, her husband had returned from Tibet a stranger. Theos was now a celebrity adventurer with strange dietary needs, novel sexual requests (Tantric sex techniques he'd learned about in Tibet), and new plans for their future, which he expected her to fund. To Viola, already a committed physician, he had carelessly revealed in letters home his "disbelief in Western medicine" along with his conviction that "there would never be any time in our lives for a home and children."

Viola had her own issues with Theos: "He deplores the fact that I don't give a damn about what he's so involved in doing, just as he doesn't give a damn about medicine. . . . He has a plan that I could set up a property in which we'd have an institute and I would sort of run it like the Clarkstown Country Club was run by DeVries for PAB and it would be full of lamas who would be deciphering and decoding and translating."

As Viola summed it up years later, "This was very far from my interests at this point . . . so we had a parting of the ways."

On April 5, 1938, three years and nine months after their wedding, Viola wrote to Theos the words she could not bear to say to him in person: "You can touch me emotionally, as you know," she explained, "and arouse a maternal aspect—the desire to help you . . . which is a part of our relationship that means a great deal to you also. But you are too much of an adult now to be satisfied with that and as a wife my feelings have ceased to function completely enough to make either of us happy." She announced that she would be traveling to Nevada to procure a divorce.

Within days Theos had packed up and moved his belongings to New York City, where he began living and working in DeVries's studio. "He was very close apparently to DeVries and she to him," Viola said, though she did not find out until much later that Theos and DeVries had fallen in love and engaged in a brief affair, despite the seventeen-year age difference.

DeVries, it seems, had found her antidote to Jeanne Powell in the form of her husband's own nephew.

As the decade ended, the three women—Vi, Di, and DeVries—were on their own. Viola moved back to Nyack, where she turned the garage and stables of her mother's estate into living quarters for herself, her home base while she began her psychiatric residency across the Hudson in Westchester. The sisters had inherited their mother's Sky Island mansion after Emma's death two years before, but neither of them wanted to live in the big house. Instead, in 1939 Viola transformed Sky Island into the first big project of her new life as a social activist and humanitarian. As one of the founders of the Non-Sectarian Committee for German Refugee Children, Viola made her mother's grand home a transitional shelter for thousands of refugee children from Nazi Germany. Her group, she later wrote, was a "key factor in the Wagner-Rogers legislation that would admit 30,000 refugee children from Germany to the United States."

Theos, too, had prospered in the wake of his divorce. While Bernard was putting Nova through his final preparation for the Baer fight, Theos's book about Tibet, *Penthouse of the Gods*, was published to wide acclaim. *Time* magazine judged the author's prose to be less than stellar, but liked the photos and applauded his yoga fortitude. "Ceremonials in the windowless temple room, lit with thousands of butter lamps, frequently lasted from sunrise to sunset, with 10,000 monks repeating one chant up to 108,000 times." And for his Tantric initiation, Theos had "braved the black chamber of horrors filled with fiendish and erotic idols [and] kept his head during four days of solitary confinement in a rock cave."

The book, of course, was a mere curtain-raiser to his long-awaited lecture tour. "The thrilling, gripping true story of the land that time forgot—Tibet," read one poster announcing his appearance. "Theos Bernard, Explorer, brings to Reno for the first time, the inside story of *Lost Horizon*, with his colored motion pictures and talk, 'Penthouse of the Gods.' Get your tickets now at Hills's Drug Store, Ramos, Reno Florist, and Southworth Cigar. Tickets 25¢ and 50¢."

According to Viola, Bernard "went nuts" after Theos's book was so well received. "He was supposed to be the great [big] shot and here was this upstart who was writing books that people were respecting," she said. At one point Bernard wrote his own unpublished review, called "In Re: Theos," in which he savaged his nephew's work, accusing him of "purloining books of modern and ancient writers, using the translation without giving credit or crediting the publishing house which printed the works, but taking credit for the text."

The rivalry continued while Theos was on tour. That summer Bernard managed to get himself crowned "American Yogi" by an enlightened set of journalists from a Chicago-based magazine called *Ken*. A vibrant but short-lived publication for a hip and progressive crowd, *Ken* was led by Arnold Gingrich, who had cofounded *Esquire* a few years before, and he was squarely on Oom's side. "In the national yoga boom that may come," the magazine wrote, "practitioners may well turn their steps to a hill in Nyack where a squire who is also treasurer of the local chamber of commerce runs a combination menagerie, training quarters, health resort and Yoga center for aspiring devotees." The piece was accompanied by a portfolio of photographs capturing the different sides of the Great Oom in his sixties: the fit, bare-chested Bernard of the Lou Nova training camp; the comically messy philosopher in his paper-strewn study; the sardonic challenger of the status quo, cigar locked in his mouth, looking as carefree as the animals around him, despite his financial, marital, and business woes. The most telling image in the portfolio: his empty dog track stadium, abandoned now to weeds and decay and the weather.

The next month Bernard took it upon himself to publish an obituary honoring forty-four-year-old Barbara Rutherfurd, who died in August 1939 at her mother's villa in Cannes. He placed the notice in the local *Journal-News*, but the obit drew city reporters to Nyack hoping for more scandal and dish. "I haven't seen or heard from the girl in a dozen years," he said to the *American Weekly*, a Hearst Sunday supplement. "People tell me I've supposed to have gotten a million dollars out of the Vanderbilts. If I could do that, I wouldn't be a mystic. I'd be a magician. A million bucks! Out of the Vanderbilts!"

When pressed to say if he was still practicing and teaching yoga, he responded, "Yoga's my bug, that's all. Like another guy will go in for gardening or collecting stamps. But I don't teach it anymore. How could I pay $15,000 a year in taxes on this place and spend my time teaching Yoga? Today, this place is a country club, just like any other country club—only better than most of them. But it's open to anybody with a check book."

The *Weekly* nonetheless reprised one last blast of scurrilous sensationalism from Hearst's yellow-press days. That Sunday in September, some 50 million Americans were told that the cause of Barbara's mental breakdown, what the *Weekly* called her "mysterious transformation," was attributable to Bernard's evil influence.

<hr />

As the new decade began, Bernard struggled hard to keep the club solvent. He owned bank stock, which paid him some small dividends, and shares in a mortgage company. The seven elephants were on the road performing, netting $700 a week this time around. But guests were few that winter and CCC records show no major activities. In his mid-sixties, the Great Oom was sinking in debt and tightly leashed to his dog track problems as the Great Depression rolled on. It must have seemed even more poignant then that in the spring of 1940 his original benefactor, Anne Vanderbilt, passed away, seven months after Barbara's death. To be sure, there was no mention of the Omnipotent Oom in the lengthy survey of Anne's life in the *New York Times* obituary. Nevertheless, Bernard attended her funeral services four days later and caught up on the family's latest developments. If he didn't already know, he learned that Margaret had dumped her French royal and married once again, to an artist named Frederick Leybourne Sprague, and that Barbara's son Rutherfurd was now attending Princeton.

To the press and those who could only see his evil influence, Bernard's generosity with his own extended family would have made for shocking headlines. That same month, his cousin George Frederic Hoffman passed away suddenly, leaving his wife, Katharin, with three teenage children to care for, and Bernard politely asked her to let him help. "Don't hesitate K to open your heart to me of troubles of whatever description and I will go to work on them," he wrote. "Cash is shy just at this moment, but I can always borrow." He offered her not only money, but his home, aid, and assistance in any way she might require. "As you know Mrs. B and I have no children of our own and we would be glad to take [Katharin's daughter] May . . . and see her through until she is settled in life. Send her to school and college . . . shoulder every expense—treating her as our own—finance her school-summer vacations to and from you for whatsoever part of every summer she may want to spend there."

Katharin did not take Bernard up on this offer, though the overture was gratefully received in Leon, Iowa. Her son, G.F. Jr., who would join and eventually take over the family's law firm there, remembered years later how touched the family had been at hearing Bernard *ask* to relieve "any burdens our family had." This strange, rich relative from the East had been good to him and his kin, said G.F., who very soon would get his own chance to know Bernard even better.

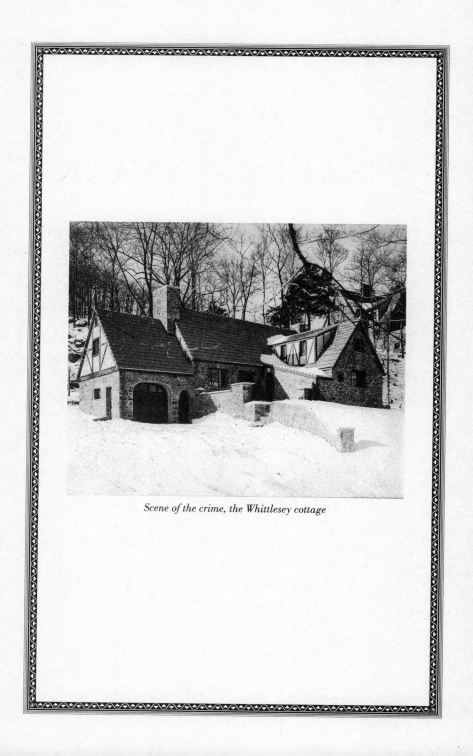

Scene of the crime, the Whittlesey cottage

Chapter 26

A NAZI IN NYACK

n late January 1941 the club was cocooned for the winter. On the grounds it was unusually quiet—off-season, wartime, post-holiday quiet. On Sunday morning, January 19, it was cold, seventeen degrees, with patches of ice and snow clinging to the ground. Inside the stone cottage of Percival Wilcox Whittlesey, Diana Wertheim's ex, a household emergency was unfolding.

"Come down immediately, something's gone wrong with the furnace," the handyman shouted. Percival pulled on some clothes to see for himself what Walter Groebli was carrying on about. The normally well-mannered merchant seaman from Atlanta had been working for him for the past four months, taking care of the house and cooking for Whittlesey and his boarder, Harry Allaire.

At first things had gone well—Allaire said he and Whittlesey both considered the young man like one of the family—but lately bad feelings had erupted between Percival and Groebli over the most galvanizing issue of the day: the war in Europe. The eighteen-year-old Groebli, an American of Swiss-German ancestry, was secretly obsessed by Nazi images of Teutonic supremacy. While Whittlesey made frequent trips to Washington, D.C., to help his new organization, Council for America, enlist high-profile support for Britain's cause against Germany, Groebli was visiting the Yorkville section of New York City, where he met pro-Hitler Germans and purchased Nazi propaganda. Groebli's diary entries during this time revealed his hatred of Jews, his sympathy for Hitler, and his growing disdain for his employer. The young man given shelter in Whittlesey's cottage had turned out to be the old spy's most paranoid fantasy—an enemy living in his own home, taking notes, making plans, most likely with the help of others.

By 1941 the war in Europe had taken on personal dimensions in Nyack, as it had in most parts of the United States. On South Mountain, just up the hill from Whittlesey, his ex-sister-in-law Viola Bernard had for two years been sheltering child refugees of the Third Reich at her mother's estate. In Upper Nyack, Alexandra Tolstoy, Leo's daughter, took in Russian refugees. A year or so earlier, in the heart of the Nyacks, someone of a different persuasion tried to sell a few acres to the German-American Bund, who were seen in the area marching around in brown shirts with swastika armbands.

As Whittlesey turned to enter the furnace room, he encountered his own .32-caliber automatic pistol pointed at his face. With no warning, Groebli began firing. He squeezed off one or two wild shots and retreated up the stairs, but not before Whittlesey got his hands on him. The teenager managed to break away and fired another shot, this time hitting Whittlesey directly in the mouth. As the struggle wheeled onto the main floor of the house, Groebli fired again and again, spraying slugs into Whittlesey's oak-paneled library of spy books. Then he fled.

"Dr. Whittlesey staggered out a door and down six ice-fringed steps, trailing blood," the *New York Times* reported on page one the following day. Whittlesey had been wounded in the mouth, neck, shoulder, and chest as well as his wrist. All the bullets but one had passed through him. The last, which punctured a lung, was his only life-threatening injury, but he was rushed to the hospital in time for the doctors to save him.

At the crime scene, the police picked up the first slug on the cellar stairs landing; at the head of the stairs, another was found in the front hall, along with two of Whittlesey's teeth. Three more slugs were lodged in the library's oak beams. Shortly after 2 p.m., the New York State police bloodhounds went yelping out the back door and picked up the trail of the assailant, who police believed still held the gun. All day, Groebli sightings were received by local police departments and phoned in to the Whittlesey home. Squad cars searched the major highways from Bear Mountain to the New Jersey state line.

Bernard, for his part, placed himself at center stage in the commotion. He acted as a welcoming committee for the reporters. He played favorites, giving better information to the *Times* man, but he provided one and all with the lay of the land, described the provenance of the Whittleseys' house on the hillside, right on the club grounds, how it was built for Diana and Percival by former CCC member Morris Whitaker, how all the involved parties were club members at one time. It was the biggest excitement at the club in quite some time.

In May, as Whittlesey was back at home recovering, Groebli was caught and confessed. Just then word came to Bernard of another ambush—nonviolent but flesh-rending in its own way. It seemed that his nephew Theos and Clara Stuart (née Thorpe), his protégée from the early days in New York, had been running a yoga school out of a plush hotel suite at the Hotel Pierre in New York—paid for by DeVries. This fact came to light when one of the trio's long-term students, a wealthy, unstable woman named Mrs. Donovan, had to be committed to an asylum by her husband. Mr. Donovan blamed her yogi and his accomplices for his wife's condition. He sued Theos for $25,000.

During pretrial testimony Theos put as much distance as possible between himself and his uncle. He insisted that he was not related to Pierre, and that he would never have gone near Nyack at all had it not been for Viola, his ex-wife. Though he attended some of his uncle's lectures, he denied that he took yoga lessons from him or learned anything of value from him. His lawyer then asked, "What were the lectures that Pierre Bernard delivered?"

THEOS: So far as I could tell, they seemed to be nothing much but personal prejudices.

Q: Against what?

THEOS: The world in general. The whole lectures were so long and involved that at the end it was impossible to say afterwards what they were about for you usually were sleeping.

Q: You slept through a number of his lectures did you?

THEOS: Every one I could, along with everyone else.

Theos's treason was detailed in Hearst's *American Weekly* Sunday magazine for the entire nation's enjoyment, and so his nephew delivered a swift and public kick to Bernard when he was already down. No amount of posturing during the Whittlesey ordeal could mask the dire financial straits both Bernard and his club had fallen into. The CCC was months behind in payments to its local vendors—butcher ($1,106), fruit and vegetable man ($402.91), fish man ($113.30), laundry ($471), drugstore ($500), and others for thousands more. Many of these proprietors, whose business once depended upon the club in thriving times, were now demanding payment in full—cash only—or they would suspend deliveries. But this was a paltry problem compared with the ever-growing mountain of back taxes—Bernard said it was upward of $36,000 at the time—that was accumulating penalties as it went unmet.

Then on October 4, 1941, DeVries officially resigned from the CCC. After twenty-four years of marriage, including a long, slow-burning separation, this act rendered the breach irreparable. She was now making a living teaching yoga at her own New York studio, the Living Arts Center. Bernard was attempting to keep the club as beautiful and welcoming a resort as it had been under her direction. Neither was entirely successful. It appeared that DeVries was also living part-time somewhere on the club grounds with her sister, Franci, declining to pay Bernard rent and siphoning off students for her own yoga school. For these and other alleged crimes—Bernard must have heard through back channels about her affair with Theos—he had rather ungallantly stopped his financial support and refused to communicate with her about arrangements for her future.

On December 7, DeVries sent a long letter to Bernard expressing her resentment at his treatment: "I have not had one single word from you as to a concrete plan as to what's what definitely about finances. I suggest you have [your lawyer] Wells sit in and try to get something clarified for me on paper." The Wertheim sisters, along with Theos and Clara and a few others, lined up on DeVries's side. Winfield Nicholls, who had remained at the club throughout these years, joined Jeanne and Martha Powell as the chief defenders of Bernard the righteous, angry husband. There was catty talk and nastiness from the Bernard faction, DeVries complained—"fools speaking out of time."

"Talk has certainly ruined and re-ruined this Club situation," she continued. "How can you afford to have your subordinates do this kind of business? This is the kind of war fare, littleness, undermining that is the human nature trait that causes the big wars."

An arrangement was reached. DeVries moved into the Farm House, the home she'd once shared with Bernard, but this time she would share it with Franci. A hundred yards or so away, Bernard made his home in the CCC clubhouse. During the years of separation (they never legally divorced), Bernard often communicated with DeVries by letters and telegrams, many sent not directly to her but to her sister. In one of these letters, he informed Franci that he expected the two of them to pay the rent on her living quarters, cobbling together the funds from subleasing other homes on the Farm House property and the profits from her yoga studio. DeVries, with a wronged spouse's righteous fury, simply refused to cooperate with this scheme and stayed in arrears, which frustrated Bernard, and in his eyes made him look like a fool to his business associates. DeVries also left Nyack for months at a time, leaving her husband no word of her whereabouts or her plans as she toured through Europe and the United States.

"It was one of those love/hate separations," explained Viola Bernard, "in which they were not divorced, and in which they continued to remain somewhat attached to each other."

Bernard and the club faced the war years with a vastly reduced roster, mostly due to fuel and food rations and travel restrictions, which meant that far-flung members or guests who'd remained loyal through the Depression could no longer easily visit. It was considered unpatriotic to travel long distances then, even if you could find the means.

President Roosevelt proclaimed to the nation that "every man, woman and child is in action. The front is right here." It certainly was in Rockland County. There were reminders every day that the country was at war. Blackouts and dim-outs were common up and down the Hudson, which was now crowded with troop ships and Coast Guard cruisers. The Hudson River Valley became known as "Last Stop USA"—more than one million soldiers marched through Nyack on their way to ship out for overseas duty. On the edge of Bernard's property, aircraft observation tower Chestnut 2-0 was manned by a local teenager named Russell McCandless, who phoned his sightings in to a central command.

By the time the United States entered the war, Bernard had waived any initiation requirements, lowered dues, and offered free admission to lectures. In the summer of 1942, he hosted a group of young actors who gave performances at night on the grounds. Will Geer's summer company, the Tower Bell Theatre, drew a curious reporter and photographer from *Life* magazine. "Summer theaters have had a bad season," *Life* reported, "but Tower Bell Theatre in Nyack, N.Y. at least had an interesting one." The editors managed to convert a bit of novelty into an uplifting tale for nervous times, as well as one that was easy on the eyes. Half a dozen or so pretty actresses in bathing suits cooled off in the elephants' swimming pool. The elephants, trained professionals that they were, sprayed the bathing beauties on the photographer's command with plumes of water.

The entire company learned a few asanas from the master. "Although about 70, Dr. Bernard can still do wonderful Yoga things with his stomach muscles, can turn a complete front flip from standing position," *Life* reported. The menagerie, which had free run of the place, kept the actors on their toes, to everyone's delight. Monkeys dropped from trees during rehearsals, and every night when lead actor Geer performed a scene that required him to raise his voice, "the lions roared, the elephants trumpeted, the chimpanzee hooted, the peacock screeched, some dogs howled and the audience grew faint with laughter."

But on July 28, a beloved member of the menagerie, Budh, died unexpectedly. Performing on the road, Budh had stepped on a spike, which penetrated his heel and allowed a fatal infection to take hold. He came home to Nyack to die. Now of Bernard's original herd of four, only Baby and Juno remained, though he was still caring for Mrs. Power's aging elephants. And there would be one last big show for his beloved pets.

* * *

Midway through the steamy night of August 21, 1942, despite stringent gasoline rationing, some 1,500 cars arrived at the Clarkstown Country Club for a benefit concert to provide food and medical supplies to the starving Russian populace. State police and local cops directed the drivers into the club grounds, where volunteers diced the lines of traffic into rows of parking spots on the lawns and roads lining Bernard's property. At 8:30, the stage lights went up, the band struck a flourish, and an electronic message board gave the club grounds the flavor of Times Square and Forty-second Street. A sellout crowd of three thousand spectators sat on folding chairs, fanning away the heat and mosquitoes on the front lawn of the club. They were here for the biggest night Rockland had seen since Bernard's sports stadium closed. Best of all for a wartime audience, it was guilt free.

U.S. Supreme Court justice Stanley F. Reed was chief among the notables in the benefit audience, but that night most of the celebrities were onstage. The show, titled the *Rockland Riot*, was the creation of Helen Hayes, event chairman, and her husband, Charles MacArthur, who staged the twelve-act variety program. Friends and collaborators Maxwell Anderson, Kurt Weill, and Lotte Lenya showed up, too. The popular comedian Ed Wynn, known to radio and Broadway audiences as "the Perfect Fool," emceed; Helen Hayes acted in a scene from Anderson's *Mary of Scotland*, along with her daughter Mary and Anderson's daughter Hesper. Donald Ross and Will Geer threw in some drama and comedy. Larry Adler, the harmonica virtuoso, played Russian love songs.

There was singing and dancing by an ad hoc group called the Rockland Rockettes, and neither rain nor a mosquito invasion squelched the good cheer. At intermission, Bernard's remaining elephants put on a show as the revelers stretched their legs. The electronic message board flashed news of further benefits for the Russian people and a few corny jokes aimed at the Axis powers. At one point it read:

ANY SIMILARITY BETWEEN DR. BERNARD'S ELEPHANT'S REAR AND
HERMANN GOERING IS PURELY CO-INCIDENTAL

The *Rockland Riot* was judged a huge success, reaping thousands of dollars for war relief, if not a cent for the generous Pierre Bernard and his failing club.

The Clarkstown Country Club limped along during the next year with no major events and no new sources of income. Eventually, Bernard was forced to part with Baby and Juno when he got an offer from Ringling Bros. Circus; he sent the Power elephants off to new homes, too. But there was some good news: 1944 also marked the twenty-fifth anniversary of the Tantriks' arrival in Nyack. Not only was practicing yoga no longer considered criminally weird—some even likened it to a patriotic duty. Cornelia Otis Skinner, a famous actress of the time, told a health columnist that "nerves are unpatriotic," and yoga helped cure hers. The year before, it had been discovered that Margaret Woodrow Wilson, the former president's daughter, had spent the last four years studying yoga at an ashram in India, where Mahatma Gandhi had also received treatments. Author Paul Brunton, who'd spent five years in the East, wrote well-received books that further spread the word about the mystical and miraculous components of yoga.

So when Bernard announced a new series of lectures that fall, he expected a somewhat higher level of familiarity with his subject than in the past. "This announcement is only for those who already have some acquaintance with Yoga and know what it means," read the printed brochure. "For this reason no effort has been made to elucidate the teachings."

He offered fifty additional memberships, with applications due in mid-September: "Club membership, one hundred dollars. Dues twenty-five dollars per year for resident members. No dues for non-resident members who come for lectures only."

Despite what he groused about to reporters just two years back—that he was too busy earning money to pay his taxes to teach yoga—he had indeed come full circle. He resumed his regular lecture series, which he'd left off more than ten years earlier, and again took up the task of his life, defining and redefining yoga for curious seekers. Yoga "insists upon the organization and adaptation of knowledge, as a preparation for complete living. Its triumphs are not over, but in and through the senses."

There it was, that old Tantric-American message of salvation not through asceticism but through the body and its portals to the world. This time Bernard had also added a snazzy new term, *Imagineering*, to describe his latest thinking on the subject of imagination. And finally, he formulated his new decalogue, or ten commandments, for the club:

KEEP PHYSICALLY FIT

CULTIVATE GOOD HABITS

REMOVE UNNECESSARY STRESS AND STRAIN . . .

ACCEPT REALITY

PLAN DAILY SCHEDULE OF ACTIVITY . . .

LIVE IN TERMS OF WE NOT I

CHERISH A SENSE OF HUMOR

KNOW YOURSELF

BE YOURSELF

IMPROVE YOURSELF

The brochure that contained this commonsense wisdom inevitably drew the attention of two women who were determined to forge reputations as this decade's witch hunters. On an undercover mission to root out quacks, Mrs. Lee Steiner presented herself to her targets as a woman with family issues. She created an imaginary husband named George, who was suffering from depression, along with a hypothetical twenty-six-year-old son named Junior, who had been forced out of the wartime military with a "psychiatric discharge." To discuss what might be done to help Junior recover, Steiner and her friend Mabelle Barrison made an appointment for lunch with Bernard at the Clarkstown Country Club.

"The site is magnificent," Mrs. Steiner wrote, "as is the stone-and-stucco clubhouse with its attractive landscaping, now somewhat neglected." The two women walked the grounds, where they ran into a few employees but no guests. They ate lunch alone in the clubhouse dining room, awaiting an audience with Bernard.

"He is a well-preserved man, but a more nervous one I have yet to meet," Steiner wrote. "The stillness of the august hall seemed too much for him." They adjourned to Bernard's office for the consultation, and the guru delivered his well-rehearsed pitch. He assured the women that yoga could cure Junior if he committed to the practice and came to live at the club full-time. In fact, Junior would be welcomed as part of the community here, and he could study, play, and join in the rowdy late-night discussions in the Cat's Whiskers.

"We kid people out of grouchy," Bernard told them.

Bernard was nervous for good reason. His instincts hadn't failed him after all these years. The interview was not a fact-finding mission at all, but a setup. The women were feigning interest in spiritual exotica, trances, and self-hypnotism to lead him on.

"No astral bunk goes on here," Bernard insisted, but they weren't buying it.

Steiner reserved her judgment for a book she published in 1945, *Where Do People Take Their Troubles?* In it she crammed Oom the Omnipotent into a single-chapter pileup of villains that included Bernard's lifelong enemies the spiritualists, along with Theosophists, Rosicrucians, black magicians, and other charlatans that she found beneath contempt. From her yellow-press portrait of Bernard's scandalous background she reached her scathing conclusion: "It was depressing to think that a man with his background should be allowed to have custody of people's personal problems."

With Bernard now close to seventy and his club an apparition of its former glory, Steiner's attack was akin to shooting at shadows. Departing the CCC, she had wandered the grounds again, looking for others to interview, and found not a single soul. "The place seemed so lonely," she wrote.

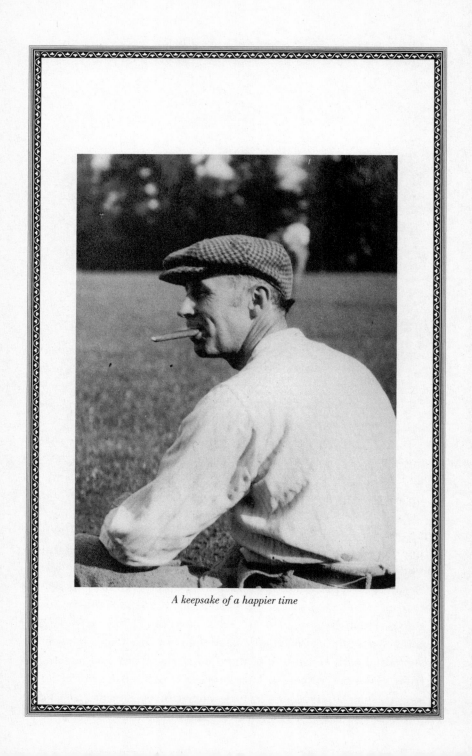

A keepsake of a happier time

Chapter 27

FAMILY MAN

y the fall of 1945, World War II had ended. Hundreds of thousands of veterans disembarked from ships up and down the East Coast, anxious to restart their lives. In Nyack as in Beckley, West Virginia, and Council Bluffs, Iowa, an immediate housing shortage followed the vets' return. "Real estate gone crazy," Bernard wrote to DeVries's sister, Franci, in 1946. "Piece of business property they had for sale for $6500 four months ago, sold for over $29,000." Bernard quickly sold off parcels of land on the Maxwell estate, the site of his original landing in Upper Nyack, but he couldn't part with the two beautiful mansions on either end of the property.

DeVries, too, was thinking about her own financial future. As November began, she was awaiting the final hammer on a three-day auction of her possessions at the Parke-Bernet Galleries in New York City. DeVries stripped her home of most anything worth selling and added to this trove the furniture, art, and bibelots given to her by clients over her thirty-year career as a decorator. "English and French furniture, tapestries, porcelains, silver, table china, Oriental rugs" was the title of the catalog, the property of "Miss Blanche De Vries, New York." Among fifty-eight separate items she auctioned were more than two dozen late eighteenth-century (and early nineteenth-century) floral engravings and aquatints, a K'ang Hsi–type Chinese peony carpet, an early eighteenth-century landscape, and a nineteenth-century watercolor by French artist Paul Gavarni. She also sold a great deal of furniture: a Louis XV decorated side table (Venetian, circa eighteenth century), a late eighteenth-century French writing table, and an assortment of other antiques, including a dining table, side chairs, a bedstead, armchairs, garden tables, a Shera-ton parrot cage, and a maroon-painted Steinway baby grand piano.

Bernard's assets by this point were decidedly less glamorous. Linger-ing lawsuits over the failed dog track tied up the potential sale of the Sports Centre, while many of his other properties, the real source of his wealth, were in receivership. Others were in the process of being sold or rented to cover unpaid taxes. He hunkered down in the clubhouse mansion with Jeanne Powell and their few guests, including Jeanne's sister Martha, who had been stricken with a degenerative neurological disease that would eventually take her life.

Bernard's publicity efforts of 1944–1945 had failed. The club attract-ed a few delegates of the just-formed United Nations and the occasional Sanskrit scholar who made use of Bernard's library or came by to lecture, but Bernard without DeVries functioned at severely diminished power. He was Shiva without Shakti, yang without yin. And without new donors and the consistent income stream necessary to maintain such a large set of luxury properties, he was forced to struggle and plot every day to keep his once mighty empire from utter diminution and disrepair.

With his uncle in this vulnerable spot, Theos Bernard cheerfully stepped in to fill his role as chief spokesman for the power and glory of hatha yoga. The White Lama, in the prime of his life, was touring, lectur-ing, writing a second book, and enjoying opening nights at the Metropoli-tan Opera with members of society's old Four Hundred. When Frederic Haskin, the popular "Questions Answered" columnist, asked on behalf of a reader, "How many postures are there in yoga?" he turned not to Uncle Pierre but to Theos, who settled the question with preposterous certainty: "Eighty-four thousand postures and exercises." Theos had even snagged a new benefactor. In 1942 he had married again, to Ganna Walska, an extremely wealthy, five-times-divorced Polish soprano. Theos convinced her to buy a thirty-seven-acre garden estate in Montecito, about ninety miles north of L.A., where they planned a spiritual retreat center called Tibetland. The venture didn't take off, however, and by 1946, the mar-riage, too, had gone south. The couple divorced after an ugly and embar-rassing public fight. Walska renamed the estate Lotusland, and Theos moved on, preparing for his second trip to Tibet with a third wife, Helen Graham Park.

But then, in search of new material for a revised version of *Penthouse of the Gods*, Theos traveled to northern India during the Hindu-Muslim blood feuds that had erupted after the Partition. He was reported missing in Pakistan in October 1947; after months of fruitless searching, he was declared dead. Though his body was never recovered, he'd left behind his academic work, three popular books, thousands of feet of color film from Tibet, and the first extended photographic record of a handsome Westerner capably demonstrating thirty-three traditional yoga asanas.

If Bernard was indifferent to his nephew's death, DeVries was devastated; she had maintained a warm spot in her emotional makeup for Theos, and his death drew her and his ex-wife Viola even closer. In fact, they remained as close as sisters—closer even than Viola and Diana—for the rest of their lives.

By 1947, the incoming tide of yoga was unstoppable. Eugenie Peterson, a former actress from the Baltic state of Livonia, opened her first yoga studio in the United States that year. Indra Devi, as Peterson became known, was the sole female to be initiated and trained by India's father of modern yoga, Krishnamacharya, in the 1930s. And though she had been in the United States since the early 1940s, she chose to teach at the center of the new crossroads of Western celebrity and Eastern culture: Hollywood. Using a gentle, flowing style of hatha yoga, she took over the education of many actors and actresses, including Marilyn Monroe, Gloria Swanson, and Greta Garbo, the last of whom had no doubt gotten an initial taste of the practice from her beau Leopold Stokowski.

Indeed, many of Bernard's original followers—Hamish and Amie McLaurin, Cheerie and Tommy Jackson, Millie and James Gillingham, among others—were already in California, studying and teaching. And in New York City, where DeVries's Living Arts Center was finally starting to take off, her yoga students came to include many powerful and influential women, like Standard Oil heiress Rebekah Harkness and socialite Sunny von Bülow. One of the original yoginis of America, Clara Thorpe, having divorced her dance partner Richard Stuart and remarried a man named Frank Spring, taught yoga with DeVries in Manhattan and also in her own studios in Chicago and Los Angeles. Charles Potter, who had lived in one of Bernard's Upper Nyack homes into the early years of the Depression, had gradually detached from the club and moved his base of operations to New York City, the home of his Humanist Society, the grand project of his life. Even the loyal and devoted Winfield Nicholls, the last of Bernard's San Francisco crew, had remarried and moved to a new home in Virginia.

The old order changeth, as Bernard himself might have put it.

<hr />

Back in Nyack, the strain of keeping the club solvent was starting to take a physical toll on Bernard, who would turn seventy-two in 1948. Sweating through a stifling Hudson Valley August with forty pounds of extra weight on his once lean frame, he began to lose his most significant personal resource: his energy. It was this nearly preternatural life force, his élan vital, that made him the master of domains as disparate as automobiles, baseball, airports, boxing, and the landscape arts. Suddenly he described himself as exhausted; on some days he could barely walk a quarter mile before he had to return to his couch, winded and grateful for a soft landing and the company of the Powell sisters.

The state of affairs at his club, in turn, shadowed his physical decline. In a letter to one of his business associates in 1948, he summed it up: "We have little or no linen, nor rugs and shy on any [and] all kinds of furniture both for the club house and our own lecture building. All stuff on second floor of billiard room building is deteriorated and ruined. Even the main pieces [of furniture on the] ground floor clubhouse [are] dried up and leather split and rotted away, so we are in the sad end there. We cannot buy these leathers today, even if you had the money and we badly need something to doll up with."

Bernard was now in a race to stay ahead of his creditors and the government. His Biophile Club Company was virtually broke, its stock worthless, though it still held some $300,000 in mortgages. After several years of warnings, on May 4, 1948, he sent a telegram to his wife, informing her that she and Franci would have to vacate their home in thirty days, as he no longer owned it. TITLE OF FARM HOUSE PASSING TO WRIGHT BROS. REAL ESTATE, the telegram read. He was forcing her hand. Would she come crawling back and live with him in the still luxurious clubhouse? The answer was an unequivocal no. Viola stepped in and rented DeVries and Franci a cottage on the western side of South Mountain (a home she purchased for them outright the next year). Neither Viola nor Blanche ever took Bernard at his word regarding the extreme state of his finances nor forgave him fully for their eviction.

Following this drama, he suffered a serious physical breakdown that brought on bronchial pneumonia and forced him into a hospital bed for the first time in his life. For two and a half days, he hovered near death, barely able to fill his lungs, utterly unable to speak without inducing a racking cough. In the hospital, he was visited by his lawyer Francis Wells, who was overseeing the dismantling of his estate and, Bernard feared, keeping the worst news from him. In a rare letter written directly to DeVries, he described his woes in a desperate-looking scrawl that barely resembled his usually elegant cursive.

> It seems I cannot get over to you an understanding of my case. You may know that I am not of the wailing type—& for two or more days just passed [it] looked bad—and that you might be saved the ordeal of seeing me again alive. I have arranged through codicil of will & otherwise to have myself put away beside my mother, etc. Wonder if you ever heard of broncho-pneumonia. Well, that is part of my condition. I am better today and may be up for a few hours today or tomorrow. All has passed away but me and I am trying to hold on. . . . I should not be making this effort writing. . . . I cannot speak yet. Could see Durand [Margaret Rutherfurd] few minutes tomorrow maybe.

Unwritten but clearly detectable between the lines, a sick and aging man desired his wife's sympathy, but could not bring himself to ask for it. His revelation that he was to be buried in Iowa beside his mother implied a threat that he had amended his last will and testament, written in 1925, which had left his entire estate to DeVries. There is no record of his wife's reply to him or her showing up at his bedside.

Happily, by the next year, Bernard had recovered somewhat and undertook another effort to get the club up and running again. It was a minor, halfhearted attempt: another printing and mailing of the "Yoga" brochure and an attempt to "doll up" the property for guests, but it was all he could muster. His energy, his health—and his weight—had not yet fully returned to normal, as he wrote to Franci.

For nearly ¾ of the last year I either spent my time lying on couches or in bed or in large armchair—spend but little time in walking and that only as far as the barn and back and a little around the house. . . . Have had three different docs pawing over me this week besides having been driven to New York Hospital for further checking, but Franc I was not born yesterday and I am telling you they're just wasting their time—there is no use.

Signing off, he mentioned to his sister-in-law that someone had recently sent him lilies, "but they were a little previous."

I'm too mean to flop yet.

Sincerely etc,

Old Doctor Gray.

PB.

This brush with mortality had a profound effect on Bernard. He began to reach out in earnest to his blood relatives in Leon, Iowa, his birthplace. He seemed more anxious than ever to forge a solid connection with this side of his family, to reveal to them parts of himself and his past, to tease them with the possibility of a small inheritance. He began a correspondence with his cousins, particularly Martha Hoffman, a fiftyish attorney who, since the death of her brother G.F. Sr. ten years before, had been running the family law firm in Leon. Bernard petitioned Martha for family news. He beseeched her to visit, offering airfare, accommodations, and big-city entertainment in return. In one letter he pleaded, "I so wished that you yourself would come East this summer to familiarize yourself with everything here. I'm just supposing that if I kick the bucket and if these properties were not left to an institution, then as the inheritor of the same, you'd have the burden of disposing of them." He sent her boxes of "old pictures, cheap snapshots, and reprints from old tintypes, the whole mess to serve your visual memory of your Uncle Dudley [Pierre] and his crazy doings."

Martha, running the office virtually alone while her nephew G.F. Jr. finished law school, informed Bernard that she was unable to get away. Undaunted, he wrote that if she wouldn't come to him, he would continue to send her little pieces of himself, of which he told her the exact value: "Since separating from the wife, I've made it a point to give away all personal effects," he wrote, including "a dozen and a half overcoats that cost from $75 to $350 each, stacks of silk socks and silk underwear made to order, never used; over four gross of the most expensive handkerchiefs, and any amount of small jewelry; I guess I have a dozen and a half watches still remaining, some are platinum case and range from $175 to $1300 a piece."

He bragged to Martha about his female conquests—"In my time I've had a great many girl and women friends" was how he put it. And he joked about destroying the evidence of his lifetime of romantic affairs: "Just finished a burning party, meaning two days time in destroying packages of letters by the hundreds," he wrote. "I believe the Statute of Limitations, including Federal[,] terminates every six years." He mused about where he might live out his last days and fibbed about his travels: "I've been around," he wrote. "Most parts of India, some of Syria, France and England."

In the end, the connections he'd hoped for were never forged. Martha, his favorite cousin, had a full enough life in Iowa and no reason to uproot to the East Coast. He understood, he wrote her, so he did the next best thing and went to Iowa to see her and the rest of the family more frequently. But Bernard, even approaching his mid-seventies, could not defeat a lifelong compulsion to conceal as much as he revealed, to blur the details of his biography and tell outright lies, even to his kin. By his own devices, he remained as mysterious a figure to his relatives in Iowa as he did to those who knew him in Nyack.

As the decade ended, a classified advertisement buried in the back pages of the *New York Times*—bearing the innocent title "Miscellaneous"—revealed more about his troubles than he ever did. It was a common enough kind of ad, the public notice of a liquidation sale to satisfy creditors and tax collectors, but the combination of items could have come from the pursuits of only one man.

Lincoln high pressure car washing machine . . . full complete equipment steam laundry for small institution or large house . . . 18,000 candlepower search light $100 . . . 25 1,000 watt globes; 4 animal cages, # 9 galvanized wire and welded angle iron size 6 x 6 x 12 and up to 25 feet . . . professional grade tap dancing mats—roll up—two of them 4'x30'. . . .

Here was an elegy in agate type, a coded obituary for an era of dreams now dimmed: the thriving, noisy club with its limousines and heiresses, its costume balls and midnight suppers. Gone now, too, were the dog track, the zoo, the airport, and the circuses once advertised in the summer skies above the Hudson Valley with a swooping white light. The Inner Circle Theatre was dark, the library and lecture hall empty. Gone were the bustling days and nights spent providing the elite of American society with yoga lessons, clean cars, and laundered sheets—none of which could be afforded now, even if the guests were to begin motoring up from New York as they once did.

In the spring of 1950, Bernard finally convinced a Hoffman to come east for a first visit. George Frederic Hoffman Jr.—now known as G.F.—had just completed law school after serving in World War II. As an amiable young relative of sturdy Iowa stock, G.F. was just what Bernard was looking for.

"He said he was involved in a lawsuit," according to G.F., "concerned with the stadium. So he thought he had plenty of legal work for me. I was honored that he would ask me—here I was just out of law school. I figured he had his own lawyers, but he just thought he ought to have one of his own. He took me down to the river to the Moorings Estate and showed me the house that he would deed to me if I'd come back and live there."

Bernard began a full-court press to win over G.F. He introduced the young man to the two pretty assistants he had recently hired: tall, silent Doris, who did his typing and office work, and Mary, who drove him around in a new blue Cadillac. The foursome motored off on a tour of Nyack, Mary behind the wheel, Bernard chewing on cigars in the back. They went to the movies and attended a Brooklyn Dodgers baseball game.

For his part, the young Iowan didn't mind being courted. He had always been fond of his first-cousin-once-removed with the twinkle in his eyes, whom he remembered visiting his home some fifteen years before. To G.F., Bernard appeared healthy and happy in the early 1950s, quite unwilling to concede his mortality and bragging that he could still do front and back flips at his advanced age. "I thought he could," said G.F. "I thought he was going to live forever."

Despite the intensity of Bernard's efforts, however, G.F. didn't succumb to the temptations of fancy cars, Eastern women, and Hudson River mansions. Besides, he told Bernard, he had a girl back home named Betty who would be waiting to pick him up at the train station in Osceola on his return. When he married Betty in June 1951, G.F. went to work with Martha at the family law firm in Leon, and Bernard gave his blessing on both counts. "Even though I wouldn't come out there and be his lawyer, he never held that against me," said G.F.

On another trip back east, G.F. said Bernard took him to the garage and showed him his collection of Packards and Cadillacs—and his pride and joy, the Belgian Minerva, the dual-wheel, nine-passenger touring car with gold-inlaid custom-made fittings. "He also had a 12-cylinder Cadillac convertible," said G.F. "Pierre said, 'I'll give you that car if you'll drive it home.' He was always offering us things, but I didn't take them. I didn't think it was a good thing, and I didn't know what the hell I'd do with a Cadillac."

During these years, Bernard circled back to the place of his birth again and again. "He never told me ahead of time he was coming," said G.F. "I'd get a call . . . 'I'm in Chicago and on my way. I'll be there at 2:30 in the morning. Pick me up.'" During the four years the two men "visited," as Iowans liked to say, they shared a series of adventures in which the older man shed a bit of his reserve and the younger man learned a little more about his elusive cousin. They drove off to nearby Humeston, Iowa, where Bernard had spent a few years in his youth, to see an old friend. On one trip, Bernard donated $10,000 to the Leon Christian Church—of which his grandfather G. W. Baker was a founding member—and then silently mocked the pastor who offered a blessing in gratitude, letting G.F. know that he had less interest in religion than in leaving behind a contribution to his family's legacy.

Bernard asked to be driven out to Lamoni, Iowa, where a few of the extended Hoffman family belonged to the Church of the Reorganized

Latter Day Saints. At a Mormon Sunday service, he chuckled and rolled his eyes at the theatrical piety of some of the elders. Then he asked, in a voice loud enough for others to hear, "I wonder which one is getting the Tony Award?"

Bernard also used these Iowa visits to continue his financial shell games, hiding his real estate gains from his creditors—and perhaps his wife. "He sold the Farm House to the Nyack school district, and he brought a cashier's check out here for $100,000," G.F. recalled. "He said, 'We're going to Des Moines to find a national bank.' He put the money in the bank, with my name on the account. Gave me the book, and the account cards and all that—just left it all with me. Then he came back and checked it out about a year later and paid his taxes with it."

On one of his last visits home, Bernard arrived with an unlikely companion: a dark-skinned young woman dressed in drab, nun-like clothing. The family thought at first that she might be one of his girlfriends, but he introduced her as his niece, which she was. Clare Baker Khan was the younger daughter of Ora Ray Baker—Bernard's "kid sister," as he called her—and Hazrat Inayat Khan, the Indian spiritual leader and founder of the International Sufi Movement.

Ora Ray had died in 1949, and Clare Khan had waited for her mother's passing before she made the decision to fully reject the religious life. She'd arrived in the United States around 1950, looking to settle in New York City. Bernard didn't quite trust her motives at first—he thought she might be angling for an inheritance—but eventually he befriended her and took her to meet the Hoffman family.

"They stayed at the hotel in Leon," G.F. recalled. "He got her a room, got himself a room. And that's when he takes me aside and says, 'Here, I want you to hold this for me.'" Bernard peeled off five $100 bills and gave them to G.F., who insisted on giving him a receipt. The next day, they all drove to the Hoffman house. "After we ate breakfast, Pierre said, 'Betty! If I can borrow some money from G.F., I want you and Clare to go to Des Moines and get her some new clothes.'" Betty was aghast. She knew nothing about Bernard's secret handoff and G.F. had forgotten to mention it. "Pierre and I went off to the bedroom. I said, 'Here's your five hundred. Give me back the receipt, okay?' He came back out, counting it, maybe even lent me some, and said, 'Well, I got the money from G.F. Tomorrow we'll go to Des Moines.'"

This strange charade about money was part of a three-day Iowa visit for Bernard and Clare. On the third day, they returned to Nyack by train. "He never stayed too long," said G.F. "Never told me in advance about coming. Oh, he'd say, 'I'll be back one of these days.' But he'd never get pinned down. Why he wouldn't call before he left . . . I don't know. He'd say, 'I'm in Chicago on business, so I'm going to come on out.' I never knew if he had business there or not."

Bernard's only significant business in the early 1950s was arranging the timely sale or rental of his remaining Nyack properties to gain the means to live out his final years in comfort. For that he turned to Homer Lydecker Jr., a young real estate agent from an old Nyack family. In the coming years Lydecker would sell all but the two homes Bernard insisted on keeping to the end: the clubhouse and the beautiful Moorings estate on the banks of the Hudson River.

"I never saw any sadness in him during these deals," Lydecker said. "He never said anything, but there were signs of relief in his eyes, because the properties weren't making money and were becoming extremely burdensome to him. He offered no resistance—when I had a buyer and we gave him an appraisal, he didn't care too much who it was. The only time I detected any sadness in him was when he talked about the animals."

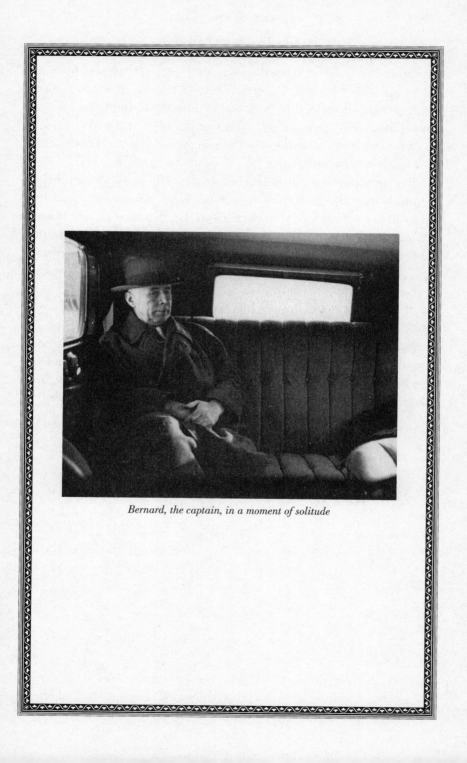

Bernard, the captain, in a moment of solitude

Chapter 28

FINAL DAYS

o life! It was always to life that Bernard turned his students' attention. During more than a half century of teaching, including four decades at the Clarkstown Country Club, Bernard had drilled his followers like soldiers in the techniques of living full and balanced lives. "Happiness is the goal of every living creature, from the lowest form of life to the highest," he said in 1912. "You can't know much about death until you know more about life," he echoed in 1927. In 1933 he said, "Life is a school. The world is a large gymnasium." He didn't have to add that he was the gym teacher.

Bernard found himself shouting at the ascetics who showed up in Nyack: "Don't give up the world! When you renounce the world, you renounce God. The spirit of Upanishadic teaching is to embrace all! We don't really own anything—we have a lease on everything that constitutes life. The purpose of Yoga is to prepare us from getting cheated; to enable us to make better bargains, and to get what we go after! Live while you can—while life is possible—don't wait until you are half-dead."

Among Bernard's admirers, Charles Potter believed that these were the words of a modern prophet, a John the Baptist for a new religion that would wake up to itself in the twenty-first century. Bernard's contribution, said Potter, was a "working synthesis, incomplete it is true, nevertheless of infinite value—a synthesis between the eastern and western philosophies of life." As anyone who listened to Bernard found out sooner or later, he filtered the sacred literature of India—the Vedas and the

Tantras—through his own point of view, that of an energetic Midwestern American. Potter labeled it a "dynamic" interpretation. Bernard himself might not have agreed with Potter's terminology or the use of so many words. He believed simply that "the only religion worthy of the name is something that is lived."

The Clarkstown Country Club was the church of the active life. Work, fun, sex, self-expression—it mattered little whether it was on the mat, the stage, the trapeze, or in the library. To Bernard, all truth was sacred and human activity was divine—when seen in the right light. "Non-expression and non-activity mean death," he said in 1927 and at various times in various ways over those four decades. "We atrophy, wither away and die. Dissolution is the result of lethargy, softness and mush. If you have no tone you rot on your feet and die. The same thing is true of the qualities of the Divine we possess."

Only on rare occasions did Bernard address the matters of death and the afterlife, and then usually as a salve for a club member who was mourning a loved one. "Try, instead of thinking of yourself as separate," he said in 1932, "thinking of yourself as Brahm. Then everything will look different. Even death. The closer you get to death, the less you fear it. Death is only a part of life. . . . Prepare yourself so that when the inevitable comes you are not shocked. You will not suffer so much if you live with that thought in mind."

Even in his late seventies and struggling with infirmities, Bernard remained cheerful and connected to life, adapting with high spirits to the minutiae of his drastically altered circumstances. When the Eastern Orthodox Archdiocese of New York leased his old Brick House mansion in Upper Nyack, Bernard made a new friend in the Russian cleric who signed the deal with him. He described the man to his cousin Martha: "Bishop wears a gold cross the dimensions of a football, has lots of whiskers and is a real guy." When the bishop then flew in twenty-two Russian Orthodox nuns, Bernard was greatly amused to find himself as landlord to a convent full of religious sisters who spoke not a word of English: "Nothing but Russian and French," he joked, "a little of which I can understand if they get to talking love." He ate dinner with his Russian tenants, but turned down their invitations to attend services. "I guess my soul, if I ever had one, is lost," he wrote to Martha.

With his old crew long gone, Bernard took pleasure in the club's few visitors—Indian diplomats and Sanskrit scholars, mostly. He marveled at the technological advancements in building maintenance. "We now use a paint gun with 250 pounds of compressed air," he wrote. All in all, he seemed pleased to conduct the day-to-day business of an elderly landlord, which was a good thing, since he had rented rooms and apartments in nearly every property he still owned.

In the summer of 1953, Bard and Meri Wiggenhorn came to inquire about a cottage for rent on the club grounds. The couple, who had two children, Julie, eleven, and Tony, sixteen, were unconventional people, according to their daughter, Julie Winslett.

Her father was an artist from the West, her mother a scholar and an English teacher. Julie recalls how her eyes widened at her first sighting of the mansion's porte cochere, a tunnel of sorts, elaborately gated, that went right through the clubhouse building to the rest of the property. This unfamiliar bit of architecture was a portent for the young girl, who sensed that there was something grand and unusual to be found on the other side of the gate. The Wiggenhorns drove up to the clubhouse, found no one there, looked at one another, and drove through the tunnel. They were shocked at what lay before them.

"There were no signs of habitation," Julie recalled. "No flower beds, no potted plants, no chairs on the terrace, no people. . . . Behind the mansion, a row of vacant buildings sagged along the drive. To the right, the rusting frame of an erstwhile solarium stood ankle deep in shattered glass." She spied a swimming pool filled with debris and an outdoor barbecue chimney turned into a weird, shapeless topiary by overgrown vines. "In the middle of a field between the grotto and the chimney," she continued, "a headless concrete dinosaur sat quietly crumbling toward its feet."

By the time the Wiggenhorns arrived, the animals had gone, guests were few, and Bernard ventured outside only on rare occasions. To the eyes of a young girl, he looked ancient and crumbling himself. "He was bald and moved stiffly," she recalled, "and because he was very stooped, it was hard to tell how tall he had been when young. He seemed short. He had a weak voice and mushed his words so that it was difficult to understand what he was saying. Even when engaged in conversation, he had an unfocused look and didn't seem to be in the present."

The house for rent, the Music Box Cottage, was charming and affordable, and the family moved in. They found themselves part of a small community of strangers who had for reasons unknown been brought together to witness the final days of a once vibrant enterprise. There were two other families living on the grounds, one local, the other a distinguished Russian clan named Saposhkov, who had arrived from the displaced persons camps of Europe in 1950.

Bard Wiggenhorn slowly started to fix his cottage up, which brought about a noticeable change in his landlord's mood. Bernard, too, began to clean up the place. He had the lawns mowed, and he permitted Wiggenhorn to fill up the swimming pool for Julie's use. He also provided access to a building next door, which then served as a painting studio for her artist father.

Bernard seemed revived by the energy of Bard and his family. When the weather was fair and mild, he came out of the mansion and sat in the shade under the elm. He engaged the Wiggenhorns in conversation and slowly walked the grounds, greeting his other tenants. "Dr. Bernard was an old school gentleman," said Helen Saposhkov. "Very reserved. When he was walking—a simple 'Hello' and 'How do you do.' He would wave and take off his hat and greet you."

Julie Wiggenhorn's curiosity led her to undertake a series of scouting trips through the empty buildings. The motivation was supplied by Diana Wertheim's picture book *Life at the Clarkstown Country Club,* which Bernard had given to Julie's parents in the hopes of impressing them with what had once been there. Julie found herself enthralled by the history of the place and its weird beauty. With some of the other children who lived on the grounds, she held make-believe cocktail parties in the old blue Belgian touring car, pretending to sip from the silver flasks that were attached by leather to the front seats. On a quiet afternoon, she sneaked into the clubhouse—Bernard's home—and by herself crept silently through the entire building. She tiptoed upstairs and downstairs, inspecting every room with an unlocked door.

"The atmosphere was hushed," she recalled, "like a museum after closing time. This was a house of greatness, filled with elegant *objets* and furniture. . . . A marvelous staircase and banister offset by lovely wall lamps graced a beautiful lobby where frescoes with mystical themes covered the walls. Unusual fountains were built into corners. . . . Unike the estate's exterior, all was perfection inside."

No one came to visit the club, it seemed to her. It was just Bernard, a secretary, and an old lady who seemed strange and disconnected from reality. The other tenants called the old lady a witch behind her back, and though her identity was not recorded, it must have been Martha Powell, in the final days of her neurological disease. Julie encountered the old woman as she sat on the ground weeding the overgrown brick walkway. "She had lived at the CCC during its heyday, she told me, and her conversation was filled with regret for the lost old days when everything had been meticulously manicured."

Aside from his small audience of renters, Pierre Bernard had fallen into total obscurity. He was no longer the darling of big-city reporters—he was in fact their worst enemy: old news. Among the locals, the high-and-mighty maestro of the CCC Sports Centre and chairman of Depression-era banks had sunk to an even lower rung: a tax cheat. The cabdriver who drove Helen Saposhkov to Bernard's club was "furious" at her landlord, she recalled. "People didn't like him in Nyack," she explained. "They said that he didn't pay taxes, though he was a wealthy man." Julie's parents heard plenty of gossip, of the past as well as the present, but most of all they were bewildered by the vaunted reputation of this man. After several conversations with him, they judged his grammar to be lacking and his observations crude. In their rented cottage the young couple laughed behind the back of the proud old man who took their monthly rent check.

Their daughter, however, remained haunted by the place. One day, she tried the lock on the studio building that housed Bernard's library and the lecture hall. She let herself in to the great room with a stone fireplace and book-lined walls, where Mrs. Vanderbilt's daughters and Paul Dukes, Cheerie Smith and Clara Thorpe and Blanche DeVries, along with hundreds of other first-generation students of hatha yoga, first heard Bernard's idiosyncratic interpretation of Eastern philosophy. The door swung open and she took in a ghostly tableau. "A gazetteer lay open on a table. A woman's fur wrap hung over the arm of one of the chairs. A player piano, covered with music rolls, stood in a corner." Behind the stage at the other end of the room was a projection room, and a projector with a reel of film still in it. "It was as though someone had just a moment before risen from his seat and stepped out."

At the back of the room she found a staircase and ascended to a darkened second story of small wrecked cubicles, the floorboards buckled with water damage, the rafters and ceiling pockmarked with large holes. This was once the storage room for the costumes that DeVries and her helpers made for the theatricals and the masked balls. Now the room was empty and "everything was covered with excrement from the pigeons which flew in through holes in the roof."

The adults on the club grounds, including the Wiggenhorns, believed the worst of what they'd heard about Bernard. Bard and Meri summed him up as a "charlatan who bamboozled silly rich women." They remained blind to what their young daughter saw—that "the place alone should have tipped them off to the fact that something extraordinary had gone on here."

In late October of 1954, Bernard heard from his old friend Edmund Dana, who had been the secretary of the Braeburn club in 1919: "Today is my birthday, and I have taken inventory," Dana wrote. "The conclusion I have reached is that the happiness I have had in my second marriage is mostly due to the philosophy I learned under your teaching in the good old days. Thought I would just drop a line to let you know how I felt, and to wish you a happy birthday on the 31st, and a long and merry life."

Bernard turned seventy-eight that Halloween. His long and merry life had spanned the horse-drawn era of Leon, Iowa, and the nuclear age. Like most Americans in the 1950s, he worried about the possibility of war with the Soviet Union or China. As the Red Scare took hold in the nation, yoga again bore the mantle of danger—bizarrely reflecting the worries and paranoia of the 1950s. Now that it was the subject of scientific inquiries, yoga was even considered in some quarters to be a high-security technology—perhaps even a Cold War weapon. Prime Minister Jawaharlal Nehru of India, wishing to calm the fears of the West, issued an official denial when asked if Indians were teaching yoga to the Soviet spacemen (though the Russians were indeed studying it). Eleanor Roosevelt, who'd performed yoga poses each morning during her time in the White House, issued a classic politician's non-denial denial when questioned about it, saying she didn't know they were called yoga exercises.

It was the buttoned-down fifties, after all, and the practice of hatha yoga was still for the few, the weird, the *nonconformists*, as they were called then. But the practice slowly attracted more early adopters who stumbled upon yoga's connection to good health. In meeting rooms and gyms at the YMCAs and YWCAs, yoga classes formed spontaneously. Friends told friends, and classes spread on both coasts and into the heartland— conformity be damned.

In 1955, Pete Seeger returned to Nyack with his mother, Constance, to visit the place that had once been such a happy part of their lives. Like everyone else, she and Pete had drifted away after the glory years and had not seen the place or its proprietor in some time.

"We knocked on the door and asked to see Dr. Bernard," said Pete. "The nurse asked who was calling, and we told her who we were. And she went away and came back and said, 'Yes, but don't make it long.'

"We went into a dark room, a room that was all closed up. There were covers on all the furniture. And Doc was sitting in a chair. He looked very old and frail. We said hello, and then, I remember, he rose like a wraith from his armchair.

"'The captain has to go down with the ship,' he said faintly, and he repeated the phrase, 'The captain has to go down with the ship.'"

It was the Seegers' last visit to the club.

Bernard stayed sequestered in the dark clubhouse. Doris Nelson, his tall, silent secretary, occasionally walked him outdoors on nice days for a little fresh air. "Sometimes I would see her helping him out to the elms, where he would sit, bent over, swaddled in a shawl," Julie recalled. There were even fewer people around the club in the summer of 1955. The old woman who seemed crazy to a thirteen-year-old's eyes had simply disappeared.

As the summer came to a close, Julie noticed that Bernard himself hadn't been seen in quite some time. Weeks of ninety-degree heat and high humidity had turned the lower Hudson Valley into a steaming soup tureen. Then two colossal hurricanes, Connie and Diana, subjected the citizens of Nyack to a weeklong deluge, and some of the worst flooding the Northeast had ever seen. Hillsides turned to waterfalls. On the rocky slopes of South Mountain, the downpour created its own culverts, crested the curbs, and soaked the wide lawns of the Clarkstown Country Club.

At the end of August, Bernard was driven down to Manhattan and checked in to French Hospital at 329 West Twenty-ninth Street, a place familiar to knowledgeable gossips as the retreat where a more famous and beloved icon of the Roaring Twenties—Babe Ruth—spent time drying out and taking treatments for his throat cancer. Bernard was attended at the hospital by an old friend and longtime club member, Dr. Anibel Zelaya, who determined in due time that his patient's condition was terminal. Whether brought on by the kidney disease that also killed his father, or the twenty or more cigars he smoked or chewed nearly every day of his adult life, Bernard's body had begun to fail.

In the end his wife, Blanche DeVries, came back to nurse him through his final days. Even the old heiress faction, represented by Margaret Rutherfurd and Diana Wertheim, returned to sit at his bedside. As the days of September ran out, and when it was clear that Bernard would not survive this stay in the hospital, Dr. Zelaya tried to find a blood relative to break the news to the family.

"I was in Minnesota on vacation," G. F. Hoffman recalled. "Dr. Zelaya told me that Pierre's vital signs weren't good. His kidneys were failing and all that. It kind of surprised me. I didn't know he had been through any ill health. My first thought was, Did somebody do him in?"

Nobody had laid a glove on him, as Bernard himself might have answered. The man who was born into the world as Perry Arnold Baker had outrun his enemies for a half century. He had outfoxed the police and outlasted the critics, and achieved the goal of his life's work: yoga had taken root in America.

At the age of seventy-nine years and eleven months, Bernard, like all creatures who exist in the illusion called maya, had run out of time. He died quietly in ward 1001 of French Hospital on the afternoon of Tuesday, September 27, 1955. According to his doctors, his death was attributed to "natural causes."

<hr />

The funeral service was held on a mild Thursday evening in Nyack. Bernard's body lay in state at his clubhouse in an open coffin, draped with a floral blanket. His face, swaddled in the coffin's white satin, looked thin and pale, as if the struggle for his last breaths had stripped him down to sinew and bone. DeVries was disconsolate at the loss of her husband, but she took charge of the arrangements. She led his remaining followers in a ritual of mourning that lasted through the night. Chanting could be heard in the clubhouse hallways, and there were incense and prayers for the dead.

Bernard's cousin G. F. Hoffman arrived in Nyack, where he was met by DeVries's attorney, the elderly Clark Jordan, the lawyer who had defended Bernard in court in 1910. Jordan appeared to Hoffman to be nervous. The question for the attorney and the widow and a few other interested people in Nyack was this: Had Bernard really changed his last will and testament, as he had threatened several times? The extant will, dated in 1925 and drawn up by Jordan, left the estate in its entirety to DeVries—or to his guru Sylvais Hamati in the event of his wife's premature death. The only person who would know the answer to the question of the will was G.F., the family's representative and an attorney himself. When DeVries and Jordan spied him in Nyack, G.F. said, "they were scared spitless."

The private funeral service was held in the clubhouse. Charles Potter officiated and friend after friend extolled the virtues of Pierre Arnold Bernard, guru, wise man, and teacher. Bard and Meri Wiggenhorn were stunned at the size of the turnout. "When my parents heard all those intellectual people talking about Bernard as though he were one of them, they were bewildered," said Julie Winslett. "They couldn't understand how any educated person could see anything in him." Also in attendance were Bernard's lawyer, doctor, real estate agent, two fellow Freemasons, and a few of his loyal friends. Di and Vi were there, as was Winfield Nicholls with his new wife. Thirteen members of the Missionary Training Institute attended, wishing their Tantric neighbor a pleasant journey into the afterlife.

On a card attached to a floral arrangement, DeVries had written in a halting, emotional scrawl: "My Darling. My Dear Pierre, you and your teaching was and is my life, the all embracing life. To try, to love, to learn, our debt to Brahm God. May we always be united in love and wisdom. Mother, Prema and Shiva."

At her husband's ceremony, DeVries read aloud an excerpt from Bernard's Red Book, the *International Journal of the Tantrik Order*. It was a strangely churchy and Victorian translation of a verse on death from the ancient Hindu hymn the Rig-Veda.

First must each several element
That joined to form thy living frame
Flit to the region whence it came,
And with its parent source be blent.
Thine eye shall seek the solar orb
Thy life breath to the wind shall fly,
Thy part ethereal to the sky;
Thine earthly part shall earth absorb.

In the end Bernard made a clean getaway. He left no large debts and his taxes were paid in full. He hadn't altered his will by a single codicil; it still named DeVries as heiress and executrix. He'd left everything to her, all the possessions he hadn't parted with, which were few and strangely enough included a large pearl necklace, assessed at $5,500. He left in DeVries's care his spiritual library, which was valued by the assessor at $1,590, and his garage full of prized cars, whose total value was appraised at not much more.

One 1930 Minerva Limousine Automobile	$40
One 1936 Cadillac Sedan Automobile	$20
One 1936 Packard Sedan Automobile	$20
One 1947 Lincoln Sedan Automobile	$50
One 1951 Cadillac Sedan Automobile	$1,500

Charlie Potter was bequeathed $150 for his final services. Some $16,000 went to Clark Jordan, attorney to Bernard and DeVries for fifty years. Bernard left funds to cover his funeral and burial plot, which sits on a rise overlooking the Hudson River in nearby Sparkill. In the end DeVries inherited an estate conservatively valued at $300,000, along with properties that would bring her wealth up to $750,000. Everything was left airtight legally, and the will went unchallenged in probate.

Three months later, on a cold and clear January day, under an empty blue sky, an anonymous filmmaker made a silent 16 mm catalog of the CCC grounds. There is no evidence of the filmmaker's purpose or motivation, but the hard, slanting shadows to the east indicate that it was late in the afternoon when he or she went to work. The trees on the grounds were bare, and the river wore an icy rime. The camera peers down from high above the club, a dry-eyed angel's point of view, and swings slowly from east to west—from the Hudson to the Ramapo Mountains—brushing the breadth of the once bustling property. The club looks stilled and shrunken in the film, like an architect's model. The clock on the bell tower had stopped on some previous day at 6:35. The only movement is a lone black sedan, as small as an insect, that drives slowly out of the frame as the film fades to black.

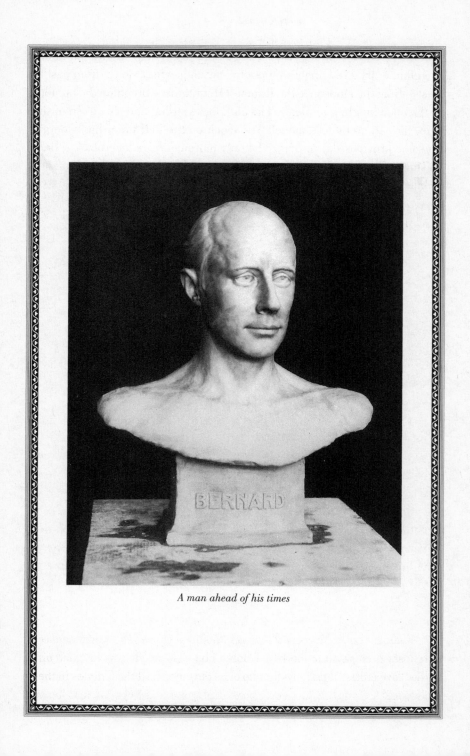

A man ahead of his times

Epilogue

GENIUS OR FRAUD?

"I can easily see why Dr. Bernard seems strange, queer, and crazy to many persons, indeed to the average citizen of the United States," wrote Dr. Charles Francis Potter in the 1940s. To the renegade minister who knew Bernard intimately for a decade, the guru of Nyack seemed to be "from another age or another planet." And Potter meant this as a compliment.

And how was such a singular, vital man remembered? Not very well, it turned out. In the years following his death, Bernard virtually disappeared from the public's memory. Dismissed as an oddity, he fell between the cracks of the onrushing decades, his story too complicated for easy telling. Even the obituarists toiled haplessly in his immediate wake. "Pierre Bernard, 'Oom the Omnipotent,' Promoter and Self-Styled Swami, Dies" was the headline that ran atop a sober farewell in the *New York Times.* The writer borrowed a few quotes from Joseph Mitchell's *World-Telegram* profile of 1931, and estimated Oom's estate to be worth at one time upward of $2 million. Readers were treated to a reprise of three of his colorful encounters with the law: the abduction arrest of 1910, the Sanskrit College showdown of 1911, and the Nyack mounted police raid of 1919.

Whatever contributions he made in his long career as a yoga teacher were lost or relegated to fodder for bored obit writers. He was laughed off as the "love cultist" and "mystic who once charmed half the females in the social register" in the *Chicago Tribune.* In Ironwood, Michigan, and Long

Beach, California, Americans read the same assortment of half-truths and mockery that had accompanied Bernard throughout his life. Fittingly, the obituaries appeared not only in the national news pages of dozens of publications, but in some cases next to Ripley's "Believe It or Not."

Then came the sacking of his Vedic temple, the CCC clubhouse. In the spring of 1956, Eva Moseley, the first lady of the Missionary Training Institute, called a taxi to take her to the deserted Clarkstown Country Club grounds. She and others from the MTI had shared South Mountain uneasily with Bernard for decades. For fifteen years she and her fellow missionaries had prayed that his property would pass on to them one day. Eva stood on Bernard's wide front lawn and offered her own plea. "Oh dear God, you know how much the college needs this wonderful property. I believe that You want us to have it, too."

Mrs. Moseley was not alone in her desire; most of Nyack had some stake in what happened to the club. The village of South Nyack preferred the idea of rezoning the remaining nineteen acres for apartment buildings. Real estate developers then saw their own version of nirvana. In the end DeVries chose the MTI as the buyer. She named her price: $250,000 for nineteen acres, including the clubhouse, theater, assembly room, music room, bell tower, and garages. On Monday, April 10, 1956, the school's trustees recognized a deal when they saw one and accepted the offer.

A three-day auction was held in the main salon of the clubhouse mansion. Curious and enthusiastic crowds arrived, bidding on twenty-nine bedroom sets, an electric Turkish bath, a billiard table, a nearly life-size marble statue of the goddess Psyche, and other stuff. Julie Wiggenhorn watched with sorrow as strangers carted off the beautiful artifacts she'd once admired. "The estate was picked clean," she said. Her parents acquired a cut-crystal rose bowl, a bedroom suite, a pair of porcelain lamps, and a cream-colored upholstered ottoman, which Bernard and DeVries had used for teaching asanas. "Now our dogs would dream there," she recalled.

The missionaries generously gave the club's tenants a year to move out and began the process of erasing Bernard's legacy. In the clubhouse, the wall-size frescoes depicting the "cosmic evolution" of man were painted over. Any remaining pagan statues were chipped out of their niches, which were left empty. The naked painted ballerinas in the dance studios were covered over. There were prayers of consecration to rid the place of what the Christian missionaries called "demon activity."

Bernard left no children, no school—only his students. His wife, Blanche DeVries—his greatest student—inherited his legacy and kept his memory alive. In her studios in New York City and Nyack, she taught a small, influential group of followers under the watchful gaze of her husband's plaster bust. For the next thirty years, the talented DeVries taught Bernard's yoga to an emerging generation of Californians and New Yorkers, including actors Frederic March, Anthony Quinn, Henry Fonda, and Claire Bloom, along with prominent women like Sunny von Bülow, Alexandra Penney, Victoria Newhouse, and Rebekah Harkness, who in turn brought the Indian yogi B. K. S. Iyengar to the United States for his first visit in 1956. And she continued the training of her old friend Leopold Stokowski.

DeVries told a reporter in 1963 that "the real Dr. Bernard was not a business man. His interests were in yoga and philosophy. The elephants, the dog track were all for show. He enjoyed the big cigar, using slang. But when he was writing or speaking about yoga, or discussing philosophy, he spoke only the most classical English. His library on Vedic literature and on Eastern philosophies was perhaps the finest of its time in the United States."

DeVries claimed that over twenty-two years, she attended thousands of her husband's lectures and passed on what she learned to her own students, who now teach in New York, California, Florida, and elsewhere. She herself remained an active teacher who was beloved by her students, many of whom considered her, with good reason, the mother of yoga in America. "DeVries for her time, was *it*," said Paula Heitzner, who studied with her in the 1960s and now teaches yoga herself in Nyack. "She was beautifully built. From the back she would look like a twenty-five-year-old. And she was very dramatic—red lipstick, full makeup, full jewelry."

DeVries taught classes well into her nineties, shuttling back and forth between yoga studios in Nyack and New York City, until she fell and fractured her skull on a staircase at the Port Authority Bus Terminal in 1982. She died two years later, just shy of her ninety-third birthday, in the care of Viola Bernard. DeVries passed away destitute; a series of bad investments had drained the savings she had accumulated from the sale of the CCC properties. Viola stepped in when the money ran out, and then she took on the care of DeVries's sister, Franci Yager, until Franci's death two years later.

Aside from Hamish McLaurin, who'd died of asthma on November 14, 1957, in his wife Amie's arms, and Percival Whittlesey, who survived the assassination attempt by a young Nazi but shot himself to death on Palm Sunday in 1945, most of Bernard's students lived long, healthy lives. Sir Paul Dukes took what he learned from Bernard in Nyack, blended it with the wisdom of his Indian gurus, and taught it in South Africa, India, Australia, and Europe. He wrote several books, including *The Unending Quest* and *Yoga for the Western World*. He made films on yoga for the BBC and joyfully spread the word about his spiritual practice in a walking trip through Tibet. He died on August 27, 1967, the same day the Beatles were called away from their Welsh retreat with the Maharishi Mahesh Yogi to mourn the sudden death of their manager, Brian Epstein.

Clara Spring, née Thorpe, opened a studio on Hollywood Boulevard in the 1950s and taught yoga to thousands of California students until her death at the age of ninety. Her influential book, *Yoga for Today*, was published in 1959, dedicated to "Blanche De Vries, pioneer teacher of Yoga in the West." Clara's friend Cheerie Jackson, happily married to Tommy Jackson for the rest of her long life, taught yoga-inspired dance to children in Santa Monica, including the young Robert Redford. She died on October 30, 1989, at the age of ninety. Marie Louise Schreiner stayed in close contact with other club members and eventually moved from the Adirondacks to Arizona, where she taught piano to support her family. She, too, lived a long and healthy life, passing away at the age of 102. The surviving Powell sister, Jeanne, moved to New York after Bernard's death and kept up a friendly correspondence with DeVries, her former rival.

Ruth Everett, first exposed to Sanskrit and Eastern philosophy at the Clarkstown Country Club in the early 1920s, became a pioneer in bringing Zen Buddhism to the West. She and her husband, Edward Warren Everett, had given lectures at the club in 1922–1923—she on Buddhism, he on litigation techniques. After his death, Ruth married a Japanese Zen monk named Sokei-an Sasaki, and she herself became the first Westerner and female to be ordained a priest at the Daitoku-ji temple in Kyoto. Her son-in-law, the writer and beat philosopher Alan Watts, described her first teacher, Bernard, as a "phenomenal rascal master" on a par with Gurdjieff and Crowley. And like his fellow minister Potter, Watts meant this in a good way.

Ida Rolf, the influential physiotherapist and inventor of the therapy known formally as Structural Integration, always credited Bernard with instilling in her the ideal of balance in the body and the importance of lengthening muscles. She took Bernard's teaching on yoga asanas, merged it with chiropractic, and came up with her "recipe," as she called it. In Rolfing, she taught the idea of stretching muscles and manipulating ligaments into place. She spread the word in the United Kingdom in the fifties, and in the sixties, like Alan Watts, became a founding fixture at Esalen, the California community that continued the serious exploration of the mind-body connection and the merging of Eastern and Western philosophies.

Viola Wertheim Bernard became a successful and respected psychiatrist, professor, and social activist. After caring for both DeVries and Franci Yager in their final years, she maintained a residence in Nyack into the 1990s, until declining health forced her to live in her New York City apartment until her death in 1998. Despite her mixed feelings about Bernard, she became the executrix of his estate and spent many years sorting and codifying the material left by him and DeVries, as well as her ex-husband Theos. These papers now exist at the Historical Society of Rockland County, the Augustus C. Long Health Sciences Library at Columbia University, Yale University Library, the University of Arizona, and other institutions. It is through her generosity of spirit that scholars and biographers have access to the records of the Clarkstown Country Club and its founder.

Though still a young man when he disappeared in 1947, Theos Bernard left behind three popular books, scholarly work, and other remarkable documentary evidence of his yogic journey. His *Hatha Yoga: The Report of a Personal Experience* (1944) remains one of the best photographic records of proper asana postures before B. K. S. Iyengar's *Light on Yoga* was published in 1966.

Viola's sister, Diana, remarried after her split from Whittlesey and lived happily in the horsy enclave of Bedford, New York. She remained loyal to Bernard and his ideas, and supported DeVries in her later years both emotionally and with decorating jobs, treating the older woman like part of her family.

Lou Nova, who went on to act in over four hundred movies, TV shows, and theatricals, kept up his yoga connection. In the 1960s, he invented, patented, and marketed a device called the Yogi Nova, a headstand-helper of sorts, that was sold in Saks Fifth Avenue and other tony stores. Another celebrated sportsman, Harold Stirling Vanderbilt, son of William K. Vanderbilt and three-time defender of the America's Cup, never forgot his introduction to yoga by Bernard in 1920. Mike, as he preferred to be called, began every morning—on land or yacht—with controlled breathing and asanas; he lived to be eighty-five years old. John Jacob Niles, whom the folk singer Bob Dylan claimed as an influence, practiced yoga throughout his life and happily posed for *Life* photographer Alfred Eisenstaedt in 1943 performing his own eccentric variation of a headstand.

Bernard's club is his bloodline. Many strands of the cultural revolution that shaped American life in the latter half of the twentieth century can be traced back to the Nyack of the 1920s. Here Bernard presented in a single, unique setting a preview of today's interests in Eastern philosophy and yoga's healing properties; our preoccupation with celebrity, diet, sex, health, and the human body; the acceptance—and even glorification—of female sexuality; and the frank recognition of the need for sex education.

Nyack was also an early center of multiculturalism. Classical music was taught and performed along with folk music. Performers from the Caribbean and the Appalachians, from the ranks of society's marginalized classes, were invited to perform on the same bill with opera stars. Bernard's students were educated in international politics, and this education often begat large-scale social action. Likewise there was an institutional respect for the religious beliefs of others: "All truth is sacred," he taught. It was the Tantriks' credo and one he lived by.

The Clarkstown Country Club was the forerunner of modern recovery institutions where hard work, spirituality, and equality form a compound antidote for addiction. As we have seen, Bernard had society women up to their elbows in hot, soapy water; there were Harvard and Yale grads gathering hay and harvesting vegetables. He believed that work of the most physical kind was not just beneficial but an important part of the cure for people fighting to regain balance after their substance abuse or depression.

The club was also a mecca of lifelong learning, an institutional bridge between the transcendentalists' Brook Farm of the 1840s and the Esalen of the 1960s. Bernard had opened his well-stocked lending library and club as a rest stop for several generations of visiting Indian scholars and holy men, some of them famous, like Yogananda and Swami Bodhananda, but many more of obscure reputation. He championed the study of Sanskrit and worked with legitimate scholars as often as he could.

And his club still stands—or at least the buildings do—looking somewhat the same as it did, though there are many more parking spaces where there once were trees and gardens. Now it is the private property of Nyack College, the renamed Missionary Training Institute, which also owns all three of the Wertheim properties on what locals call "the hillside." Bernard's pride and joy, the new clubhouse, is now the men's dormitory, and from this spot on South Mountain, on certain nights, students can easily see the glow of the light towers from Bernard's Sports Centre, which now illuminate the playing fields down at the old Nyack High School.

Everybody in town, it seems, has a story about Bernard. He is remembered there chiefly for his animals—the escape of Mr. Jimmer, the lions roaring in the night, the elephants that paraded through the downtown streets and delighted the children who are grandparents today. Most Nyackers will preface their stories with "I don't know if it's true or not . . ." but it doesn't stop anyone from repeating a good tale.

***

Ten years after Bernard's death, the American counterculture was emerging into the mainstream. In July of 1965, Jess Stearn, a *Newsweek* editor, published *Yoga, Youth and Reincarnation*, a best-selling how-to, history, and personal journey. Stearn was inspired by Clara Spring's *Yoga for Today* and Blanche DeVries's classes in Nyack and went on to become a serious practitioner and advocate for yoga. His book remained wildly popular, with twenty paperback printings over the next eight years. With its flower-power cover and youth-oriented approach to the subject, the book handed off hatha yoga to the exultant energies of the baby boomers: "Come alive—you're in the yoga generation," one cover line beckoned. (Bernard would have been proud of that one.) "The amazing key to physical, sexual and spiritual harmony—a modern step-by-step approach to the ancient art of yoga."

<hr />

So: Was Bernard a fraud or a genius? He taught and defended a single idea for more than fifty years, even when it was downright dangerous to do so. He was the leader of a cultural vanguard that transformed hatha yoga from a loathed "Oriental" practice into something vigorous and healthy and American in outlook. He started the first yoga classes in the nation and trained the teachers who kept the knowledge flowing—here and abroad. These innovations alone would make him worthy of consideration in any history of yoga.

But to his critics, Bernard's flaws overwhelmed his accomplishments. He seemed to show little regard for the truth as others knew it, dismissing it as an unhealthy obsession with "name and form." He was capable of using others for money and support, of unleashing great cruelty, of having an unbridled ego, of allowing others to overstate his qualifications, of overstating his own qualifications, of piling up an alphabetical train wreck of honorary degrees and affiliations out of deep-seated insecurity. He was materialistic, arrogant, selfish, and, worst of all, he profited greatly from his spiritual pursuits.

In the end, perhaps his biggest battle was not with the press or the clergy or his rebellious students but with himself. His powerful ego was the engine that propelled him to his greatest worldly successes. It made him a master in a stunning variety of endeavors; without it he could never have accomplished what he did. But his ego also led him to develop a fatal case of "founder's disease," which ultimately killed the club and hampered his influence. In the final decades of his life he pushed away those who could have carried on his agenda. Since he had no heirs and no successor, the CCC—with its wonderful resources, history, location, and library—was sold off piecemeal by DeVries to support herself in her declining years.

In the end, it was his business. He asked no one's permission to live as he did. He rarely felt the need to explain himself to outsiders. He believed in what he taught and in the power of time to prove its correctness. Let the seekers come to him, he said, and they did. They would find their own truth among the sunlight and the shadows on a pretty hillside in Nyack.

Acknowledgments

I am grateful to my wife, Nichol, who throughout this seven-year journey traveled by my side every step of the way. She haunted archives, libraries, and bookstores, scorched her retinas searching online databases, kept the faith and kept the files in impeccable order. Without her diligence, skill, and integrity, I could never have written this book. I am likewise indebted to Suzanne Gluck and Rick Kot, who were there from the beginning and never lost confidence during the long gestation period. And a deep bow of gratitude to my supremely talented editor, Liz Van Hoose, whose tireless efforts unearthed the narrative from a mountain of factual material.

For contributions and support beyond the call of duty, I must acknowledge the following people: Joan Wofford, who graciously gave her time, wisdom, family photos, and documents—along with encouragement and advice; Sara Hale, who sat for hours of interviews and provided me with her mother's papers and photos; Peter Rubi and Barbara Junge, who granted me access to Llellwyn Jackson's memoirs and photos; Dennis Prindle, who shared the story of his family's interaction with Pierre Bernard; and finally to Julie Winslett, whose memoir of life at the Clarkstown Country Club animated the last chapters of the book.

To the generous scholars who never failed to answer my e-mails, my humble thanks: Paul Gerard Hackett, who shared his research and dissertation on Theos Bernard; Brad Verter, whose work guided me through a history of the occult in America; Stefanie Syman, who swapped tales of yoga's early history in America; and Hugh Urban, who answered countless questions. A special thanks to Jeffrey J. Kripal, who offered encourage-ment and knowledge of India's religious and cultural traditions, and read multiple drafts with an expert's eye. Likewise, I owe a great debt of grati-tude to Rick and Suellen Stringer-Hye, who shared with me their passion for all things Oom, along with research and material they had gathered for their own project.

My great appreciation to G. F. Hoffman, for his assistance and thought-ful recollections, and Dr. John P. Viner, for his Bernard family research, correspondence, and artifacts. A special thanks to the late Marjorie Nem-itz, who provided family details and moral support. I regret that she could not have seen the book in its final form.

A hearty thanks to Andrew P. Bradbury, who fact-checked an ever-changing mansuscript; to researchers Marty Miller and Missy Melinger, who cheerfully turned up new material just when it was needed; to Matt Steigbigel, who organized the photographs. To my friends Robert Wal-lace, Lisa Henricksson, Fred Allen, Mary Billard, and Richard and Edith Hanley, who read early drafts and kept my spirits up through dark days and nights, my humble appreciation.

To Stephen Novak, my guide at the Columbia University Health Sci-ences Library Archives and Special Collections, my great appreciation. Thanks also to that institution's talented and dedicated Henry Blanco, who always came through, as did Brian Jennings of the Nyack Library. To Erin Martin, director of the Historical Society of Rockland County, as well as her able curators, Jessica Kuhnen and Rebecca Streeter, I owe a debt far greater than can ever be enumerated here.

For granting interviews, I thank: Homer Lydecker, David Whittlesey, Belle Zeck, Helen Saposhkov, Addie Osuch, Greta and Dick Smolowe, Grace Gordon, Molly Scott, Paul Glaziek, Marvene Gordon, Don Hanlon Johnson, Rosemary Feitis, Pete Seeger, and John Seeger, among others. Finally, to H.S.T, J.S.W, P.J, T.W, and all my journalistic and literary gurus, past and present, my humble hopes that the book delivers on its promise.

Notes

PROLOGUE: A MAN IN LOVE WITH BEAUTY

1 **"I look out"**: F. Scott Fitzgerald, *The Notebooks of F. Scott Fitzgerald*, ed. Matthew J. Bruccoli (New York and London: Harcourt Brace Jovanovich/Bruccoli Clark, 1978), 332.

1 **"A place of mystery"**: Joseph Mitchell, "Oom Is Booster of His County, His Proud Boast," *New York World-Telegram*, December 15, 1931, 18.

1 **"English countryside estates"**: Ibid.

2 **next to Katharine**: William Engle, "Hepburn . . . Hertz . . . Bernard" Dramatic Personalities in the Week's News, *New York World-Telegram*, November 18, 1933, Pierre Arnold Bernard (PAB) Collection, Historical Society of Rockland County (HSRC).

3 **"You are the first"**: Mitchell, "Oom Is Booster," 18.

3 **"more concerned with"**: Ibid.

3 **"I wouldn't care to"**: Ibid.

3 **"the Guru of Nyack"**: Eckert Goodman, "The Guru of Nyack," *Town & Country*, April 1941, 52.

3 **"all the earmarks"**: "Oom Is a Sound Theologian, Not a Charlatan, Says Dr. Potter," *New York World-Telegram*, May 31, 1931, HSRC.

4 **as familiar to**: Goodman, "The Guru of Nyack," 52.

4 **"Dr. Bernard seems"**: "Evolution," *Fortune*, July 1933, Off the Record, 4.

4 **"Dr. Pierre Bernard"**: "Where Are They Now? Oom's Guests," *New Yorker*, July 16, 1938, 32.

4 **a cartoon character**: "The Omnipotent Oom Gets Two Customers," *Hairbreadth Harry, Lincoln Sunday Star*, April 15, 1917, color section, 1.

4 **"the Omnipotent Oom"**: "The Screen," *New York Times*, July 14, 1934, 15.

4 **"Of all the natural"**: F. Scott Fitzgerald, "The Crack-Up," in *The Jazz Age* (New York: New Directions Publishing, 1996), 61.

4 **"We take sufferers"**: Mitchell, "Oom Is Booster," 18.

4 **"The safety valve"**: PAB lectures, February 20, 1927, HSRC.

5 **"the modern 'jazz life' ":** PAB lectures, March 4, 1928, HSRC.

5 **"There's nothing high-brow":** Mitchell, "Oom Is Booster," 18.

CHAPTER 1: FIRST SON OF A FIRST SON

9 **never at ease:** Confusion about Bernard's birthplace can be traced to his numerous obfuscations. In his own voice he listed as his birthplace Chicago (statement to Vanderbilt attorneys), Paris (self-published prospectus for yoga lessons), and Des Moines (*San Francisco Call*, January 27, 1898, 1, and *New York Times*, January 29, 1898, 1).

9 **"May be alright":** PAB (Pierre Arnold Bernard), letter to Martha Hoffman, 1950, 5, HSRC (Historical Society of Rockland County).

9 **Bernard's forebears arrived:** Family tree, PAB collection, HSRC, and personal communication with Dr. John Viner, family historian.

10 **Dr. George Washington Baker:** "An Old Pioneer Passes Away," *Decatur County Journal*, January 21, 1909, HSRC.

10 **Catherine C. Givens:** Kittie's name was sometimes spelled Givans. PAB's date of birth, another disputed fact, was confirmed to me by Marj Nemitz, a relative, who read the inscription in a family Bible: "Perry A. Baker was born Oct. 31st 1876."

10 **Kittie was a:** United States Census, 1880. Kittie, 26, lists her occupation as housekeeper, living with her parents and son, age three, born in Leon, Iowa.

11 **There he opened:** "Omnipotent Oom Held," *Humeston New Era*, May 11, 1910, 1.

11 **"eighteen hours a day":** PAB "statement," his response to a deposition taken by Vanderbilt attorneys, HSRC.

11 **Mormons' persecution and flight:** "Early," chap. 7, "History and the Constitution," *Iowa Official Register* 2007–2008 (Iowa General Assembly, Legislative Services Agency, Dennis Prouty, director, vol. 72), 319.

11 **from 13,000 to 52,000:** *1994 Lincoln City-Lancaster County Comprehensive Plan*, chap. 1, "History of Planning and Development," 1. PDF found online at www.lincoln.ne.gov/City/plan/complan/1994/chap1.pdf on February 8, 2007.

12 **Sylvais Hamati:** The meeting is related firsthand in the transcription of PAB "deposition," in response to questions from a set of attorneys who were investigating his past on behalf of the Vanderbilt family. Though it includes some seventy pages of interrogatories, it is incomplete, missing the first twelve pages, HSRC.

12 **fewer than eight hundred:** Padma Rangaswamy, *Namasté America* (University Park: Pennsylvania State University Press, 2000), 41: United States Immigration and Naturalization Service data. Also "A Brief History of Indian Immigration to America," American Immigration Law Foundation, published on its Web site, www.ailf.org.

12 **Who was Sylvais Hamati?:** Physical description from photograph, HSRC.

12 **"Professor Craig of Hebron":** "Nebraska Notes," *Fairfield Independent*, March 24, 1889, 3.

13 **an itinerant tutor:** PAB statement.

13 **"Hamati made it very":** Ibid.

13 **"The time that I did":** Ibid.

14 **"every authoritative Tantra":** Shiva Nath Katju, "Pierre Arnold Bernard: A Tribute," *Sunday Amrita Bazar Patrika* (Allahabad, India), December 18, 1955, page unknown, HSRC. Katju was a distinguished lawyer, judge, and professor of law at

Allahabad University in India, who became interested in Bernard and Tantrik yoga in the 1950s.

14 **connection to the bedrock:** *Vira Sadhana: International Journal of the Tantrik Order,* external issue, vol. 5, no. 1 (New York: Tantrik Order in America, 1906), 95. Hereafter referred to as *IJTO.*

14 **"blood transfusion":** PAB lecture notes, undated, HSRC.

14 **"To the very best":** PAB statement and deposition. As for guru lineage, Perry Baker's guru had his own guru, a yogi-monk-ascetic named Mahidhar, who trained the young Hamati from the age of seven until he turned twenty-six, as Bernard recounts in PAB statement and PAB deposition. Hamati's guru is acknowledged by Swami Ram Tirath, a legitimate Hindu monk who said that he knew of two great Tantrik masters in India, in "Mahidhar and Yogi Gyanananda," in an interview in the *IJTO* conducted by D. J. Elliott.

15 **"He appeared to":** "Colton," *Los Angeles Times,* May 13, 1895, 9.

CHAPTER 2: KALI MUDRA

19 **wildest week:** *Los Angeles Times,* January 19–24, 1898.

20 **a rare simulation of death by mental power:** "Sewed His Lip to His Nose," *San Francisco Call,* January 28, 1898, 1. Also, "Puzzle to Physicians," *Washington Post,* May 1, 1898, 25. Technically the name "Kali Mudra" as used by Bernard for "death trance" is at least an idiosyncratic translation.

20 **"sensitive in nature":** "Puzzle to Physicians." This piece explains the mechanics of how PAB (Pierre Arnold Bernard) did it.

21 **"telepathically":** "Sewed His Lip to His Nose."

21 **"Professor P. A. Bernard":** Ibid.

22 **William Kissam Vanderbilt:** "Mr. Depew May Retire: A Possible Outcome of W. K. Vanderbilt's Scheme of New York Central Reorganization," *New York Times,* January 29, 1898, 1.

22 **"The use of":** "Doctors Differ on Hypnosis," *Chicago Daily Tribune,* January 29, 1898, 6.

22 **"Self-induced hypnosis":** Ibid.

22 **Americans were fascinated:** In the *New York Times, Los Angeles Times, Chicago Daily Tribune,* and *Washington Post* between 1895 and 1905, 2,993 articles mentioned "hypnotism." In addition there were 3,334 articles in the same newspapers that mentioned the "occult" in some form.

22 **Nearly eight hundred books:** Beryl Satter, *Each Mind a Kingdom* (Berkeley and Los Angeles: University of California Press, 1999), 51.

22 **schools teaching:** Ibid.; "College to Teach Hypnotism," *New York Times,* August 1, 1900, 5.

23 **"wonderful":** "Puzzle to Physicians."

23 **"outclasses anything I":** Ibid.

23 **"far outweighs the":** "The Use of Hypnotism in Medicine," *San Francisco Call,* July 14, 1901, magazine, 1.

23 **"I will say":** "Puzzle to Physicians."

23 **more than twice:** The average annual wage in the United States at the time was $400–$500. See http://historicaltextarchive.com/sections.php?op=viewarticle&artid=594.

24 **"Vedic philosophy and":** PAB statement, HSRC.

24 **"practical" Hinduism:** Personal communication Jeffrey J. Kripal, chair of the religion department at Rice University. Re Vivekananda's faith: "It was basically an eclectic synthesis of Western social thought and Indian yoga and Advaita Vedanta—a very unstable mix, but an effective one, at least for a time."

24 **"The science of Yoga":** From Vivekananda's lecture on "Concentration," transcribed on the scene by a follower and found in full at www.vivekananda.net. Accessed February 14, 2009.

25 **"perfect understanding of Tantrik doctrine":** *IJTO*, 95. PAB gave Ram a place to live for an entire winter in San Francisco. C. F. Potter, notes for a PAB biography.

25 **"I always made":** PAB statement, HSRC.

25 **misrepresenting his medical credentials:** PAB deposition, 45, HSRC. It could have been that Bernard was claiming to be his uncle or an honest mix-up, as PAB later claimed.

26 **arrest in April 1902:** "Illegally Practices Medicine," *San Francisco Call*, April 30, 1902, 7.

26 **brotherhood of Tantrik lodges:** "Puzzle to Physicians."

CHAPTER 3: TANTRIK NIGHTS

29 **"Kaula Rite, Chakra":** Classified advertisement, undated, HSRC (Historical Society of Rockland County), from a San Francisco newspaper. Judging from the street address and Bernard's known whereabouts, it has to be 1900, since these initiations were held at the full moon, and the only year during his time in S.F. with a full moon on October 8 was 1900.

30 **suicide, illness, early death:** "Hugh Tevis Dead," *New York Times*, June 8, 1901, 9; "L. T. Breckenridge a Suicide," *New York Times*, July 27, 1901, 3; "Disposing of Tevis Millions: New Apportionment of Great Wealth Necessitated by Little Girl's Death," *New York Times*, January 18, 1903, 13. Hugh Tevis, age forty, died suddenly in Yokohama in 1901 on a world trip with his second wife, just two years after his father died. Hugh's daughter Alice died suddenly in 1903. His sister's son, Lloyd Tevis Breckenridge, a nephew to Harry, committed suicide at the age of twenty-three at Harry's house.

30 **Tevis men:** PAB deposition, HSRC.

30 **Lansing Kellogg and Major Henry Farnsby Bulwer:** "How Many Wives Had Gay Major Bulwer?" *Los Angeles Times*, July 3, 1904, A1; Lansing Kellogg: "Coronado Beach, Dinner Party and a Dance," *Los Angeles Times*, November 14, 1898, 9; also "Coronado Brevities," *Los Angeles Times*, October 30, 1898, A15.

30 **Winfield Jesse Nicholls:** "Faker's Slave a Coast Lad," *Los Angeles Times*, May 6, 1910, 19. Also "Police Are Taking Look into Occult Affairs," *San Francisco Call*, June 6, 1905, 1.

30 **Florin Howard Jones:** "Faker's Slave a Coast Lad."

30 **among Irish and German:** U.S. Census reports, 1900, for the mix of neighborhoods frequented by the Tantriks.

31 **"life school":** PAB (Pierre Arnold Bernard) letter to followers, undated, HSRC.

31 **"seven years working":** Ibid.

31 **"blood taints":** Ibid.

31 **"Bernard seemed to":** "Faker's Slave a Coast Lad."

31 **"thousands of all"**: PAB letter to Tantrik Order, HSRC.

32 **"Our yoga rooms"**: Ibid. In this letter PAB refers to hatha yoga by another Sanskrit name, Ghatastha-yoga, literally "pot based" yoga, designating the body as a pot to be fired to hardness by the discipline of yoga. Georg Feuerstein, *The Shambhala Encyclopedia of Yoga* (Boston: Shambhala Publications, 1997), 105.

32 **women who came along:** Membership roll of the T.O., HSRC.

32 **Howard Petterson:** "Police Are Taking Look into Occult Affairs."

32 **Eugenie Charbonnier:** "Marriage Licenses," *San Francisco Call*, October 29, 1905, 45.

32 **perils that their association:** "Police Are Taking Look into Occult Affairs."

33 **73,000 pounds of books:** James Petersen and Hugh Hefner, *The Century of Sex* (New York: Grove Press, 1999), 11.

33 **"turbanned Syrian":** "Faker's Slave a Coast Lad."

34 **"The neighbors complained":** Ibid.

34 **Glen was welcomed:** Glen A. Bernard, letter, from Theos Bernard Collection, University of California at Berkeley; cited in Paul Gerard Hackett, "Barbarian Lands: Theos Bernard, Tibet, and the American Religious Life" (doctoral thesis, Columbia University, 2008).

35 **into the millions:** Theda Skocpol, *Diminished Democracy: From Membership to Management in American Civil Life* (Norman: University of Oklahoma Press, 2003), 6.

35 **Third Great Awakening:** Robert William Fogel, *The Fourth Great Awakening and the Future of Egalitarianism* (Chicago: University of Chicago Press, 2000), 22. For first New Age, see Philip Jenkins, *Mystics and Messiahs* (New York: Oxford University Press, 2000), 70.

35 **morphed and borrowed:** Brad Verter, "Dark Star Rising" (doctoral thesis, Princeton University, 1999), 28. Catherine L. Albanese, *A Republic of Mind and Spirit* (New Haven and London: Yale University Press, 2007).

36 **Tantrism, a mix of:** My understanding of the history and meaning of Tantra and Tantrism is based on these readings: Georg Feuerstein, *Tantra: The Path of Ecstasy* (Boston: Shambhala Publications, 1998) and *The Shambhala Encyclopedia of Yoga* (Prescott, AZ: Hohm Press, 1998); Hugh B. Urban, *Tantra: Sex, Secrecy, Politics and Power in the Study of Religion* (Berkeley, CA: University of California Press, 2003), as well as discussions with Jeffrey J. Kripal and other sources.

37 **Ice Age rituals:** Nik Douglas, *Spiritual Sex* (New York: Pocket Books, 1997), 25.

37 **extreme forms of:** Translation by Professor Hugh Urban, Ohio State University, direct communication with author. For this section, I am indebted to many discussions of Hinduism and Tantra with Jeffrey Kripal.

37 **"marry by mutual choice":** *IJTO*, 48.

38 **"In this day and age":** "Tantrik Worship: The Basis of Religion," *IJTO*, 71.

38 **"The animating impulse":** Ibid.

38 **"is the most":** Ibid.

39 **Nicholls on the front page:** "Police Are Looking into Occult Affairs."

39 **Bernard came to:** "Police Still Hold Nichols [*sic*]," *San Francisco Call*, June 6, 1905, 16.

39 **"a rare student":** Ibid.

40 **"men dressed in long black gowns":** "Wild Orgies in the Temple of 'Om,'" *San Francisco Chronicle*, May 5, 1910, 1; "Faker's Slave a Coast Lad."

40 **Chinese opium addicts and prostitutes:** On the preponderance of commercial sex and social degradation as well as the selective harassment of the Chinese and Latin American women, see Jacqueline Baker Barnhart, *The Fair but Frail: Prostitution in San Francisco, 1849–1900* (Reno: University of Nevada Press, 1986).

40 **police made it:** "Faker's Slave a Coast Lad."

CHAPTER 4: DOWNFALL AND DISGRACE

43 **"The whole man":** PAB (Pierre Arnold Bernard) lecture notes, 1906, HSRC (Historical Society of Rockland County). Also see PAB deposition and PAB statement. The events and timing of the New York episode are based on court documents related to his arrest in 1910 and newspaper clippings from a dozen or so New York City newspapers, along with a scattered few from across the country. I am indebted to Professor Brad Verter of Bennington College for the New York City court documents, which he shared with me.

43 **yoga schools and health clinics:** PAB deposition, HSRC.

43 **"During my stay":** Ibid.

43 **Judge John Stanley Webster:** Known in the lodge as Lassen, John Stanley Webster (1877–1962) was a Washington state supreme court justice from 1916 to 1918, a representative from the Fifth District of Washington State from March 4, 1919, to May 8, 1923. His lodge name is found in the Tantrik list; his biographical info was found online at Washington State University Libraries: www.wsulibs.wsu.edu/Holland/masc/finders/cg459.htm.

43 **Walter A. Keene:** He was known in the lodge as Hathaway. For bio see H. James Boswell, *American Blue Book Western Washington* (Seattle: Lowman and Hanford, 1922), 190. He was a Mason and a member of the Seattle, Washington State, and American bar associations. The Boswell book can be found at http://freepages.genealogy.rootsweb.com/~jtenlen/wkeene.txt. Accessed August 13, 2009.

43 **W. W. French:** There were two members of the French family active in the Seattle lodge, with the lodge names of Leighton and Moffatt.

44 **became Pierre's ward:** PAB statement.

44 **Hindu lecturer:** www.mozumdar.org/yesterdaysevangelist.html. Accessed February 24, 2009.

45 **Lillian Russell:** Membership roll of the T.O. (Tantrik Order), HSRC

45 **taught a few:** PAB deposition.

45 **"Calcutta and other points in India":** Notarized bill of sale, HSRC. Inflation calculator: www.westegg.com/inflation/infl.cgi.

45 **Gertrude, who was living:** For her joining the T.O., see her various statements to several New York City newspapers, May 1910, HSRC.

46 **Gertrude Leo arrived in New York:** For the date, see "Nautch Girl Tells About Om; He Lured Her Here to Become His Consort," *New York Sun*, May 8, 1910, 1. For details, see "Dread of Death or Insanity Made Miss Leo a Slave," *New York World*, May 8, 1; for weather, see *New York Times*, May 8, as well as the *Chicago Daily Tribune* and the *Los Angeles Times*, same date.

46 **to be a nautch girl:** "Dread of Death or Insanity Made Miss Leo a Slave—'Nautch Girl' Tells of Strange Rites and Queer Influences That Held Her Long in the Power of 'Oom,'" *New York World*, May 8, 1910, 1; "Nautch Girl Tells About Om."

47 **"All priests have nautch girls"**: "Ruin Brought to This Woman by High Priest," *Atlanta Constitution*, May 8, 1910, B1.

47 **"I am not a real man"**: Ibid.

47 **"I became a novitiate"**: "'Oom' to Grand Jury," *New York Tribune*, May 8, 1910, 14.

47 **"As lightning from the womb"**: Tantrik Oath, HSRC.

48 **"guard my speech"**: Ibid.

48 **Duval, who was now pregnant**: Lodge name. There is no other record of a Duval in the T.O. documents.

48 **Opulence was the order**: "Girls in Weird Rite," *Washington Post*, May 4, 1910, 1; " 'Hindoo Priest' Lures Girls," *Chicago Daily Tribune*, May 4, 1910, 7; "Secret Revels of Oom's Pretended School Told for the First Time by Girl Dupes," *New York Evening World*, night edition, May 4, 1910, 1.

49 **Hopp family were introduced**: "Girl 'Yogi Wife' of 'Om' Tells How Faker Lured Her," *New York Evening World*, May 6, 1910, 1. Also see *New York Sun*, May 7, 1910, HSRC.

49 **average American worker**: American Cultural History, http://kclibrary.nhmccd .edu/decade00.html. Accessed January 8, 2009.

49 **"sanitarium"**: PAB often used this description to refer to one or another of his operations.

49 **Several nights later**: It was November 10th, according to her testimony to the court, p. 12 of the complaint.

50 **The weather was severe**: *New York Times*, February 27, 1910, 1.

50 **Nicholls skipped meals**: "Defying Wrath, Girl Discloses Secrets of Cult," *New York World*, May 5, 1910, and combined newspaper reports from that time, HSRC.

50 **Bernard's mother had married**: Bureau of Census, 1910, reports list them as a married couple in Fillmore, California, as of April 25–26.

50 **full $100 fee**: From enrollment form, HSRC.

51 **"Yogi suits"**: "Secret Revels of Oom's Pretended School Told for the First Time by Girl Dupes."

51 **"ethical culture"**: "Pleading Guilty, Bares Details of 'White Slave' Traffic in City," *New York Evening World*, May 3, 1910, 1.

51 **convinced both women**: "Dread of Death or Insanity Made Miss Leo a Slave."

52 **She wrote to**: "Pleading Guilty." Also see "Great God Oom Accused by Girls, Lands in Cell," *New York World*, May 3, 1910, 1.

52 **On May 2, Mrs.**: "Grent God Oom Accused by Girls"; complaint of Zelia Hopp, May 3, 1910.

52 **mild spring evening**: See *New York Times*, May 3, 1910, 1, for temperature that night, and *Washington Post*, May 3, 1910, for no rain.

52 **beneficial to bathe**: "Om Still Willing to Wed," *New York Sun*, May 7, 1910, HSRC.

52 **"a long, two short"**: Zelia Hopp statement to detectives, PAB indictment.

52 **the detectives rushed**: "Mystic Held as Abductor," *New York Journal* (Night Extra), May 3, 1910, 1. For the presence of the butler, see "Hindoo Mystic Is Accused by Girls," *New York Herald*, May 3, 1910.

52 **sounds of chanting**: "Weird Dance in Hindu Den." *Gettysburg Times*, May 4, 1910, 2.

53 **"A young man"**: "Arrest Hindu Seer," *New York Times*, May 3, 1910, 3.

53 **"What means this"**: "Weird Dance in Hindu Den."

53 **"For God's sake"**: "Girls in Weird Rite"; "Court Aghast at Her Story of Hindu Den," *New York Evening Mail*, May 3, 1910, 1.

53 **"Zim-zim-zim"**: "Weird Dance in Hindu Den."

53 **"So that's the"**: "Bernard the Oom Comes to Grief," *New York Evening Sun*, May 3, 1910, 1.

53 **Together they set**: "Police Break In on Weird Hindu Rites," *New York American*, May 3, 1910, 1.

53 **"I know all"**: "'Oom' Waits in Court as Girl Devotees Describe 'Rites,'" *New York World*, May 5, 1910, 1.

54 **"Keep my name out"**: Ibid.

54 **"Arrest Hindu Seer"**: "Arrest Hindu Seer."

54 **"Says He's a Swami"**: "Hindoo Mystic Is Accused by Girls."

54 **"His Students in"**: *New York Tribune*, May 3, 1910, HSRC.

54 **"'Great God Oom'"**: *New York World*, May 3, 1910, 1.

54 **wispy "sideboards"**: "Girls to Reveal Mysteries of Oom's School," *New York Evening World*, May 4, 1910, 1.

54 **"Oom, the self-styled"**: Ibid.

55 **Quakers, Shakers, Mormons**: Catherine L. Albanese, *A Republic of Mind and Spirit* (New Haven and London: Yale University Press, 2007). Also, Philip Jenkins, *Mystics and Messiahs* (New York: Oxford University Press, 2000) for the scandals that attached themselves to new or emerging American religions and "cults."

CHAPTER 5: "WHAT IS THIS MAN?"

57 **"inveigled and enticed"**: PAB (Pierre Arnold Bernard) indictment.

57 **$25,000 bail**: "White Slave Traffic Shown to Be Real," *New York Times*, April 30, 1910, 1.

57 **"What is this"**: "Bernard the Oom Comes to Grief," *New York Evening Sun*, May 3, 1910, 1.

58 **"No, he's not"**: Ibid.

58 **the grim details**: "'Omnipotent Oom' Held as Kidnapper," *New York Times*, May 4, 1910, 7; also see "Bernard the Oom Comes to Grief"; "Court Aghast at Her Story of Hindu Den," *New York Evening Mail*, May 3, 1910, 1; and "Arrest Hindu Seer," *New York Times*, May 3, 1910, 3.

58 **"When we got"**: "'Omnipotent Oom' Held as Kidnapper."

58 **"Fixed up swell"**: "Bernard the Oom Comes to Grief."

58 **Bail was set**: "'Omnipotent Oom' Must Scurry for $15,000 Bail," *New York Evening World*, May 3, 1910, 1.

58 **"That man ought"**: "Court Aghast at Her Story of Hindu Den."

58 **"unmarried and of"**: Complaint No. 77371, City Magistrates Court. This is the original complaint, handwritten and signed by Judge Breen and the other principals on May 3, 1910.

59 **"I am not guilty"**: Ibid.

59 **"No, I never"**: "Court Aghast at Her Story of Hindu Den."

59 **"a higher order"**: "Pleading Guilty, Bares Details of 'White Slave' Traffic in City,"

New York Evening World, May 3, 1910, 1; "White Slaver Will Lay Bare the Trade," *New York Times*, May 4, 1910, 6.

59 **"my sister has"**: Ibid.

59 **"comely"**: "Court Aghast at Her Story of Hindu Den."

59 **"sumptuously furnished"**: "Pleading Guilty." Also see "Hindoo Mystic Is Accused by Girls."

59 **"most exclusive"**: "Girls Tell How Hindoo Held Them Captives," *New York American*, May 4, 1910, HSRC.

59 **"scanty bathing suits"**: " 'Omnipotent Oom' Must Scurry for $15,000 Bail."

59 **"mesmerizing"**: "Pleading Guilty"; "White Slaver Will Lay Bare the Trade," which covered the confession the next day.

60 **out-of-town newspapers**: "Ruin Brought to This Woman by High Priest," *Atlanta Constitution*, May 8, 1910, B1. Also see "Girls in Weird Rite," *Washington Post*, May 4, 1910, 1; " 'Hindoo Priest' Lures Girls," *Chicago Daily Tribune*, May 4, 1910, 7; " 'Oom' Says Stories Are Exaggerated," *Trenton Evening Times*, May 5, 1910, 1; "Weird Dance in Hindoo Den," *Gettysburg Times*, May 4, 1910, 2; "Great 'God Oom' Locked in Jail," *Evening Telegram* (Elyria, OH), May 4, 1910, 6; "Scientific Seduction," *Nevada State Journal* (Reno), May 9, 1910, 6.

60 **"Wild Orgies in"**: "Wild Orgies in the Temple of 'Om,' " *San Francisco Chronicle*, May 5, 1910, 1.

60 **"He was beautiful"**: "Secret Revels of Oom's Pretended School Told for the First Time by Girl Dupes," *New York Evening World*, May 4, 1910, 1.

60 **"Tantriks' Worship Calls"**: "Tantriks' Worship Calls for Dead Bodies and Young Girls," *New York World*, May 5, 1910, HSRC.

60 **compendium of abridged**: Ibid.

60 **"salacious in nature"**: "Two Girl Victims Face 'Oom' with Fear in Court," *New York World*, May 5, 1910, HSRC.

60 **"He didn't look"**: "Testify Against the Om, Zelia Hopp and Miss Leo Begin Their Stories," *New York Sun*, May 6, 1910, 1.

61 **not terribly well**: See "Court Aides Shifted, Felled by Colds," *New York Times*, January 22, 1943, 40, for the history of the West Side Court and its condition. It was christened "Pneumonia Hall" by one chief justice before he closed it. Also see "Court on West Side to Close Its Doors," *New York Times*, December 22, 1942, 21; and "Two Courts to Quit 'Pneumonia Hall,' " *New York Times*, February 13, 1943, 7.

61 **"One of the"**: "Girl Dupes in Court Quail at Sight of 'Oom,' " *New York Evening Journal (Extra)*, May 6, 1910, 1.

61 **"Oom began kissing"**: "Girl 'Yogi Wife' of 'Om' Tells How Faker Lured Her," *New York Evening World*, May 6, 1910, 1.

61 **"He embarrasses me"**: "Girl Tells Magistrate of Heart Treatment by Oom," *New York Herald*, May 6, 1910, 1.

61 **"would rather have"**: "Om and Three of His Girl Accusers As They Appeared in Court Today," *New York Evening World*, May 6, 1910, 1 (story also has additional headline, "Girl 'Yogi Wife' of 'Om' Tells How Faker Lured Her." Also see "Oom Still Willing to Wed," *New York Sun*, May 7, 1910, HSRC.

62 **"Sex worship as"**: "Tantriks' Worship Calls for Dead Bodies and Young Girls."

62 **blood oaths and:** "Girl Fascinated by Oom Until She Heard of Orgies," *New York Sun*, May 7, 1910, HSRC.

62 **would indeed marry:** Ibid.

62 **"I both feared":** "Ruin Brought to This Woman by High Priest."

62 **"kaula rites":** Ibid.

63 **"Ruin Brought":** Ibid.

63 **sharing the same:** "Dread of Death or Insanity Made Miss Leo a Slave," *New York World*, May 8, 1.

63 **"I find that":** "Ruin Brought to This Woman by High Priest."

63 **"I shan't!"** Ibid.

63 **Comstock made an:** "Girl Reveals How 'Hindu' Won Her Love," *New York Evening Mail*, Wall Street Edition, May 6, 1910, HSRC.

63 **Tombs, a notorious:** "Overcrowding in the Tombs," *New York Times*, December 3, 1911, 14; "Tombs a Disgrace," *New York Times*, December 10, 1907, 7; "City Prisons Pack Beyond Legal Limit," *New York Times*, November 17, 1911, 10.

64 **"The Pierre Bernard":** "Omnipotent Oom Held," *Humeston New Era*, May 11, 1910, 1. This story was labeled "special," picked up from the *Chicago Daily Inter Ocean* a few days before.

64 **His followers had scattered:** "Testify Against the Om."

64 **"Let me go!":** Ibid.

65 **"previously chaste character":** Jordan, motion to reduce bail, June 6, 1910.

65 **"do no harm":** Affidavits and motion to dismiss, August 9, 1910.

65 **"nearly driven insane":** Ibid.

66 **no intention of:** Ibid.

66 **Bernard walked out:** "Oom, the Self-Named Free," *New York Times*, August 26, 1910, 2; also see "Oom out of Prison," *Washington Post*, August 26, 1910, 3.

CHAPTER 6: YOGA AT LARGE

69 **"A yogi is":** Marguerite Merington, "Oriental Definitions: Yogi," in *The Critic*, February 1906, 48.

69 **first English transcription:** Richard Leviton, "Celebrating 100 Years of Yoga in America," *Yoga Journal*, June 30, 1993, no. 110, 67–70.

70 **"It was as":** Joel Porte, ed., *Emerson in His Journals* (Cambridge, MA: Harvard University Press, 1984, 394). http://books.google.com/books. Accessed October 10, 2009.

70 **"to some extent":** Letter, Henry David Thoreau to H. G. O. Blake, November 20, 1849. Found at the Thoreau Institute at Walden Woods Library's online site.

71 **first Hindu cleric:** J. Gordon Melton, ed., *The Encyclopedia of American Religions*, 6th ed. (Detroit: Thomson Gale, 2002), chap. 23, 183.

71 **five hundred active chapters:** H. S. Olcott, "Theosophy and Theosophists," *Overland Monthly* and *Out West Magazine*, May 1901, 992.

71 **"over men and natural phenomena":** "Yogis in Their Own Land," *New York Times*, May 27, 1889, 3.

72 **"injurious to the"** H. P. Blavatsky, *The Secret Doctrine*, vol. 1, 1888, 95–96. Theosopical University Press Online Edition, www.theosociety.org/pasadena/sd/sd1-1-05.htm. Accessed October 13, 2009.

72 **"nothing but a":** *The Complete Works of Swami Vivekananda*, Volume Six, Epistles, Second Series, XXVII. Vivekananda, letter to his follower, Akhandanada, March 1890. "Our Bengal is the land of Bhakti and of Jnana, where Yoga is scarcely so much as talked of even. What little there is, is but the queer breathing exercises of the Hatha-Yoga—which is nothing but a kind of gymnastics." *www.ramakrishnavivekananda .info/vivekananda/volume_6/vol_6_frame.htm.* Accessed October 15, 2009.

73 **"a strange compound":** Monier Monier-Williams, *Indian Wisdom: or, Examples of the Religious, Philosophical, and Ethical Doctrines of the Hindus* (London: William H. Allen, 1875), 103. The lone defender among American philosophers was William James, who wrote approvingly of physical yoga in an essay called "The Energies of Men" in 1907.

73 **"Body and soul":** PAB lecture notes, August 13, 1912, HSRC.

73 **"The first duty":** Ibid.

74 **"The ascetics are":** Ibid.

74 **"The only way":** Ibid.

74 **"parlor talks":** Pandit, prospectus for his classes.

74 **"only decidedly original":** William James, *Varieties of Religious Experience* (New York: Longman Green, 11th impression, 1905), 98.

75 **"I am utterly":** "Under Yoga Spell," *Washington Post*, May 3, 1908, 1.

76 **"dangerously ill":** "Declares Yogis Diverted $500,000," *Chicago Daily Tribune*, May 26, 1911, 5.

76 **"animalistic":** "'Yoga' Followers Shut Out of Hall," *Chicago Daily Tribune*, September 20, 1909, 8.

76 **"seems to suggest":** Ibid.

76 **"immorality":** Ibid.

76 **"yogaistic tendencies":** "Yoga Divides Theosophy Ranks," *Chicago Daily Tribune*, September 19, 1909, 3.

76 **"it will be":** Ibid.

77 **Evelyn Arthur See:** "See Found Guilty of the Abduction of Bridges Girl," *Chicago Daily Tribune*, July 14, 1911, 1.

77 **"a bullet hole":** "Doctor Found Shot in Riverside Flat," *New York Times*, May 1911, 1.

77 **"typifies the sensual":** "This Soul Destroying Poison of the East," *Washington Post*, May 28, 1911.

77 **"to which nearly":** Ibid.

77 **divorce of Mr.:** "Quits Husband for Yoga Cult," *Los Angeles Times*, June 20, 1911, 11.

78 **"various swamis and":** "A Hindu Apple for Modern Eve," *Los Angeles Times*, October 22, 1911, III, 20; "The Heathen Invasion of America," *Current Literature*, November 1911, vol. 51, no. 5, 538.

CHAPTER 7: PARTNERS

81 **courts dismissed the:** Clark Jordan, letter to Clerk of the Court, April 4, 1923, asking for proof of the dismissal of the indictment many years later.

81 **The day after:** PAB statement, 13. Also see Viola W. Bernard (VWB) transcripts for references to New Jersey days. For description of Leonia, see "Panoramic View of Leonia Heights, N.J.," *New York Times*, December 18, 1910, RE-1.

82 **"Comfortable seats, cool":** Classified ad, *New York Times*, June 10, 1911, 19.

82 **Homer Stansbury Leeds:** Bernard's pseudonym is mentioned in "Night Revels Held in Sanskrit College," *New York Times*, December 15, 1911, 22.

82 **"to enable young":** Pierre Arnold Bernard (PAB) statement, HSRC (Historical Society of Rockland County).

82 **"The money which":** Ibid.

82 **"giving them instruction":** Ibid.

83 **He tutored the wife:** Ibid.

83 **"physiological yoga":** Classified ad, *New York Times*, April 30, 1911, 13.

83 **Sundays, Vedic Philosophy:** Ibid.

83 **far less glamorous space:** Photograph of classroom, HSRC.

83 **"Mysticism of the Orient":** Classified ad, *New York Times*, May 14, 1911, 13.

84 **"very dark, good looking":** "American Women Victims of Hindu Mysticism," *Washington Post*, February 18, 1912, Sunday Magazine, 1.

84 **who always knew:** Llellwyn Smith Jackson, notes for "The Adventures of a Girl from Seattle on Stage and Screen" (unpublished memoir, Santa Barbara, CA, 1988). DeVries describes Ora Ray as a graceful woman with an ordered mind.

84 **a sage from:** International Sufi Movement Web site: www.sufimovement.org/special_message.htm. Accessed August 14, 2009.

84 **"I do not hesitate":** Hazrat Inayat Khan, letter to PAB, June 5, 1911, HSRC.

85 **"What my wife":** "Night Revels Held in Sanskrit College," *New York Times*, December 15, 1911, 22.

86 **"I am conducting":** Ibid.

86 **"good looking man":** Ibid.

86 **"violating the educational law":** "Warrant out for 'Oom,'" *New York Times*, December 22, 1911, 11.

86 **Here Bernard set:** PAB deposition, 69–70.

87 **"The Tantrik Order":** PAB lecture notes, August 13, 1912, HSRC.

87 **"My definition of":** Ibid.

88 **Dace Shannon Charlot:** VWB statement, 184, item number 20. According to VWB's notes, by the time Bernard moved back to West End Avenue in Manhattan, both DeVries and her sister, Franci, were living with him.

88 **lovely, outsize features:** Dace's eye color and her physical appearance and size are from her passport application; for the critique of her teenage performance, see *Detroit Free Press*, October 12, 1908, HSRC.

88 **represented her in:** "Decision for Mrs. Dace Charlot," *New York Times*, August 19, 1913, 18.

89 **"quiet, unobtrusive, a":** Marian Dockerill, *My Life in a Love Cult* (Dunellen, NJ: Better Publishing Company, 1928), 64.

89 **"Look at our":** Ibid.

89 **"We can teach":** Ibid.

89 **"nodded solemnly":** Ibid.

90 **civil ceremony in:** Jean Overton Fuller, *Noor-un-nisa Inayat Khan* (London: East-West Publications Fonds, 1971). There are many errors in the short bios of Ora Ray Baker, including the date of her marriage to Khan and her alleged relationship to Mary

Baker Eddy. Fuller quotes reliably from the marriage certificate. As for the Baker Eddy connection, it does not appear to exist.

91 **more than fifty:** *Rockland County Red Book 1927* (Nyack, NY: Rockland County Trust Company, 1927), 112—for PAB's claimed degrees and membership in learned societies.

91 **"that marvelous intimacy":** PAB lecture notes, May 9, 1915.

91 **"Ninety-nine percent":** Ibid.

91 **"Orgasm is prolonged":** Ibid.

91 **"Thirty-five hundred years ago":** Ibid.

92 **"If sex is right":** Ibid.

CHAPTER 8: EXPANSION

95 **Llellwyn Delores Smith:** Llellwyn Smith Jackson, "The Adventures of a Girl from Seattle on Stage and Screen" (unpublished memoir, Santa Barbara, CA, 1988), 112. For her appearance in *Miss 1917*, Ms. Jackson seems to be mistaken in her memoir, referring to it as "Miss 1918." *Miss 1917* ran for forty-eight performances at the Century Theatre; Ziegfeld coproduced this attempt to follow up on the success of the previous year's *Century Girl*.

95 **"I didn't understand":** Jackson, "The Adventures of a Girl . . . ," 112.

96 **"The papers might":** Ibid.

96 **"He warned me":** Ibid., 121.

97 **bewildered by Jones:** Ibid., 124.

97 **an offer for a five-year contract:** "Daring Directors Chase Girl in Taxi to Get Her to Pose," *Pittsburgh Gazette Times*, October 14, 1917, HSRC (Historical Society of Rockland County). Also see Jackson, "The Adventures of a Girl. . . ."

97 **"a strange mistake":** Jackson, "The Adventures of a Girl . . . ," 143.

97 **"a saint in":** Ibid., 124.

97 **"I saw a":** Ibid.

97 **eight studios:** "Twelve Cult Worshippers Taken in a Raid upon the Home of the 'Great Oom,'" *New York American*, May 1, 1918, 1; "New Raid on 'Great Oom's' Cult Shrines," *New York American*, May 2, 1918, 1.

98 **best undercover officers:** Ibid.

98 **"Dr. Bernard shook":** Ibid.

99 **"He said there":** Ibid.

99 **"Will I meet":** Ibid.

99 **"psychics, soothsayers, cryptic":** Ibid.

99 **"Twelve Cult Worshippers":** "Twelve Cult Worshippers. . . ."

99 **"The disciples of":** Ibid.

101 **symbolized Vanderbilt wealth:** Cornelius Vanderbilt Jr., *Queen of the Golden Age* (New York: McGraw-Hill, 1956), 40.

101 **wooed in Paris:** "Young Roosevelt in Paris," *New York Times*, July 31, 1910, 17; "Mrs. Mills in Sanitarium," *New York Times*, June 18, 1916, 14.

101 **"You don't know":** Amanda Mackenzie Stuart, *Consuelo and Alva Vanderbilt* (New York: HarperCollins, 2005), 1.

102 **"Made quite a little":** PAB deposition, 74.

CHAPTER 9: FOR LOVE AND MONEY

105 **"introduced by Miss"**: PAB (Pierre Arnold Bernard) statement, 7, HSRC (Historical Society of Rockland Country).

105 **faithfully attended his:** Ibid., 8.

106 **"Through the lips":** *IJTO*, 52.

106 **outrageous falsehoods:** Marriage certificate of PAB and DeVries, August 27, 1918, HSRC.

107 **"I want to tell":** Margaret Rutherfurd, letter to PAB, November 21, 1918, HSRC.

108 **Margaret, Harold:** PAB statement, 9.

108 **Paris couture and:** Alfred Allan Lewis, *Ladies and Not-So-Gentle Women* (New York: Penguin Group, 2000), 373.

109 **West Side schools:** "Landmarks," a CCC chronology, HSRC.

109 **"Then they were":** Eckert Goodman, "The Guru of Nyack," *Town & Country*, April 1941, 52.

109 **"Cleanliness Is Next":** Ibid.

110 **"affected me deeply":** Llellwyn Smith Jackson, "The Adventures of a Girl from Seattle on Stage and Screen" (unpublished memoir, Santa Barbara, CA, 1988), 125–126.

110 **"used no ponderous":** Ibid.

111 **"gathered like a":** Jackson, notes for memoir, 3.

111 **"woman who had":** Ibid.

111 **its main sponsor:** Anne gave generously, as the trail of her checks shows. One, dated January 11, 1919, for $5,000, was signed over to PAB and DeVries. A second, dated January 18, 1919, for $5,000 was made out to Blanche DeVries from A. H. Vanderbilt. A third, dated January 20, 1919, for $100, was made out to PAB from AHV. A fourth, dated March 14, 1919, for $10,000, was made out to PAB from AHV. All signed checks found at HSRC.

111 **a society dilettante:** Society, *Washington Post*, June 15, 1919, A7.

111 **suffered financial reverses:** Lewis, *Ladies and Not-So-Gentle Women*, 349.

111 **jealousy of her:** Ibid., 312.

112 **another realm:** Jackson, memoir, 135–136

112 **"so listless, [it]":** Ibid., 136.

113 **"Some folk like":** Sir Paul Dukes, KBE, *The Unending Quest* (London: Cassell, 1950), 131.

113 **"Since my job":** Jackson, memoir, 134.

113 **she arrived early:** Ibid.

113 **"sometimes seen by":** Goodman, "The Guru of Nyack," 52: "Among the female teachers were two of social prominence: Mrs. Loring Andrews and Mrs. Hannah Prince . . . who were known by their lodge names of Miss Hawley and Miss Raleigh."

113 **"He understood how":** Jackson, memoir, 134.

113 **"beauty, cleanliness, and":** Ibid., 127.

114 **"the Sunday comics":** "The Omnipotent Oom Gets Two Customers," *Hairbreadth Harry, Lincoln Sunday Star*, April 15, 1917, color section, 1.

114 **Two young policemen:** Jackson, memoir, 129.

115 **"He thought this":** Ibid.

115 **"Beloved! My love":** Margaret Rutherfurd letter to PAB, undated, HSRC.

116 **"Good bye dear"**: Anne Vanderbilt letter to DeVries, undated, HSRC.

116 **"Dear DeVries"**: Ibid., April 4, 1919, HSRC.

CHAPTER 10: THE PROMISED LAND

121 **"It took us less"**: Llellwyn Smith Jackson, "The Adventures of a Girl from Seattle on Stage and Screen" (unpublished memoir, Santa Barbara, CA, 1988), 138.

122 **"bypassed and ignored"**: Ibid.

122 **"On account of"**: Benson J. Lossing, *The Hudson from the Wilderness to the Sea* (New York: Virtue and Yorston, 1866), 435.

122 **late as 1855**: Historic marker, Main Street and Route 9W, Nyack, HSRC (Historical Society of Rockland County).

122 **Zukor had purchased**: Linda Zimmerman, *Rockland County, Century of History* (New City, NY: HSRC, 2002), 84. Also, the Dominican nuns were in Sparkill, and the Marydell center in Upper Nyack would be opened in 1922, three years later.

123 **three-story, eighteen-room**: Grace Gordon, "Pierre Bernard and the Clarkstown Country Club," *South of the Mountain*, vol. 44, no. 1, January–March 2000, 3–18. Also see the *Rockland County Red Book* for 1927.

123 **"For our labors"**: Jackson, memoir, 140.

124 **"renounced her Episcopalian"**: "Was the Club Yoga Colony?" *Los Angeles Times*, November 28, 1919, III 4.

124 **"the strange things"**: Ibid.

124 **"You can be"**: Jackson, notes on PAB (Pierre Arnold Bernard) lectures, July 12, 1924, 13.

124 **"Live dangerously"**: Jackson, notes for memoir, "PA Bernard a Success," 1.

125 **largest private pleasure**: Arthur T. Vanderbilt II, *Fortune's Children: The Fall of the House of Vanderbilt* (New York: William Morrow, 1989), 147.

125 **"Things are very"**: Margaret Rutherfurd letter to PAB, June 17, 1919, HSRC.

125 **"the propitious moment"**: Ibid.

125 **"Needless to say"**: Ibid.

125 **"She is very"**: Ibid.

126 **seemed to care**: According to VWB (Viola Wertheim Bernard), recalled in her transcript, HSRC.

126 **"Am now going"**: Margaret Rutherfurd, letter to PAB, June 17, 1919, HSRC.

127 **"Cannot Understand Why"**: Margaret Rutherfurd, cable to PAB, June 21, 1919, HSRC.

127 **"Tantrikam, Thanks for"**: Ibid., July 1919, HSRC.

127 **"overpowering force"**: Margaret Rutherfurd, letter to PAB, undated, HSRC.

127 **"I assured Mrs. Vanderbilt"**: PAB statement, 17, HSRC.

128 **"in every way"**: Margaret Rutherfurd letter to PAB, November 21, 1918, HSRC.

CHAPTER 11: WELCOME TO NYACK

131 **150 members strong**: "Fakir Driven from City Has Country Club," *New York American*, October 20, 1919, 1.

131 **wives of prominent**: Charles B. Alexander's daughter served in France during the war, and in 1918 she married a decorated soldier and Yale man named Captain

Arnold Whitridge, which was noted in the *New York Times*: "Miss Alexander to Marry in Wartime," January 24, 1918. Hattie Crocker, daughter of a railroad magnate, was a leader in San Francisco society. She was married in that city to C. B. Alexander, an attorney, in 1887, according to the *New York Times*, April 27, 1887. One of her ushers was Harry Tevis, son of a San Francisco tycoon, who was coached by Bernard during the years 1900–1906.

132 **an army of spies:** Ibid.

132 **"queer antics":** Ibid.

132 **"yoga colony":** Ibid.

133 **"A cult here?":** Ibid.

133 **"As for Sister":** Ibid.

134 **Chalmers Wood Jr.:** "Miss K. Turnbull Weds C. Wood, Jr.," *New York Times*, October 1, 1916, 23. He was pronounced "one of the best known young men in New York society." Wood was a Wall Street and society clubman—he belonged to the Racquet and Tennis Club, among others—and a graduate of Columbia in 1905.

134 **"yoga ritual":** "Oom Is Defended by Chalmers Wood," *New York World*, October 21, 1919, 3.

134 **"women devotees of":** "Fakir Driven from City Has Country Club."

134 **"one of the":** Ibid.

134 **"nothing queer about":** "Oom Is Defended by Chalmers Wood."

134 **patients of Dr. Brewster:** Ibid.

134 **"a great man":** Ibid.

135 **personally investigate:** Ibid.

135 **"Bernard in Seclusion":** "Bernard in Seclusion; Society Women Vanish," *Nyack Evening Journal*, October 21, 1919, 1.

135 **"The women and":** "State Police Swoop Down on 'Oom' Club," *New York American*, October 22, 1919, 8.

135 **Morton Lexow attested:** Ibid.

135 **leading his own:** "Sheriff Merritt to Quiz Society Flock of 'Oom,'" *Nyack Evening Journal*, October 23, 1919, 1.

136 **female captives:** "Sheriff Will Quiz Society Flock of 'Oom,'" *New York American*, October 23, 1919, 6.

136 **three Nyack clergymen:** Ibid.

136 **Thursday night meeting:** "Oom's Flock Flies Before Sheriff," *New York American*, October 24, 1919, 1.

136 **"find some way":** Ibid.

136 **"a committing magistrate":** Ibid.

136 **"not the place":** Ibid.

136 **to be in hiding:** Ibid.

136 **"Oom's Flock Flies":** Ibid.

136 **"The greatest possession":** PAB (Pierre Arnold Bernard) lecture, undated, HSRC.

136 *buying* **the Maxwell:** "Chief of Police of Upper Nyack Gives 'Oom the Omnipotent' Clean Bill," *Nyack Evening Journal*, October 28, 1919, 1.

136 **$6,000 a month:** Ibid.

137 **"about $50,000 worth"**: Ibid.

137 **"They didn't get"**: Ibid.

137 **that all of:** Eckert Goodman, "The Guru of Nyack," *Town & Country*, April 1941, 52.

137 **soon be elected:** "Judge A. S. Tompkins Heads N.Y. Masons," *New York Times*, May 5, 1922, 2.

137 **"he and the"**: Goodman, "The Guru of Nyack," 52.

137 **stream of limousines:** Ibid.

138 **"After each visit"**: Llellwyn Smith Jackson, "The Adventures of a Girl from Seattle on Stage and Screen" (unpublished memoir, Santa Barbara, CA, 1988), 155.

138 **purchased the Maxwell:** "Country Club Property Sold; Price $100,000," *Nyack Evening Journal*, January 29, 1920, 1.

138 **"one of the"**: Ibid.

139 **purchased the Bradley:** "Dr. P. A. Bernard Buys the Bradley Property," *Nyack Daily News*, May 7, 1920, HSRC.

139 **series of checks:** Copies of checks, HSRC.

139 **a dance pantomime:** Program notes from the club's Oriental Bazaar, "The 400 at Rossiter," April 1920, HSRC.

139 ***The Fakir of:*** Ibid.

139 **Sanskrit, Imagination, and:** Ibid.

140 **"He stood out"**: Jackson, memoir, 154.

140 **Charles Ezra Scribner:** His most important contribution was the development of the multiple switchboard, an important component of telephone networks.

140 **flirted with abandon:** Jackson, memoir, 152, for Stokowski's hijinks. For Povla Frijsh, see Alfred Allan Lewis, *Ladies and Not-So-Gentle Women* (New York: Penguin Group, 2000), 387. For Cyril Scott, see his very English appreciation of DeVries in his autobiography, *Bone of Contention* (New York: Arco Publishing, 1969), 168.

141 **"Get a knowledge"**: Jackson, lecture notes, January 3, 1920.

141 **"The pleasure, peace"**: PAB lecture undated.

141 **"We can't all"**: Ibid.

142 **"We get yoga"**: Ibid.

142 **teach private yoga lessons:** Mildred Ryder, 1924 worksheets.

142 **"I can truthfully"**: Scott, *Bone of Contention*, 163–168.

142 **"For some time"**: Jackson, memoir, 173.

CHAPTER 12: INTERROGATION

146 **"Was Eldest Male"**: "W. K. Vanderbilt Dies in France in His 71st Year: Was Eldest Male Survivor of Family That Built Fortune in New York Central," *New York Times*, July 23, 1920, 1.

146 **the Supreme Court:** *Vanderbilt v. Eidman*, 196 U.S. 480 (1905) 196 U.S. 480, went to trial over a disputed clause of the Commodore's will and subsequent tax issues. Willie K. was the executor, and the case was argued before the U.S. Supreme Court, October 13–14, 1904. Decided February 20, 1905; Howard Taylor, Henry B. Anderson, and Chandler P. Anderson for the Vanderbilts. Later Anderson & Anderson became Anderson, Ferris, Gasser and Anderson. Chandler P. Anderson served as counsel to the U.S. State Department under President Taft and until 1915 under Woodrow Wilson.

146 **His investigation into Bernard's:** The remnant copy of Bernard's deposition in this investigation contains eighty-two pages, the first eleven of which are missing, as are the ending pages. It leaves slightly open to interpretation exactly when some of the investigation and the interrogation took place. I pinpoint the interrogation to 1921 after a lengthy investigation that was begun in the latter half of 1920, as mentioned in the text. The clients, except for Mr. Wood, are not named, though the Vanderbilt and the Mills families are clearly referred to.

147 **"unfair at this":** Anne Vanderbilt, telegram to PAB (Pierre Arnold Bernard), HSRC (Historical Society of Rockland County).

147 **"Understand You Had":** Ibid.

147 **"Anderson Cables Investigation":** Anne Vanderbilt, telegram to Barbara Hatch, HSRC.

148 **"It is stated":** PAB deposition, 13.

151 **"I promised you":** Ibid., 35.

153 **"And we are":** Ibid., 39

153 **"You were correctly":** Ibid., 41.

154 **E. O. Anderson: "Well, leaving out the sex":** Ibid., 76.

156 **"The morality?":** Ibid., 80.

156 **"I will guarantee":** Ibid., 80.

157 **"I am not":** Ibid., 81.

157 **"My name is":** PAB statement, 1, HSRC.

157 **"a former pupil":** PAB statement, 1–12.

157 **"I should very":** Investigative Reports of the Bureau of Investigation 1908–1922, Publication Number: M1085, Publication Title: Investigative Case Files of the Bureau of Investigation 1908–1922. Publisher: NARA. Series: Bureau Section Files, 1909–1921. Case Number: 218352. Roll Number: 954. Pages: 1–3.

159 **"complete mental breakdown":** Alfred Allan Lewis, *Ladies and Not-So-Gentle Women* (New York: Penguin Group, 2000), 373.

CHAPTER 13: BODY AND MIND

161 **"Tantrik Yoga, a":** Cyril Scott, *Bone of Contention* (New York: Arco Publishing, 1969), 166.

162 **"God re-appears with":** Ralph Waldo Emerson, *The Collected Works of Ralph Waldo Emerson,* vol. 2, Essays First Series, "Compensation" (Cambridge, MA: Belknap Press, 1979), 60.

162 **"What are we":** PAB (Pierre Arnold Bernard) lecture notes, undated, HSRC (Historical Society of Rockland County).

163 **"God consciousness":** PAB lecture notes, March 11, 1928, HSRC.

163 **"Consciousness of names":** Ibid.

163 **"The idea or":** PAB lecture notes, March 17, 1928, HSRC.

163 **R. Tait McKenzie:** www.archives.upenn.edu/faids/upt/upt50/mckenziert.html. Accessed August 10, 2009.

164 **"Most people use":** PAB lectures, March 4, 1928, HSRC.

164 **"The Yogis have":** Ibid.

164 **"All the divinity":** Ibid., April 22, 1928.

164 **"Our formal study":** Ibid., February 19, 1928.

CHAPTER 14: ENTER SIR PAUL

167 **"the man of a hundred"**: "Sir Paul Dukes, a Secret Agent," *New York Times*, August 28, 1967, 31. Also see Paul Dukes, *Red Dusk and the Morrow* (Garden City, NY: Doubleday, Page, 1922).

168 **"You don't have"**: Sir Paul Dukes, KBE, *The Unending Quest* (London: Cassell, 1950), 126.

168 **several side trips**: Ibid., 125–126.

168 **"curt and uncommunicative"**: Ibid., 127–129.

169 **bought the boat**: Ibid., 117. For a synopsis of Dukes's spy career, see Phillip Knightley, *The Second Oldest Profession* (New York: Norton, 1986—First American ed., 1987), 65–69.

169 **"We met before"**: Dukes, *Unending Quest*, 129.

169 **"Good many books"**: Ibid.

170 **walls were decorated**: Ibid.

170 **"If you stick"**: Ibid.

170 **"to their delight"**: Ibid., 130.

170 **"The background of"**: Ibid., 131.

171 **"I understood of"**: Ibid.

171 **"He was the"**: Ibid., 132.

171 **"a salutary revolution"**: Ibid.

172 **"one of the"**: "Review," *New York Times*, March 19, 1922, Book Review and Magazine, 54.

172 **"We immediately fell"**: "Dukes and Bride Settle in Paris," *New York Times*, October 22, 1922, 20.

173 **"Married Durand"**: Dukes diary, October 3, 1922, Dukes papers, Hoover Museum of War and Peace, Stanford University.

173 **"Sir Paul has"**: "Mrs. Ogden L. Mills Weds Sir Paul Dukes," *New York Times*, October 18, 1922, 1.

173 **"any move Mrs. Mills"**: Ibid.

173 **"has known Sir"**: Ibid.

174 **"Sir Paul may"**: Ibid.

174 **"inestimable privilege"**: "Dukes Champions 'Omnipotent Oom,'" *New York Herald*, October 23, 1922, 1.

174 **"It is not"**: Ibid.

174 **Bernard was being**: Ibid.

174 **"All I fear"**: Ibid.

CHAPTER 15: BACH, BASEBALL, AND BUDDHA

179 **"With no warning"**: Llellwyn Smith Jackson, "The Adventures of a Girl from Seattle on Stage and Screen" (unpublished memoir, Santa Barbara, CA, 1988), 149.

179 **"open invitation for"**: Ibid.

179 **"This hurt me"**: Ibid.

180 **Diana's $750,000 trust**: "Two Girls Ask for $50,000 Income from Estate," *New York Times*, May 3, 1922, 8. For growing up rich in New York, see "Alwyn Court Fire; Maids Aid in Rescue," *New York Times*, March 5, 1910, 1; for Jacob's $9 million legacy, see "Wertheim Left $8,895,478," *New York Times*, June 20, 1922, 16; for context see "Girl, 20, Needs

$25,000 Yearly to Live, Heiress Says; $1200 Says YWCA," *Decatur (IL) Review*, May 14, 1922, 1. The average American teacher was paid $1,166 a year in 1922, according to *The Chicago Daily News Almanac and Year Book*, 1926, 320. See www.historicaltextarchive .com/sections.php?op=viewarticle&artid=420. Accessed August, 10, 2009.

180 **sweet music of:** The actual James quote is "We all have some ear for this monistic music: it elevates and reassures. We all have at least the germ of mysticism in us." William James, "The One and the Many," lecture 4 in *Pragmatism: A New Name for Some Old Ways of Thinking* (New York: Longman Green, 1907), 59. James, of course, later rejected monism in favor of pluralism, though he seemed to maintain a soft spot for the romance of the former.

180 **"The girls were":** Interview with Joan Wofford, Diana's daughter.

181 **"I owe the":** Diana Hunt, "The Twice-Born," *Reveries,* self-published limited edition, copyright 1925 by Diana Hunt (Diana Wertheim).

181 **offered to donate:** Theos Bernard (TCB), letter to Glen Bernard (GAB), June 20, 1934, 5. Theos writes that Viola "once offered to give all she had to P.A. and he refused." Theos Bernard papers, Bancroft Library, University of California, Berkeley; thanks to Paul Hackett.

182 **"The Mechanicals seldom":** Dennis Prindle, "The Prindle Family History," unpublished family history. Dennis is the son of Charles Jr.

182 **"with a submarine":** Ibid.

182 **green-dyed costumes:** Ibid.

182 **"the enemy of":** Jackson, lecture notes.

182 **"Insipid playing and":** Ibid.

183 **"It will be":** "Braeburn Club Circus Pronounced a Thriller," *Nyack Evening Journal,* September 1, 1922, 1.

183 **"The scenery, props":** Ibid.

184 **midway of booths:** "Big Circus of Braeburn Club on Saturday," *Nyack Evening Journal,* September 7, 1922, 1; "Braeburn Club Circus Pronounced a Thriller"; "Club Circus Is Remarkable Success Here," *Nyack Evening Journal,* September 11, 1922, 1.

184 **"I was three":** Interview with Pete Seeger.

185 **"had very strong":** Charles Seeger, "Reminiscences of an American Musicologist," oral history transcript: www.archive.org/stream/reminiscencesofaooseeg/ reminiscencesofaooseeg_djvu.txt. Accessed August 1, 2009.

185 **"The doctor is":** Interview with Pete Seeger.

185 **"I was always":** Ibid.

185 **"Yes, We Have":** Frederick Lewis Allen, *Only Yesterday and Since Yesterday* (New York: Bonanza Books, 1986), 3; "Doyle Recites Talk with Stead Spirit," *New York Times,* April 9, 1923, 9.

185 **"It was an":** F. Scott Fitzgerald, "Echoes of the Jazz Age," *Scribner's,* November 1931, 459–465.

186 **Doyle's paranormal conversations:** "Hints of Seances at White House," *New York Times,* May 19, 1926, 26.

186 **"As an excuse":** From "Buddhamas" brochure, HSRC (Historical Society of Rockland County).

186 **"a place where":** Ibid.

187 **"Oh brethren, let":** Ibid.

187 **"wild orgies of":** Ibid.

187 **"willing to have":** Ibid.

188 **"My older brother":** Interview with Pete Seeger.

188 **sneak into Sir:** "Sir Paul Dukes' Auto Is Stolen and Dynamited," *Nyack Evening Journal*, September 24, 1923, 1.

189 *two* **masked balls:** "P.A.'s Birthday Only Comes Once in Every Year," *Nyack Evening Journal*, November 10, 1923, 1.

189 **Professional costumers from:** Eckert Goodman, "The Guru of Nyack," *Town & Country*, April 1941, 52.

189 **Amateur enthusiasts from:** "Widely Known Folks Arrive for 'Big Top,'" *Nyack Evening Journal*, August 26, 1924, 1.

189 **"initiated" into the:** "Armed Guards Surround Tent for CCC Show," *Nyack Evening Journal*, August 30, 1924, 1.

190 *The Jazz:* "Annual Orgies of Oom Witnessed by Hundreds in Big Top on Club's Grounds," *Nyack Evening Journal*, September 4, 1924, 1 and 4

190 **"Annual Orgies of Oom":** Ibid.

CHAPTER 16: THE VANDERBILT KNOT

193 **an altogether different remedy:** Alfred Allan Lewis, *Ladies and Not-So-Gentle Women* (New York: Penguin Group, 2000), 387.

194 **On August 11:** Ibid., 387–388, for Barbara pregnant by Nicholls before the marriage.

195 **"Vanderbilts Join Cult":** *Gettysburg Times*, August 27, 1924, 2.

195 **"September 18th, 1924":** Barbara Nicholls, letter to Anne Vanderbilt, HSRC (Historical Society of Rockland County).

196 **"Mrs. Nichols [sic] and":** *Nyack Evening Journal*, May 2, 1925, 1.

196 **"Sir Paul and":** Ibid.

196 **amount of ridicule:** Lewis, *Ladies*, 375.

197 **deteriorated further:** Dukes, diaries, February 1926.

198 **"must see P.A.":** Dukes, diaries, February 1927.

198 **"Now understand that":** Ibid.

198 **"She rather expressed":** Ibid.

199 **"that man's clutches":** Ibid.

199 **after her money:** Dukes, diaries, April 1927.

199 **"A hard, strange look":** Ibid.

199 **found a new target:** "Lady Dukes Wins Divorce," *New York Times*, January 10, 1929, 27.

199 **"it is quite":** *American Weekly* Sunday magazine, in *San Antonio Light*, May 15, 1927, 71.

200 **dying tragically young:** *Kingston Daily Freeman*, August 8, 1939, 1. For Barbara's marriage, see *Los Angeles Times*, July 9, 1929, 3; for Nicholls, see "Oom Aide Seeks to Be Free Again," *Rockland County Evening Journal*, July 8, 1929, 1.

CHAPTER 17: THE SHOW GOES ON

204 **first annual Spring:** "Spring Gambol of Club Inner Circle Is Colorful Event," *Nyack Evening Journal*, May 1925, 1.

205 **"We harvested the":** Llellwyn Smith Jackson, "The Adventures of a Girl from Seattle on Stage and Screen" (unpublished memoir, Santa Barbara, CA, 1988), 166.

205 **a funeral cortege:** "Two Coffins Used at Wedding Fete," *New York Times*, December 21, 1925, 14.

205 **"We'll make this":** Marian Dockerill, *My Life in a Love Cult* (Dunellen, NJ: Better Publishing Company, 1928), 70.

206 **an old "twister":** "Club Members Turn to Circus Stunts in Preparing for Show," *Nyack Evening Journal*, June 24, 1926, 1.

206 *CCC Male Orgies:* From festival brochure and production notes.

206 **"and even dared":** Jackson memoir, 179.

207 **$5 million in:** "Oom Will Help U.S. to Poison Alcohol," *Washington Post*, October 29, 1926, 1.

207 **"Until one has":** PAB (Pierre Arnold Bernard) lecture notes, undated, HSRC (Historical Society of Rockland County).

208 **"Again not trusting":** Jackson, memoir, "Adventures of a girl . . . ," 170.

208 **"I sensed his":** Ibid.

208 **"Cheerie, anyone can":** Ibid.

208 **"Cheerie, I'm going":** Ibid.

CHAPTER 18: BLUE SKIES, BIG PLANS

211 **a baby elephant:** "Country Club 'Zoo' Gets a Baby Elephant," *Nyack Evening Journal*, June 1, 1925, 1.

211 **"oceans of upturned":** Charles A. Lindbergh, "Lindbergh Says His Mind Is Ablaze with Noise and an Ocean of Faces," *New York Times*, June 14, 1927, 1.

212 **Cheerie's turn at the altar:** Llellwyn Smith Jackson, "The Adventures of a Girl from Seattle on Stage and Screen" (unpublished memoir, Santa Barbara, CA, 1988), 190–192.

212 **"Two factors in":** James Thurber and E. B. White, *Is Sex Necessary? Or Why You Feel the Way You Do* (New York: Harper and Brothers, 1929; Garden City, NY: Blue Ribbon Books, 1944), xi.

212 **"An airport in":** "H. J. Robertson President of Aircraft Club," *Nyack Evening Journal*, February 17, 1928, 2.

212 **Bernard was persuaded:** "Dr. Bernard New Leader of Aero Club," *Nyack Evening Journal*, March 5, 1928, 1.

213 **applause at the:** "Aero Club Members View Flight Films," *Nyack Evening Journal*, March 31, 1928, 1.

213 **in Bernard's hands:** "Aero Club to Keep Up Drive for Members," *Nyack Evening Journal*, March 24, 1928, 1; "Dr. Bernard New Leader of Aero Club"; "Aero Club Hears Talk on Piloting," *Nyack Evening Journal*, March 17, 1928; "German Baron at Clarkstown Country Club," *Nyack Evening Journal*, March 2, 1928, 1.

214 **"Bernard's insight into":** Major Francis Yeats-Brown, letter to CCC, December 15, 1925.

214 **"transport pilot, limited":** "Aero Club Plans to Seek License for Flying School," *Nyack Evening Journal*, March 21, 1928, 1.

214 **Bernard was reelected:** "Dr. Bernard Retains Post in Aero Club," *Nyack Evening Journal*, April 14, 1928, 1.

214 **"all departments are"**: PAB (Pierre Arnold Bernard) lecture notes, January 29, 1928, HSRC (Historical Society of Rockland County).

215 **Rockland Airport opened:** "Stunt Flying to Embellish Airport Opening," *Nyack Evening Journal,* May 26, 1928, 1.

215 **young parachutist, slipped:** "Parachute Jumper Killed in Fall at Airport Opening," *Nyack Evening Journal,* May 31, 1928, 1.

215 **Bernard helped take:** "Club Denies Blame for Air Tragedy: Death of Clausen, Parachute Jumper at Airport Opening, Laid to His Hurried Action," *Nyack Evening Journal,* June 2, 1928, 1.

216 **informal passenger service:** "Passenger Flying and Instruction Under Broad Schedule Is Proposed by Aero Club Technical Committee," *Nyack Evening Journal,* June 16, 1928, 1.

216 **"Dr. Pierre Bernard":** "Air Notables on Program of Aero Club," *Nyack Evening Journal,* July 12, 1928, 1.

216 **"the power tube":** PAB lecture notes, March 4, 1928, HSRC.

216 **"Auto-intoxication, in":** Ibid.

217 **"An enema, thoroughly":** Ibid., March 10, 1928.

217 **"Under the terms":** "Airport Leased to Government," *Sparkill Herald,* November 2, 1928, 1.

217 **"It will put":** Ibid.

217 **Charles Francis Potter:** "Rev. C. F. Potter Addresses Nyack Congregation," *Nyack Evening Journal,* April 30, 1928, 1.

218 **First India Conference:** Stefanie Syman, *Practice: A History of Yoga in America,* forthcoming.

CHAPTER 19: A LEAP OF FAITH

221 **The Museum of Modern Art opened:** Edward Alden Jewell, "The New Museum of Modern Art Opens," *New York Times,* November 10, 1929, X14.

221 **the "sexual revolution":** James Thurber and E. B. White, *Is Sex Necessary? Or Why You Feel the Way You Do* (Harper and Brothers, 1929). The edition I used is Blue Ribbon Books, 1944, same pagination. Chapter 4 is "The Sexual Revolution: Being a Rather Complete Survey of the Entire Sexual Scene," 73. Bernard read this book and kept a copy in his library. In David Allyn's *Make Love, Not War* (Boston: Little Brown, 2000), 4, the term *sexual revolution* is said to have been coined by Wilhelm Reich in Germany in the 1920s.

221 **"We advise you":** From typewritten pamphlet, "The Clarkstown Country Club Presents the Summer Season of 1929," HSRC (Historical Society of Rockland County). Also see "Circus Rider Back from Convention," *Nyack News,* September 1929, page unknown, HSRC.

222 **Miss Jessie Fowler:** Allen Gribben, "Mark Twain, Phrenology and the 'Temperaments': A Study of Pseudoscientific Influence," *American Quarterly,* vol. 24, no. 1, March 1972, 45.

222 **"More than average":** PAB (Pierre Arnold Bernard) lecture notes, January 19, 1929, HSRC.

222 **"Very conscientious—has":** Ibid.

223 **"Came to deliver applejack"**: "Police Chief Held After Clarkstown Club Invasion; Nyack and South Nyack Policemen Accused of Attempt to Suppress News; Bernard Won't Talk; Nutter Held for Hearing on Charge of Driving While Intoxicated," *Rockland County Evening Journal*, February 15, 1929, 1. The *Tribune* story was reprinted in full as a shirttail to the *RCEJ* report.

225 **"She was very tall"**: Interview with Joan Wofford.

225 **took the plunge**: "Miss Wertheim Wed at Country Home," *New York Times*, May 31, 1929, 26. For quote, see interview with Joan Wofford.

225 **"have incorporated as"**: From typewritten pamphlet, "The Clarkstown Country Club Presents the Summer Season of 1929," HSRC. PAB lecture notes, March 16, 1929, for quote on Unitarians.

225 **"Yoga doesn't present"**: Ibid.

226 **Potter had been**: Charles Francis Potter, *The Preacher and I* (New York: Crown, 1951), 191. Potter's success in the debates led to his being crowned a "doctor" by the press, though he had only a master's degree. So, like Bernard, he was an unaccredited doc.

226 **"Strange tales were"**: Ibid., 339.

226 **"It was said"**: "Oom Is a Sound Theologian, Not a Charlatan, Says Dr. Potter, Promising to Explode Accounts of Nyack Cults and Orgies," *New York World-Telegram*, May 31, 1931, HSRC.

226 **"He always liked"**: Potter, *The Preacher and I*, 339.

226 **"He was both"**: Ibid., 341.

227 **"particularly successful with"**: Ibid., 336.

227 **"In yoga training"**: PAB lecture notes, March 16, 1929, HSRC.

228 **"As darkness falls"**: "Gilded Dowagers, Sacred Elephants Among Features," *New York Daily News*, September 5, 1929.

228 **"colored ballet dancers"**: Ibid.

228 **fewer than 1 million**: John Kenneth Galbraith, *The Great Crash 1929* (Boston: Houghton Mifflin, 1961), 133.

229 **largest and most**: Details on the Minerva from the Western Reserve Historical Society, which has one.

CHAPTER 20: GOOD TIMES, BAD TIMES

231 **"It feels funny"**: "Dr. Bernard's Elephants Return from a Show Debut," *Rockland Life*, August 13, 1931, HSRC (Historical Society of Rockland County).

232 **ISVAR soon collapsed**: Charles Potter, notes for PAB bio, "Introducing East and West," 1–5. Also see Chatterji and Joshi letters. Thanks to Stefanie Syman.

232 **capacity crowd**: "5,000 Roosevelt Lead Foreseen in Rockland," *New York Times*, November 2, 1930, N2.

233 **Kittie Martin, died**: "Bernard Is Made Executor of His Mother's Estate," *Rockland County Evening Journal*, September 26, 1931, 1.

233 **Potter comforted Bernard**: Charles Francis Potter, *The Preacher and I* (New York: Crown, 1951), 348.

234 **"Oom Is a"**: "Oom Is a Sound Theologian, Not a Charlatan, Says Dr. Potter, Promising to Explode Accounts of Nyack Cults and Orgies," *New York World-Telegram*, Thursday, May, 7, 1931, HSRC.

234 **"all the earmarks":** Ibid.

234 **"There are groups":** Ibid.

234 **gave up his:** "Claim Bernard in Plan to Break Airport Lease, Fears Schomberg Will Decision," *Rockland County Evening Journal*, June, 6, 1931, 1.

235 **Bernard purchased a:** "The Clarkstown Country Club Properties Debt Free."

235 **"It feels funny":** "Dr. Bernard's Elephants Return from a Show Debut."

235 **two more elephants:** "Third Elephant Chaperone to 'Baby' and 'Budh,'" *Nyack Daily News*, September 19, 1931, 1; "This Is How They'll Look Tomorrow," *Nyack Daily News*, November 7, 1931, 1.

237 **"my boy":** Joseph Mitchell, "Oom Is Booster of His County, His Proud Boast," *New York World-Telegram*, December 15, 1931, 18.

237 **"He has become":** Ibid.

237 **"curious combination of":** Ibid.

237 **"Nobody knows if":** Ibid.

CHAPTER 21: CITIZEN OOM

239 **Mom, Baby, Budh:** "Many Odd Gifts Received by Nyackers but with Delight," *Nyack Daily News*, December 26, 1931, HSRC (Historical Society of Rockland County).

240 **shown in theaters:** "Film Made of Bernard's Elephants Is Released," *Nyack Daily News*, June 6, 1932, HSRC.

240 **John Ringling was:** "Elephants Go to Ringlings," *Rockland Evening Journal*, April 8, 1932, 1. A description of the elephants' tricks is in this story.

240 **"best elephant act":** "Dr. Bernard's Elephants Achieve Circus Triumph," *Nyack News*, May 1932, HSRC. "Bernard Elected Member of Saints and Sinners Club," *Rockland Evening Journal*, May 16, 1932, 1.

240 **"The old Vedic":** PAB (Pierre Arnold Bernard) lecture notes, January 28, 1934, HSRC.

240 **"experimented not on":** Ibid.

241 **"Here, take this":** Charles Francis Potter, *The Preacher and I* (New York: Crown, 1951), 342.

241 **"Eleven per minute":** Ibid.

241 **Potter's observation, was:** Ibid., 342–343.

242 **"War on Depression":** "Nyack Legion to Begin 'War on Depression,'" *Rockland County Evening Journal*, March 18, 1932, 1; "Nyack Tea Garden Owner Files Bankruptcy Petition," *Rockland County Evening Journal*, January 16, 1932, 2.

242 **visionary thinking in:** The first professional night game was in 1935. "Apples for a Nickel, and Plenty of Empty Seats," *New York Times*, January 7, 2009, B11. Also see www.baseball-almanac.com/firsts/first10.shtml. Accessed August 3, 2009.

243 **first night baseball:** "Bernard's Field Being Prepared with Floodlamps," *Rockland County Evening Journal*, July 6, 1932, 7; "Clarkstown Country Club Field Being Improved," *Rockland County Evening Journal*, July 7, 1932, 7.

243 **Bernard met the:** "Detroit Clowns to Play Monday," *Rockland County Evening Journal*, August 11, 1932, 7.

243 **two thousand paying spectators:** "Grandstand to Seat 2,000," *Rockland County Evening Journal*, July 22, 1932, 2.

243 **Rockland County Chamber:** "Night Games Are Endorsed: Member of Chamber of Commerce Says Events Put County on Map," *Rockland County Journal*, July 25, 1932, 1.

244 **Major Jimmy Doolittle:** Ewen Mee, "Elephants Lend New Zest to Night Baseball Game," *Rockland County Evening Journal*, July 26, 1932, 7.

245 **"to P.A.B. with":** Hamish McLaurin, *Eastern Philosophy for Western Minds: An Approach to the Principles and Modern Practice of Yoga* (Boston: Stratford, 1933), front matter. Francis Yeats-Brown, Preface, v–xiii.

246 **Monday night football:** "Night Football Season to Start in Nyack Oct. 7th," *Rockland County Evening Journal*, September 28, 1932, 1.

246 **"Without the club":** Ibid.

246 **Viola Wertheim had:** VWB (Viola Wertheim Bernard), archive, notes to collection, HSRC.

247 **"Isn't it just":** VWB transcript, 159–163, HSRC.

247 **Viola went off :** Interview with Joan Wofford.

247 **"I don't know":** "County Must Plan Wisely, Bernard Idea; Reckless Disregard for Neighbors in 'Wide Open Spaces' Curbed by Forethought," *Rockland County Evening Journal*, November 27, 1932, 4.

248 **"must be shown":** Ibid.

248 **"philosophy reduced to":** "Yoga Theory Is Unfolded: Dr. Bernard Gives History of Tribal Movements in Dinner Talk," *Rockland County Journal-News*, January 17, 1933, HSRC.

248 **"Its teachings in":** Ibid.

249 **solvent and profitable:** "100 Men Work on Club Lands," *Rockland County Journal-News*, March 20, 1933, 3; "Nation's Banks Close Doors," and "Banks Closed in Rockland," *Rockland County Journal-News,* March 4, 1933, 1.

249 **army of men:** "100 Men Work on Club Lands," *Rockland County Journal-News*, March 20, 1933, 3.

249 **convinced the engineering:** Kenneth MacCalman, "Impressions of Dr. Bernard and the C.C.C. As Viewed by a Nyack On-Looker," *South of the Mountain*, vol. 14, no. 4, October–December 1970, 2. I've also been told that the light towers were built by the New York Central Railroad (which was still in the hands of the Vanderbilt family) in a direct communication from Richard Helmke, former mayor of South Nyack.

250 **"I have noticed":** Charles Francis Potter, "Second Article," unpublished biography of Bernard, 3. Thanks to Frank Potter, Regina Dasilva, Richard and Suellen Stringer-Hye.

250 **Bernard presented his:** "Dr. Bernard Holds Favor of Lady Luck."

250 **"I don't know":** Ibid.

250 **In the audience:** Ibid.

250 **"near beer":** a malt-based brew with an alcohol content below 0.5 percent.

250 **"rocked in the":** "Dr. Bernard Holds Favor of Lady Luck."

250 **"He has thrown":** "North End Extension of Playing Field at Clarkstown Country Club Sports Center Now Being Completed."

251 **"a shrewd and":** "Evolution," *Fortune*, July 1933, Off the Record, 4.

251 **"speed the return":** *Time*, July 3, 1933, cover photograph.

251 **four-acre extension:** "North End Extension of Playing Field at Clarkstown Country Club Sports Center Now Being Completed."

251 **NRA marches:** "Employers of 100,000 Sign for NRA Parade," *New York Times*, September 7, 1933, 12; "NRA Parade in Tarrytown," *New York Times*, October 7, 1933, 5; "Monroe NRA Parade Over Mile in Length," *Atlanta Constitution*, October 14, 1933, 10; "Mom, Huge Elephant, Dies in 92nd Year," *New York Times*, November 11, 1933, 2; "Lehman Sets Navy Day," *New York Times*, October 26, 1933, 20.

252 **clearly in physical:** "Now It's Clear Mom Was Too Ill to Parade," *Rockland County Journal-News*, November 7, 1933, 12; "Rockland in Gay Dress for Motorcade," *Rockland County Journal-News*, November 1, 1933, 1.

252 **"'Mom' lies on":** "Now It's Clear Mom Was Too Ill to Parade."

252 **"Treatment of the":** Ibid.

252 **several books:** Courtney Ryley Cooper, "Old Mom, Queen of the Elephants," *Billings* (MT) *Gazette*, November 26, 1933, Sunday supplement, 8.

252 **"There's life in":** "Twenty Men, Nurses and Keepers, Strive to Save Pachyderm," *Rockland County Journal-News*, November 9, 1933, 1; "As the World Wags," *Charleston Daily Mail*, November 16, 1933, 6; Courtney Ryley Cooper, "Old Mom, Queen of the Elephants."

253 **"Never mind old":** Winifred Van Duzer, "Mom's Fight for Life Ends at CCC Home," *Rockland County Journal-News*, November 10, 1933, 1.

253 **"With a final":** Ibid.

253 **"whatever aspect the":** "Bernard Tells of New Plans for C.C.C.," *Rockland County Journal-News*, December 19, 1933, 1.

CHAPTER 22: THE MESSAGE GETS OUT

255 **Yale Club luncheon:** "Dr. Bernard Guest Speaker at Luncheon at Yale Club," *Rockland County Journal-News*, February 1, 1934, 12.

255 **"a lot of converts":** Alma Whitaker, "Weird Occult Creeds Thrive Among Stars," *Los Angeles Times*, October 21, 1934, A1.

256 **"introduced to me":** Elsie de Wolfe, *After All* (New York: Harper and Brothers, 1935), 233–235; Gary Cooper reference from Hector Arce, *Gary Cooper: An Intimate Biography* (New York: William Morrow, 1979), 135; also in here is a description of the success and popularity of the film *Lives of a Bengal Lancer*, and the fact that de Wolfe was one of the "status designers of the day" out in Hollywood. For those movie stats, see www.ils.unc.edu/dpr/path/goldenhollywood. Accessed August 13, 2009.

256 **Mae West, Greta:** Bildad, "Theatre News," syndicated column in the (Madison) *Wisconsin State Journal*, September 26, 1933, 6.

256 **"Scientists Study Yoga":** "Scientists Study Yoga Breathing," *El Paso Post*, April 10, 1934, 11; "Oddities," *Vidette Messenger*, November 19, 1934, 1.

256 **"Yoga for You":** Francis Yeats-Brown, "Yoga for You," *Hearst's International—Cosmopolitan*, April 1935, 56, courtesy of the Hearst Corporation.

257 **"Yoga Is Helpful":** "Yoga Is Helpful to Mental, Physical Powers," *Chester Times*, April 25, 1935, 16, among other sources; "What Is This Thing Called Yoga?" *American Weekly* magazine, published in the *San Antonio Light*, October 7, 1952, 8.

257 **"dean of American":** "Dean of Playwrights Tells of His Career," *Rockland County Journal-News,* May 8, 1933, HSRC.

258 **"Noël Coward is":** James Aswell, "My New York Becomes My Nyack," *Rockland County Journal-News,* November 25, 1933, HSRC.

258 **"unique quality of":** Ibid.

258 **"crackled with celebrity":** Ibid.

CHAPTER 23: CHANGE IN THE AIR

261 **old grievances very:** VWB (Viola Wertheim Bernard), interview with Carol Ling-ham, 12–13, HSRC (Historical Society of Rockland County).

262 **Theos Bernard had:** Theos Bernard's life story is taken from the preface and first two chapters of his book *Heaven Lies Within Us* (Durban, South Africa: Essence of Health, 1970), along with Viola Bernard's interviews from HSRC and Columbia. I am indebted to the work of TCB scholar Paul G. Hackett, who has produced a Columbia University Web site on TCB, and questions the veracity of Theos's account of this period in his life. See Paul Gerard Hackett's PhD dissertation, "Barbarian Lands: Theos Bernard, Tibet, and the American Religious Life," Columbia University, Department of Religion, 2008. For Glen's extended absence, see Viola W. Bernard's taped interviews, 21, HSRC.

262 **"He was a":** Bernard, *Heaven Lies Within Us,* 19. Also see Hackett, "Barbarian Lands."

262 **"All action without":** Ibid., 20.

262 **"through the practice":** Ibid., 21.

262 **"Live free from":** Ibid., 25.

263 **"to be economically":** Ibid., 26.

263 **"Patience and perseverance":** Ibid., 36.

263 **"family guru":** Theos Bernard, *Penthouse of the Gods* (New York: Charles Scribner's Sons, 1939), 29; interview with Paul G. Hackett.

263 **"He was young":** VWB transcript, HSRC.

263 **"He was handsome":** Ibid.

264 **"We were drawn":** Ibid.

264 **"considerable zinc holdings":** VWB letter to Maurice Wertheim, July 23, 1934. VWB Archive, Columbia University.

265 **"He was a":** VWB transcript, HSRC.

265 **"It is a little":** TCB (Theos Casimir Bernard) letter to GAB (Glen Agassiz Bernard), July 20, 1934, quoted in Hackett, "Barbarian Lands."

266 **"Bernards Flee to Oom":** *New York Daily Mirror,* August 3, 1934, 13.

266 **"Viola Wertheim, Disciple":** "Viola Wertheim, Disciple of Oom, Weds a Bernard," *New York Daily News,* August 8, 1934, HSRC.

266 **founding member of:** "Nyack Society Leader Participating in Southern Sports," *Rockland County Journal-News,* January 30, 1934, HSRC; "Dr. Potter, Magazine Editor," *Rockland County Journal-News,* March 7, 1934, HSRC.

267 **a book about:** *Life at the Clarkstown Country Club,* 1935, copyright the CCC.

267 **"doubled in the":** Property taxes rose from 5.4% of national income in 1929 to 11.7% in 1932. David T. Beito, *Taxpayers in Revolt: Tax Resistance During the Great Depression* (Chapel Hill: University of North Carolina Press, 1989), 6; quoted in the paper "The

Success of the Great Depression Tax Revolts" by Mark Thornton and Chetley Weise, www .mises.org/journals/scholar/Thornton1.PDF. For top tax rates see www.hyperhistory.com/ online_n2/connections_n2/great_depression.html. Both accessed August 3, 2009.

268 **leased the Rossiter:** "Private School for Boys Will Be Opened in Nyack," *Rockland County Journal-News*, June 3, 1937, 1. For $1,000 salary for the elephants, see "Evolution," *Fortune*, July 1933, Off the Record, 4.

268 **"In the apartment":** Sara Hale, letter to author and interview.

268 **waited overnight in:** *New York Evening Post*, August 28, 1935, HSRC.

268 **"baseball game of":** Paul Harrison, "In New York," *Lowell Sun*, November 3, 1934, 11.

269 **lineup included gossip:** "Broadway Stars to Stage Baseball Game Sunday to Benefit Nyack Y: Chorus Beauties to Head Rooters," *Rockland County Journal-News*, October 25, 1934, 1.

269 **included Humphrey Bogart:** Ibid.

269 **"A consensus of":** Harrison, "In New York."

269 **"There were, in":** Ibid.

270 **"Billy Rose of music":** "Film and Stage Stars Clash with Writers in Winter Baseball Game," *Rockland County Journal-News*, October 29, 1934, 1; "Broadway Stars to Stage Baseball Game."

CHAPTER 24: RUNNING OUT OF TRICKS

273 **fully engulfed in:** "19 Boy Students Are Led to Safety as Flames Destroy School," *Rockland County Journal-News*, March 10, 1936, 1.

274 **seventeen-year-old Pete:** Interview with Seeger, 2002. For donkey ball, see "The House of David Baseball Team" by Joel Hawkins and Terry Bertolino at www .baseballlibrary.com/excerpts/excerpt.php?book=house_of_david&page=18. Accessed August 13, 2009.

274 **"another kind of":** "Big Stadium to Be Dog Track," *Rockland County Journal-News*, July 9, 1936, 1; "Oom Sidetracks Cult for Dog Racing," *New York Evening Post*, July 30, 1936, HSRC (Historical Society of Rockland County).

274 **new oval track:** Ibid.

275 **popular with working:** "Many in Nassau Back Dog Racing Measure," *New York Times*, May 24, 1936, 8.

275 **closed the place:** "Nyack Dog Track Raided," *New York Times*, September 2, 1936, 23.

276 **shut the place:** "Dog Races Are Raided," *New York Times*, September 13, 1936, 12.

276 **liens were filed:** "Court to Sift Sale of Dog Track Stock," *New York Times*, August 15, 1936, 30; "Jailed over Dog Track," *New York Times*, September 14, 1936, 16; "Receiver for Dog Track," *New York Times*, October 15, 1936, 7; "Lessees Face 3 More Liens," *Rockland County Journal-News*, October 21, 1936, 1; G. F. Hoffman Jr. interview.

276 **seek the counsel:** Interview with G. F. Hoffman Jr.

276 **"What the hell":** "Weird Echo (from a Dog-Track!) of the Mysterious Epic of 'Oom,'" *New York Sunday Mirror*, December 6, 1936, magazine, 9.

276 **"In all there":** "Clarkstown Club Members Give Halloween Party for Dr. Bernard on Birthday," *Rockland County Journal-News*, November 15, 1936, 1.

277 **"You Must Never"**: Ibid.

277 **"The club is"**: M. L. Schreiner, letter to Mildred Gillingham, 1936, Sara Hale personal papers. For studio in New York City, see *Rockland County Journal-News*, November 11, 1934; Ruth is joined there by her sister, Cabot, in 1936.

277 **"I guess you"**: M. L. Schreiner, letter to Mildred Gillingham, November, 8, 1936.

278 **"Our Xmas intention"**: Notes from "The Pill," December 1936.

278 **graduation from Cornell**: "Medical Degrees to 64," *New York Times*, June 17, 1936, 26. Also see http://library.cpmc.columbia.edu/hsl/archives/findingaids/bernard.html for other details.

278 **"Be careful on"**: PAB (Pierre Arnold Bernard), letter to TCB (Theos Casimir Bernard), June 1, 1936, HSRC.

278 **"I'd pay a good"**: Ibid.

279 **training and initiation**: Theos Bernard, *Penthouse of the Gods* (New York: Charles Scribner's Sons, 1939), 238.

278 **"vitally interested in"**: TCB letter to Viola Bernard, March 6, 1937, VWB (Viola Wertheim Bernard), Columbia.

279 **"lives on his"**: Ibid.

280 **"I would become"**: Bernard, *Penthouse of the Gods*, 320.

280 **"I got a"**: VWB, letter to TCB, June 2, 1937.

280 **"P.A. got mad"**: Ibid.

280 **"I told him"**: Ibid.

280 **"He sputtered about"**: Ibid.

280 **"P.A. is doing"**: DeVries, letter to TCB, undated, 1937, HSRC.

281 **"The present movement"**: Memo to PAB, March 3, 1937, unsigned, HSRC.

281 **"the concentration of"**: Ibid.

281 **"at one time"**: Edmund Pearson, "A Reporter at Large—The Left Bank II," *New Yorker*, September 4, 1937, 37.

282 **"Buddhist Worship in"**: "Buddhist Worship in Tibet Pictured," *New York Times*, November 2, 1937, 1. Also see George Ross, "In New York," *Lowell* (MA) *Sun*, December 4, 1937, 4.

CHAPTER 25: THE COSMIC PUNCH

285 **"an almost rabid"**: "Where Are They Now? Oom's Guests," *New Yorker*, July 16, 1938, 40–42.

285 **"Bring them right"**: Ibid.

286 **"I remember there"**: Interview with Pete Seeger.

286 **"The big opening"**: DeVries, diary fragment, weeks of July 25 and August 8–13, 1938, HSRC (Historical Society of Rockland County), 1998, 1.

287 **"Tantric yog in Nyack"**: Jeffrey J. Kripal, *Esalen: America and the Religion of No Religion* (Chicago: University of Chicago Press, 2007), 236.

287 **"the cornerstone of"**: Rosemary Feitis, "Ida Rolf Talks About Rolfing and Physical Reality," in *Bone, Breath and Gesture*, ed. Don Hanlon Johnson (Berkeley, CA: North Atlantic Books, 1995), 156; Don Hanlon Johnson e-mail message to author. Also see DeVries diary fragment, weeks of July 25 and August 8–13, 1938, HSRC.

287 **"Worship the body!"**: Ibid., 238.

287 **"a constant stream"**: "Yoga for Nova," Talk of the Town, *New Yorker*, May 19, 1939, 17.

288 **"What a joint!"**: "Nova Will Train in Clarkstown for Fight," *Reno Evening Gazette*, March 30, 1939, 13.

288 **"You ought to"**: Frank Graham, "Setting the Pace," *New York Sun*, May 5, 1939, HSRC.

288 **"Sweat-shirted men"**: Elliot Arnold, "Oom Tries to Unite Mysticism and Cult of Tony Galento," *New York World-Telegram*, March 31, 1939, 16.

289 **"He is stronger"**: Henry McLemore, "Today's Sports Parade," *Logansport Pharos-Tribune*, May 23, 1939, 9.

289 **"It is not"**: Ibid.

289 **"'Oom the Omnipotent'"**: Paul Ross, "'Oom the Omnipotent' Works Yoga Wonders on Lou Nova," *Sheboygan Press*, May 18, 1939, 17.

289 **"I believe athletics"**: Arnold, "Oom Tries to Unite Mysticism."

290 **"I'll give him"**: "Heavyweight Challenger Took Tunney as Model," *Lowell Sun*, May 16, 1939, 12. Also see Ross, "'Oom the Omnipotent' Works Yoga Wonders on Lou Nova."

290 **"Not for nothing"**: John Lardner, "Mighty Oom and Trainer Praise Nova," *Hartford Courant*, May 19, 1939, 13.

291 **"Baer took the"**: "16,738 See Nova Batter Baer and Score Knockout Victory," *New York Times*, June 2, 1939, 33.

291 **TKO for Nova:** Ibid.

291 **"one of the"**: Mark Kram, "The Fighter," *Sports Illustrated*, December 12, 1966, 66.

291 **The challenge was:** Ibid.

292 **"will never be"**: Art Cohn, "Cohning Tower," *Oakland Tribune*, October 8, 1941, 42. Also see Cohn columns July 27, 1940, 30, and September 17, 1941, 38.

292 **spending much of his:** Abram Chasins, *Leopold Stokowski: A Profile* (New York: Hawthorn Books, 1979), chap. 1; for the details of his collaboration with Disney and the timeline of 1938–1939, see chap. 10.

292 **slim down in:** "Notes by Jean Duncan on 'Super-Sunday' at the Song House," September 18, 1977, tells the tale in DeVries's view of Stokowski's visit to the club in 1939, HSRC.

293 **"Dear Stokowski"**: DeVries, letter to Stokowski, April 24, 1939, HSRC.

293 **"I feel we"**: Stokowski, letter to DeVries, April 26, 1939, HSRC.

293 **"I thought he"**: VWB (Viola Wertheim Bernard) interview with Carol Lingham of Arizona Historical Society, June 25, 1991, 4, Columbia, Box 1, 1.2.1.

294 **"disbelief in Western"**: VWB, "Notes re: Letters from Theos Bernard from India to VWB," dictated July–August 1996 by VWB, 3–14, HSRC.

294 **"He deplores the"**: Ibid.

294 **"This was very"**: Ibid.

294 **"You can touch"**: Letter from VWB to TCB (Theos Casimir Bernard), April 5, 1938. VWB archive 11.3; VWB interview with Carol Lingham of Arizona Historical Society, June 25, 1991, 17, from Columbia Archive, Box 1, 1.2.1.

294 **"He was very"**: VWB interview with Carol Lingham, 20; communication from Paul Hackett, Theo Bernard scholar.

295 **"key factor in"**: "Note About the Use of Sky Island as a Summer Hostel for Refugees from Nazi Persecution, 1939–1945, Inclusive," dictated by VWB, April 1981. VWB Papers, Columbia, Box 1, 1.2.2.

295 **"Ceremonials in the"**: "White Lama," review of *Penthouse of the Gods*, *Time*, April 3, 1939, www.time.com/time/magazine/article/0,9171,771641,00.html. Accessed August 13, 2009.

295 **"braved the black"**: Ibid.

295 **"The thrilling, gripping"**: Ad in the *Reno Evening Gazette*, March 19, 1939, HSRC.

295 **"Theos Bernard, Explorer"**: Ibid.

295 **"went nuts"**: VWB interview with Carol Lingham, 33, HSRC.

295 **"He was supposed"**: Ibid.

295 **"In Re: Theos"**: PAB, notes for an unpublished review, HSRC.

296 **"American Yogi"**: "American Yogi," *Ken*, July 20, 1939, HSRC. See F. L. Allen, *Only Yesterday and Since Yesterday: Two Volumes in One* (New York: Bonanza Books, 1986), 274, for *Ken* description. Also see "The Press: Ken's End," *Time*, July 10, 1939, www.time.com/time/printout/0,8816,761662,00.html. Accessed August 4, 2009.

296 **"In the national"**: Ibid.

296 **most telling image**: Ibid.

296 **an obituary honoring**: "Oom the Omnipotent Inserts Obituary Notice of Mrs. Vanderbilt's Daughter," *Kingston Daily Freeman*, August 8, 1939, 1; Alfred Allan Lewis, *Ladies and Not-So-Gentle Women* (New York: Penguin Group, 2000), 450–453.

296 **"I haven't seen"**: "Mystery of Barbara Rutherfurd's Strange Change of Character," *San Antonio Light*, September 10, 1939, *American Weekly*, Sunday supplement, 49.

296 **"People tell me"**: Ibid.

296 **"Yoga's my bug"**: Ibid.

297 **"mysterious transformation"**: Ibid.

297 **"Don't hesitate K"**: PAB letter to Katharin Hoffman, circa April 1940, HSRC.

297 **"Cash is shy"**: Ibid.

298 **"any burdens our"**: Interview with G. F. Hoffman, 2006.

CHAPTER 26: A NAZI IN NYACK

301 **a household emergency**: "Pro-British Banker Shot by Houseboy," *Washington Post*, January 20, 1941, 16.

301 **"Come down immediately"**: "'Oom' Ex-Aide Shot, Bloodhounds Used to Hunt Young Nazi," *New York Times*, January 20, 1941, 1; "Advocate of British War Aid Shot by His German Houseboy," *Los Angeles Times*, January 20, 1941, 2.

302 **Bund, who were**: "Two Rockland Towns Oppose Camp of Bund," *New York Times*, April 30, 1939, 26. Also see Alice Beal Parsons's *The Mountain* (New York: E. P. Dutton, 1944), 210–211. Yorkville was home to Fritz Kuhn's German-American Bund, the most notorious pro-Nazi group of the 1930s.

302 **"Dr. Whittlesey staggered"**: "'Oom' Ex-Aide Shot."

302 **at center stage**: "Ex-Aide to Omnipotent Oom Shot; Hunt Boy," *Chicago Daily Tribune*, January 20, 1941, 6; "'Oom' Ex-Aide Shot."

303 **sued Theos for**: "Wealthy Mrs. Donovan (Now in the Asylum) and her Yogi Teacher," *San Antonio Light*, May 4, 1941, 69 (in *American Weekly* Sunday supplement, 3).

303 **"What were the"**: Ibid.

303 **"So far as":** Ibid.

304 **months behind in:** Memo to PAB (Pierre Arnold Bernard), July 17, 1941 re: finances, HSRC (Historical Society of Rockland County). The sum of $36,000 was reported in PAB letter to Katharin Hoffman, circa April 1940, HSRC.

304 **"I have not":** DeVries, letter to PAB, December 7, 1941, HSRC.

304 **"fools speaking out":** Ibid.

304 **"Talk has certainly":** Ibid.

305 **"It was one":** VWB (Viola Wertheim Bernard) transcript, 264.

305 **rations and travel restrictions:** "Bids Americans Take Vacations Near Home," *New York Times*, June 10, 1942, 12; Irving S. Cutter, "How to Keep Well," *Chicago Daily Tribune*, July 23, 1944, 12; "ODT to Remove All Sports Travel Bans Today," *Chicago Daily Tribune*, August 17, 1945, 21; Peggy Preston, "War Influence Evident at Sea Shore Resorts," *Washington Post*, July 8, 1943, B7. Also see Eckert Goodman, "The Guru of Nyack," *Town & Country*, April 1941, 52.

305 **"every man, woman":** FDR address to the nation, April 1942, http://library .thinkquest.org/15511/index.htm. Accessed August 13, 2009.

305 **observation tower Chestnut:** Linda Zimmerman, *Rockland County: Century of History* (New City, NY: Historical Society of Rockland County, 2002), 165–171.

306 **"Summer theaters have":** "Oom's Animals," *Life*, August 17, 1942, 53–56.

306 **"Although about 70":** Ibid.

306 **"the lions roared":** Ibid.

307 **"Any Similarity Between":** Ibid.

307 **a huge success:** Ibid.

308 **"nerves are unpatriotic":** "Nerves Are Unpatriotic, Says Actress," *Washington Post*, April 11, 1942, 13.

308 **Margaret Woodrow Wilson:** Herbert L. Matthews, "Margaret Woodrow Wilson Finds Peace as Disciple of Yoga in India," *New York Times*, January 28, 1943, 21; "Gandhi to Undergo Two Months Yogi Health Treatment," *Washington Post*, August 1, 1938, 4.

308 **"This announcement is":** From "Yoga," pamphlet published in 1945 by Bernard and the CCC, HSRC.

308 **"Club membership, one":** Ibid.

308 **"insists upon the":** Ibid.

308 **"Keep physically fit":** Ibid.

309 **"The site is":** Lee R. Steiner, *Where Do People Take Their Troubles?* (Boston: Houghton Mifflin, 1945), 179.

309 **"He is a":** Ibid.

309 **"We kid people":** Ibid., 180.

309 **"No astral bunk":** Ibid.

310 **"It was depressing":** Ibid.

310 **"The place seemed":** Ibid.

CHAPTER 27: FAMILY MAN

313 **"Real estate gone":** PAB (Pierre Arnold Bernard), letter to Franci Yager, February 15, 1946, HSRC (Historical Society of Rockland County); for housing shortages see "Even Without Limit on Prices, Wyatt Says There Would Be Material Shortages,"

Council Bluffs (IA) *Nonpareil*, April 26, 1946, 4; "Find Homes for Veterans," *Raleigh Register*, Beckley, WV, March 22, 1946, 4.

313 **"Piece of business":** PAB, letter to Franci Yager, February 15, 1946.

313 **"English and French":** "English and French furniture, tapestries, porcelains, silver, table china, Oriental rugs," Catalogue 801, Parke-Bernet Galleries, Inc., October 30– November 2, 1946.

313 **fifty-eight separate items:** Ibid.

314 **with Jeanne Powell:** Letter from "Melvin," Jeanne Powell's club name, to Bernard, undated. VWB (Viola Wertheim Bernard) transcripts, September 26, 1987, 156, HSRC.

314 **attracted a few delegates:** PAB, letter to Martha Hoffman, December 2, 1949, for presence of UN delegates.

314 **enjoying opening nights:** "Brilliant Throng at Metropolitan," *New York Times*, November 28, 1944, 27.

314 **"How many postures":** Frederic J. Haskin, "Questions Answered," *Hartford Courant*, March 13, 1944, 5.

314 **a new benefactor:** "Yogi Charm Dead; Walska Cleans House," *Washington Post*, July 26, 1946, 8; "Enemy of the Average," *New York Times*, April 14, 2002, G80; "Ganna Walska Fights Mate's Support Suit," *Los Angeles Times*, July 9, 1946, A1; "Sued by 6th Mate," *Chicago Daily Tribune*, May 26, 1946, 17.

315 **was reported missing:** "U.S. Tibetan Scholar Is Missing in Punjab After a Tribal Attack; Theos Bernard, Author, Feared Dead by Wife Who Reports Incident in New Delhi," *New York Times*, October 31, 1947, 17.

316 **could barely walk:** PAB, letter to "Max," August 27, 1948, HSRC.

316 **"We have little":** Ibid.

316 **"Title of Farm House":** PAB, telegram to DeVries, May 4, 1948, HSRC.

316 **a cottage on:** VWB transcripts, 220, for chronology of Sunstone Hill, HSRC.

317 **"It seems I":** PAB, letter to DeVries, undated, summer 1948, HSRC.

318 **"For nearly ¾":** PAB, letter to Franci Yager, undated, 1949, HSRC.

318 **"but they were":** Ibid.

318 **"I so wished":** PAB, letter to Martha Hoffman, July 12, 1950, HSRC.

318 **"old pictures, cheap":** Ibid., December 2, 1949.

319 **"Since separating from":** Ibid., July 12, 1950, HSRC.

319 **"In my time":** Ibid.

319 **"Just finished a":** Ibid.

319 **"I've been around":** Ibid.

319 **"Miscellaneous":** Classified ad, *New York Times*, September 4, 1949, 162.

320 **"Lincoln high pressure":** Ibid.

320 **"He said he":** Interview with G. F. Hoffman.

321 **"I thought he":** Ibid.

321 **"Even though I":** Ibid.

321 **"He also had":** Ibid.

321 **"He never told":** Ibid.

322 **"'I wonder which'":** Ibid.

322 **"He sold the":** Ibid.

322 **"They stayed at"**: Ibid.

322 **"After we ate"**: Ibid.

322 **"Pierre and I"**: Ibid.

323 **"He never stayed"**: Ibid.

323 **"I never saw"**: Interview with Homer Lydecker Jr.

CHAPTER 28: FINAL DAYS

325 **"Happiness is the"**: PAB (Pierre Arnold Bernard) lecture notes, 1912, HSRC (Historical Society of Rockland County).

325 **"You can't know"**: PAB lecture notes, February 28, 1927, HSRC.

325 **"Life is a"**: PAB lecture notes, April 16, 1933, HSRC.

325 **"Don't give up"**: PAB lecture notes, February 28, 1927, HSRC.

325 **"working synthesis, incomplete"**: C. F. Potter, "The Place of Pierre A. Bernard," manuscript for unpublished biography, thanks to Frank Potter, Regina Dasilva, Richard and Suellen Stringer-Hye.

326 **"the only religion"**: Ibid.

326 **"Non-expression and"**: PAB lecture notes, February 28, 1927.

326 **"Try, instead of"**: "Excerpts from lecture by P. A. Bernard," August 24, 1932, thanks to Richard and Suellen Stringer-Hye.

326 **"Bishop wears a"**: PAB, letter to Martha Hoffman, December 2, 1949, HSRC.

326 **"Nothing but Russian"**: Ibid.

326 **"I guess my"**: Ibid.

327 **"We now use"**: Ibid.

327 **cottage for rent**: Julie Winslett, unpublished memoir of her years at the Clarkstown Country Club (copyright J. T. Winslett). This section is based on her memoir, along with her recollections shared in our personal correspondence over six years. My thanks to her for her generosity and sharp memory.

327 **"There were no"**: Winslett, memoir.

327 **"In the middle"**: Ibid.

327 **"He was bald"**: Interview with Julie Winslett.

328 **distinguished Russian clan**: Interview with Helen Saposhkov.

328 **"Dr. Bernard was"**: Ibid.

328 **"The atmosphere was"**: Winslett, memoir.

329 **"She had lived"**: Ibid.

329 **"People didn't like"**: Interview with Helen Saposhkov.

329 **"A gazetteer lay"**: Winslett, memoir.

329 **"It was as"**: Ibid.

330 **"everything was covered"**: Ibid.

330 **"charlatan who bamboozled"**: Ibid.

330 **"the place alone"**: Ibid.

330 **"Today is my"**: Edmund T. Dana letter to PAB, October 25, 1954, HSRC.

331 **"We knocked on"**: Interview with Pete Seeger.

331 **"Sometimes I would"**: Interview with Julie Winslett.

332 **"I was in Minnesota"**: Interview with G. F. Hoffman.

332 **"natural causes"**: PAB death certificate, HSRC.

332 **"funeral service was":** "Deaths," *New York Times*, September 29, 1955, 33.

332 **thin and pale:** color photo of PAB in casket, HSRC.

333 **"they were scared":** Interview with G. F. Hoffman.

333 **"When my parents":** Interview with Julie Winslett.

333 **Also in attendance:** PAB funeral register, HSRC.

333 **"My Darling. My":** Card accompanying funeral flowers, September 1955, HSRC.

334 **"First must each":** *IJTO*, 101.

334 **"One 1930 Minerva":** PAB, last will and testament, HSRC.

334 **16 mm catalog:** Untitled film, HSRC.

EPILOGUE: GENIUS OR FRAUD?

337 **"I can easily":** C. F. Potter, "Second Article," notes for a Bernard biography, 5. Also see C. F. Potter, "Miscellaneous Notes," 1. Thanks to Frank Potter, Regina Dasilva, Richard and Suellen Stringer-Hye for Potter material.

337 **"from another age":** Potter, "Second Article."

337 **"Pierre Bernard, 'Oom'":** "Pierre Bernard, 'Oom the Omnipotent,' Promoter and Self-Styled Swami, Dies," *New York Times*, September 28, 1955, 35.

337 **"love cultist":** "Obituaries," *Chicago Tribune*, September 28, 1955, B7.

337 **In Ironwood, Michigan:** "'Oom' the Mystic Dies in New York," *Ironwood* (MI) *Daily Globe*, September 28, 1955, 6; "Mystic 'Oom' of '20s Fame Dead at 80," *Long Beach Press-Telegram*, September 28, 1955, A-23. Also see "Mystic 'Oom' of the 1920s Dead at 80," *Washington Post*, September 29, 1955, 22; "Noted Society Mystic of Roaring '20s Dies," *Corpus Christi Times*, September 28, 1955, 3-B; "Pierre Bernard Dies, Mystic 'Oom' of 1920's," *Syracuse Herald-Journal*, September 28, 1955, 40.

338 **For fifteen years:** "The School That Vision Built: The Expansion Years 1940—Until Christ Returns," www.nyackcollege.edu/?page=Vision05. Accessed August 10, 2009.

338 **"Oh dear God":** "Moseley Hall," *Bailey Library Historic Buildings Collection*, Nyack College, Nyack, NY, http://74.125.95.132/search?q=cache:B6VaFbRTUgEJ:www.nyackcollege.edu/library/RC_Historical_Photos.pdf+Bailey+Library+Historic+Buildings+Collection,%E2%80%9D&cd=1&hl=en&ct=clnk&gl=us. Accessed August 13, 2009.

338 **April 10, 1956:** William D. Carlsen, "Two Institutions on a Hill," *Alliance Magazine Centennial Edition*, October 13, 1982, 6. Also see "The School That Vision Built."

338 **twenty-nine bedroom:** Surrogate's Court Appraisal of . . . the Estate of Pierre A. Bernard, January 6, 1957.

338 **Julie Wiggenhorn watched:** Julie Winslett, unpublished memoir.

338 **"The estate was picked":** Ibid.

338 **"Now our dogs":** Ibid.

339 **"demon activity":** Carlsen, "Two Institutions on a Hill," 6.

339 **brought the Indian:** "Cover Biography: B. K. S. Iyengar," *Current Biography*, June 2007. "In 1956 the Standard Oil heiress Rebekah Harkness invited Iyengar to travel to the United States, where he was shocked by American life and its incompatibility with the teachings of yoga." www.hwwilson.com/currentbio/cover_bios/cover_bio_6_07.htm. Accessed August 16, 2009. Also see DeVries biographical materials, HSRC.

339 **"the real Dr. Bernard":** Virginia Parkhurst, "The Real Yoga of Dr. Pierre Bernard: Wife Cites Usage as Modern Therapy," *Rockland County Journal-News*, April 7, 1963, 40.

339 **"DeVries for her":** Interview with Paula Heitzner.

340 *Yoga for Today:* Clara Spring and Madeleine Goss, *Yoga for Today* (New York: Holt, Rinehart and Winston, 1959).

341 **"phenomenal rascal master":** Alan Watts, *In My Own Way: An Autobiography* (New York: Pantheon Books, 1972), 126.

342 **Harold Stirling Vanderbilt:** George Plimpton, "House of Cards: The Vanderbilt Story, Part IV," *Sports Illustrated*, November 5, 1956, 69.

344 **"Come alive—you're":** Jess Stearn, *Yoga, Youth and Reincarnation* (New York: Bantam Books, 1965), back cover.

344 **"The amazing key":** Ibid., front cover.

Sources and Bibliography

LIBRARIES, ARCHIVES, PAPERS, AND LETTERS

Alan Mason Chesney Medical Archives, The Johns-Hopkins Medical Institutions
Bernard Collection, Historical Society of Rockland County, New City, NY
Charles Francis Potter papers, personal collection of Frank Potter
Columbia University Butler Library
Columbia University Journalism Library
Dennis Prindle, "Bernard in the Prindle Oral Family History," personal collection
Hoover Institution Library and Archives at Stanford University
Joan Wofford, papers and letters of Diana and Viola Wertheim, personal collection
Julie Winslett, unpublished memoir, copyright J. T. Winslett
Llellwyn Jackson, unpublished memoirs and notes, personal collection of Barbara Junge
New York City Public Library
New-York Historical Society Library
Nyack Public Library History Room, Nyack, NY
Richard and Suellen Stringer-Hye, CCC personal collection
San Francisco Public Library
Sara Hale, papers of Marie Louise Schreiner and Morris Whitaker, personal collection
University of California at Berkeley Special Collections
University of Texas, Austin: Institute of American Culture
Viola W. Bernard Papers, Archives and Special Collections, Columbia University Health
    Sciences Library, New York, NY

SELECTED NEWSPAPERS

Atlanta Journal-Constitution
Boston Globe
Chicago Daily Tribune
Los Angeles Times
New York Herald

New York Sun
New York Times
New York World
Nyack Daily News
Nyack Evening Journal
Rockland County Journal-News
Washington Post

WORKS CONSULTED

Albanese, Catherine L. *A Republic of Mind and Spirit: A Cultural History of American Metaphysical Religion.* New Haven and London: Yale University Press, 2007.

Allen, Frederick. *Secret Formula: How Brilliant Marketing and Relentless Salesmanship Made Coca-Cola the Best-Known Product in the World.* New York: Harper Business, 1994.

Allen, Frederick Lewis. *Only Yesterday and Since Yesterday: Two Volumes in One.* New York: Bonanza Books, 1986.

Allyn, David. *Make Love, Not War: The Sexual Revolution: An Unfettered History.* Boston: Little, Brown, 2000.

Alter, Joseph S. *Yoga in Modern India: The Body Between Science and Philosophy.* Princeton, NJ: Princeton University Press, 2004.

Anonymous. *Life at the Clarkstown Country Club.* Nyack, NY: Clarkstown Country Club, 1935.

Arce, Hector. *Gary Cooper: An Intimate Biography.* New York: William Morrow, 1979.

Barnhart, Jacqueline Baker. *The Fair but Frail: Prostitution in San Francisco, 1849–1900.* Reno: University of Nevada Press, 1986.

Bernard, Theos. *Hatha Yoga: The Report of a Personal Experience.* New York: Columbia University Press, 1944.

———. *Heaven Lies Within Us.* Durban, South Africa: Essence of Health, 1970.

———. "Introduction to Tantrik Ritual." Master's thesis, Columbia University, 1936.

———. *Penthouse of the Gods: A Pilgrimage into the Heart of Tibet and the Sacred City of Lhasa.* New York: Charles Scribner's Sons, 1939.

Braden, Charles S. *Spirits in Rebellion: The Rise and Development of New Thought.* Dallas, TX: Southern Methodist University Press, 1963.

Brandon, Ruth. *The Life and Many Deaths of Harry Houdini.* New York: Random House, 1993.

Breen, Matthew P. *Thirty Years of New York Politics—Up to Date.* New York: Privately printed, 1899.

Bridges, Hal. *American Mysticism: From William James to Zen.* New York: Harper and Row, 1970.

Chasins, Abram. *Leopold Stokowski: A Profile.* New York: Hawthorn Books, 1979.

Clark, Tom. *The World of Damon Runyon.* New York: Harper and Row, 1978.

Cohan, Tony. *Native State: A Memoir.* New York: Broadway Books, 2003.

Cope, Stephen. *Yoga and the Quest for the True Self.* New York: Bantam Books, 1999.

Danielou, Alain, translator. *The Complete Kama Sutra.* Rochester, VT: Park Street Press, 1994.

Delano, Sterling F. *Brook Farm: The Dark Side of Utopia.* Cambridge, MA: Belknap Press, 2004.

De Michelis, Elizabeth. *A History of Modern Yoga: Patanjali and Modern Esotericism*. London: Continuum, 2004.

Devi, Indra. *Yoga for Americans*. Englewood Cliffs, NJ: Prentice-Hall, 1970.

De Wolfe, Elsie. *After All*. London: William Heinemann, 1935.

Diamond, Sander. *The Nazi Movement in the United States, 1924–1941*. Ithaca and London: Cornell University Press, 1974.

Dockerill, Marian. *My Life in a Love Cult: A Warning to All Young Girls: My True Life Story by Marian Dockerill, Priestess of Oom*. Dunellen, NJ: Better Publishing Company, 1928.

Douglas, Ann. *Terrible Honesty: Mongrel Manhattan in the 1920s*. New York: Noonday Press, Farrar, Straus and Giroux, 1995.

Douglas, Nik. *Spiritual Sex, Secrets of Tantra from the Ice Age to the Millennium*. New York: Pocket Books, 1997.

Dukes, Sir Paul, KBE. *Red Dusk and the Morrow: Adventures and Investigations in Red Russia*. Garden City, NY: Doubleday, Page, 1922.

———. *The Unending Quest: Autobiographical Sketches*. London: Cassell, 1950.

———. *The Yoga of Health, Youth and Joy*. London: Cassell, 1960.

Dunaway, David King. *How Can I Keep From Singing: Pete Seeger*. New York: McGraw-Hill, 1981.

Ellwood, Robert S., ed. *Eastern Spirituality in America: Selected Writings*. New York: Paulist Press, 1987.

Ernst, Robert. *Weakness Is a Crime: The Life of Bernarr Macfadden*. Syracuse, NY: Syracuse University Press, 1991.

Ferguson, Charles W. *Fifty Million Brothers: A Panorama of Lodges and Clubs*. New York: Farrar and Rinehart, 1937.

———. *The New Books of Revelations: The Inside Story of America's Astounding Religious Cults*. Garden City, NY: Doubleday, Doran, 1929. (Plain Talk Edition of *The Confusion of Tongues* by Charles W. Ferguson).

Feurstein, Georg. *The Shambhala Encyclopedia of Yoga*. Prescott, AZ: Hohm Press, 1998.

———. *Tantra: The Path of Ecstasy*. Boston: Shambhala Publications, 1998.

———. *The Yoga Tradition*. Boston: Shambhala Publications, 1997.

Fitzgerald, F. Scott. *The Jazz Age*, a compilation of previously published essays and articles. New York: New Directions Publishing, 1996.

Fogel, Robert William. *The Fourth Great Awakening and the Future of Egalitarianism*. Chicago: University of Chicago Press, 2000.

Fronc, Jennifer. "I Led Him On: Undercover Investigation and the Politics of Social Reform in New York City, 1900–1919." PhD diss., Columbia University, 2005.

Fuller, Jean Overton. *Noor-un-nisa Inayat Khan*. London: East-West Publications Fonds, 1971.

Gay, Peter. *Modernism: The Lure of Heresy*. New York: W. W. Norton, 2007.

Gilfoyle, Timothy J. *City of Eros*. New York: W. W. Norton, 1992.

Goodman, Eckert. "The Guru of Nyack: The True Story of Father India, the Omnipotent Oom," *Town & Country*, April 1941, 50, 53, 92–93, 98–100.

Gordon, Grace. "Pierre Bernard and the Clarkstown Country Club." *South of the Mountains*, vol. 44, no. 1, January–March 2000. New City, NY: Historical Society of Rockland County, 2000.

Hackett, Paul Gerard. "Barbarian Lands: Theos Bernard, Tibet, and the American Religious Life." PhD diss., Columbia University, 2008.

Hanna, Thomas, ed. *Explorers of Humankind.* "Ida Rolf," essay by Don Hanlon Johnson. New York: Harper and Row, 1979.

Hunt, Diana. *Reveries.* City unknown, privately printed, 1925. Collection of Joan Wofford.

Isherwood, Christopher, and Swami Prabhavananda. *How to Know God: The Yoga Aphorisms of Patanjali.* Hollywood, CA: Vedanta Press (The Vedanta Society), 1953.

Jackson, Llellwyn Smith. "The Adventures of a Girl from Seattle on Stage and Screen." Unpublished memoir, Santa Barbara, CA, 1988.

————. Notes for an unpublished memoir, collection of Barbara Junge.

James, William. *The Varieties of Religious Experience: A Study in Human Nature.* New York: Modern Library, 1994.

Jenkins, Philip. *Mystics and Messiahs: Cults and New Religions in American History.* New York: Oxford University Press, 2000.

Johnson, Don Hanlon. "Ida Rolf," in *Explorers of Humankind,* ed. Thomas Hanna. New York: Harper and Row, 1979.

King, Francis. *Sexuality, Magic and Perversion.* London: Neville Spearman, 1971.

Knightley, Phillip. *The Second Oldest Profession.* New York: Norton, 1986 (first American ed., 1987).

Kripal, Jeffrey J. *Esalen: America and the Religion of No Religion.* Chicago: University of Chicago Press, 2007.

Kripal, Jeffrey J., ed., with Glenn W. Shuck. *On the Edge of the Future: Esalen and the Evolution of American Culture.* Bloomington: Indiana University Press, 2005.

Lewis, Alfred Allan. *Ladies and Not-So-Gentle Women.* New York: Penguin Group, 2000.

MacCalman, Kenneth R. "Impressions of Dr. Bernard and the C.C.C. as Viewed by a Nyack On Looker," *South of the Mountains,* vol. 14, no. 4. New City, NY: Historical Society of Rockland County, 1970.

McLaurin, Hamish. *Eastern Philosophy for Western Minds: An Approach to the Principles and Modern Practice of Yoga.* Boston: Stratford, 1933.

Melton, J. Gordon. *Biographical Dictionary of American Cult and Sect Leaders.* New York: Garland Publishing, 1986.

Melton, J. Gordon, ed. *The Encyclopedia of American Religions,* 7th ed. Detroit: Thomson Gale, 2002.

————. *New Age Almanac.* Detroit: Visible Ink Press, 1991.

————. *Religious Leaders of America: A Biographical Guide to Founders and Leaders of Religious Bodies, Churches, and Spiritual Groups in North America.* Detroit: Gale Research, 1991.

Miller, Fred S. *Fighting Modern Evils That Destroy Our Homes: A Startling Exposure of the Snares and Pitfalls of the Social World.* Chicago: L. W. Walter, 1913.

Mitchell, Leslie. *Bulwer Lytton: The Rise and Fall of a Victorian Man of Letters.* London and New York: Hambledon Continuum, 2003.

Morris, James McGrath. *The Rose Man of Sing Sing.* New York: Fordham University Press, 2003.

Nasaw, David. *The Chief: The Life of William Randolph Hearst.* Boston: Houghton Mifflin, 2000.

Norris, Frank. *McTeague: A Story of San Francisco.* New York: Vintage Press, 1990.

Parsons, Alice Beal. *The Mountain*. New York: E. P. Dutton, 1944.

Patterson, Jerry E. *The Vanderbilts*. New York: Harry N. Abrams, 1989.

Perrett, Geoffrey. *America in the Twenties, Days of Sadness, Years of Triumph*. New York: Simon & Schuster, 1982.

Petersen, James R., and Hugh Hefner. *The Century of Sex*. New York: Grove Press, 1999.

Potter, Charles Francis. *The Preacher and I*. New York: Crown, 1951.

Randall, Monica. *Phantoms of the Hudson Valley: The Glorious Estates of a Lost Era*. Woodstock, NY: Overlook Press, 1995.

Rangaswamy, Padma. *Namasté America: Indian Immigrants in an American Metropolis*. University Park: Pennsylvania State University Press, 2000.

Reed, Elizabeth A. *Hinduism in Europe and America*. New York: G. P. Putnam's Sons, 1914.

Remarque, Erich Maria. *All Quiet on the Western Front*. New York: Random House, 1958.

Rodrigues, Santan. *Life of Shri Yogendra, The Householder Yogi*. Bombay, The Yoga Institute, 1995.

Rosen, Ruth. *The Lost Sisterhood*. Baltimore: Johns Hopkins University Press, 1983.

Rosenblum, Constance. *Gold Digger: The Outrageous Life and Times of Peggy Hopkins Joyce*. New York: Metropolitan Books, Henry Holt, 2000.

Said, Edward. *Orientalism*. New York: Vintage Books, Random House, 1979.

Sann, Paul. *Fads, Follies and Delusions of the American People*. New York: Crown, 1967.

Satter, Beryl. *Each Mind a Kingdom: American Women, Sexual Purity, and the New Thought Movement, 1875–1920*. Berkeley and Los Angeles: University of California Press, 1999.

Scott, Cyril. *Bone of Contention*. New York: Arco Publishing, 1969.

Seabrook, William. *Witchcraft: Its Power in the World Today*. New York: Harcourt Brace, 1940.

Shepard, Leslie, ed. *The Encyclopedia of Occultism and Parapsychology*. Detroit: Gale Research, 1991.

Sinclair, Mick. *San Francisco: A Cultural and Literary History*. New York: Interlink Books, 2004.

Sinh, Pancham, trans. *The Hatha Yoga Pradipika*. New Delhi: Munshiram Manoharlal Publishers, 2002 (first published 1914–1915).

Skocpol, Theda. *Diminished Democracy: From Membership to Management in American Civil Life*. Norman: University of Oklahoma Press, 2003.

Soderlund, Gretchen. "Covering Urban Vice: *The New York Times*, 'White Slavery,' and the Construction of Journalistic Knowledge." *Critical Studies in Media Communications* (vol. 19, no. 4, December 2002), 438–460.

Spectorsky, A. C. *The Exurbanites*. Philadelphia: J. B. Lippincott, 1955.

Spring, Clara, and Madeleine Goss. *Yoga for Today*. New York: Holt, Rinehart and Winston, 1959.

St. Denis, Ruth. *Ruth St. Denis: An Unfinished Life, an Autobiography*. New York: Harper and Brothers, 1939.

Stearn, Jess. *Yoga, Youth and Reincarnation*. Garden City, NY: Doubleday, 1965.

———. *Yoga, Youth and Reincarnation*. New York: Bantam Books, 1976.

Steiner, Lee R. *Where Do People Take Their Troubles?* Boston: Houghton Mifflin, 1945.

Sterling, Isabel. *Zen Pioneer: The Life and Works of Ruth Fuller Sasaki*. Emeryville, CA: Shoemaker and Hoard, 2006.

Stuart, Amanda Mackenzie. *Consuelo and Alva Vanderbilt*. New York: HarperCollins, 2005.

Sutin, Lawrence. *Do What Thou Wilt: A Life of Aleister Crowley*. New York: St. Martin's Griffin, 2000.

Tantrik Order in America. *Vira Sadhana: International Journal of the Tantrik Order*. American Edition, vol. 5, no. 1. New York: Tantrik Press, 1906.

Taylor, Eugene. *Shadow Culture: Psychology and Spirituality in America*. Washington, D.C.: Counterpoint, 1999.

Taylor, Kathleen. *Sir John Woodroffe, Tantra and Bengal*. Richmond, Surrey, U.K.: Curzon Press, 2001.

Thurber, James, and E. B. White. *Is Sex Necessary? Or Why You Feel the Way You Do*. Garden City, NY: Blue Ribbon Books, 1944 (originally published under the same title in New York, Harper and Brothers, 1929).

Turner, Hy B. *When Giants Ruled: The Story of Park Row, New York's Great Newspaper Street*. New York: Fordham University Press, 1999.

Twain, Mark. *Following the Equator*, vols. 1 and 2. New York: Harper and Brothers, 1897 and 1899.

Urban, Hugh B. *Tantra: Sex, Secrecy, Politics and Power in the Study of Religion*. Berkeley: University of California Press, 2003.

Vanderbilt, Arthur T., II. *Fortune's Children: The Fall of the House of Vanderbilt*. New York: William Morrow, 1989.

Vanderbilt, Cornelius Jr. *Queen of the Golden Age: The Fabulous Story of Grace Wilson Vanderbilt*. New York: McGraw-Hill, 1956.

Verter, Brad. "Dark Star Rising." PhD diss., Princeton University, 1999.

Viner, John. *A Visit to Nyack, 1953*. Personal home movie.

Vivekananda, Swami. *The Yogas and Other Works*. New York: Ramakrishna-Vivekananda Center, 1953.

Worthington, Vivian. *A History of Yoga*. London: Routledge and Kegan Paul, 1982.

Yeats-Brown, Francis. *Yoga Explained*. New York: Viking Press, 1937.

Zimmerman, Linda. *Rockland County, Century of History*. New City, NY: Historical Society of Rockland County, 2002.

Index

Page numbers in *italics* refer to photographs.